Ethical Decision Making in Therapy: Feminist Perspectives

SECTION EDITORS

Gail Anderson, MA, Park Rapids Medical Clinic, Park Rapids, MN

Mary Ballou, PhD, Northeastern University, Boston, MA

Maryka Biaggio, PhD, Pacific University, Forest Grove, OR

Jane Close Conoley, PhD, University of Nebraska–Lincoln Teachers College, Lincoln, NE

Susan Contratto, EdD, University of Michigan, Ann Arbor, MI

Kristin Glaser, PhD, Private Practice, Montpelier, VT

Beverly Greene, PhD, St. John's University, Queens, NY

Judy Harden, PhD, Goddard College, Plainfield, VT

Jane Hassinger, MSW, ACSW, Private Practice, Ann Arbor, MI

Marcia Hill, EdD, Private Practice, Montpelier, VT

Paula Larson, MS, Millard Public Schools, Omaha, NE

Rosemary Liburd, PhD, University of Alberta, Edmonton, Alberta, Canada

Ruth Parvin, JD, PhD, Private Practice, Portland, OR

Natalie Porter, PhD, University of New Mexico School of Medicine, Albuquerque, NM

Esther Rothblum, PhD, University of Vermont, Burlington, VT

Rachel Josefowitz Siegel, MSW, BCSW, Private Practice, Ithaca, NY

Theo B. Sonderegger, PhD, University of Nebraska–Lincoln, Lincoln, NE

Denise C. Webster, PhD, University of Colorado Health Sciences Center, Denver, CO

ETHICAL DECISION MAKING IN THERAPY

FEMINIST PERSPECTIVES

Edited by

Elizabeth J. Rave, EdD

Carolyn C. Larsen, PhD

THE GUILFORD PRESS
New York   London

©1995 The Guilford Press
A Division of Guilford Publications, Inc.
72 Spring Street, New York, NY 10012

Printed in the United States of America

This book is printed on acid-free paper.

Last digit is print number: 9 8 7 6 5 4 3 2 1

Library of Congress Cataloging-in-Publication Data

Ethical decision making in therapy : feminist perspectives / edited by
Elizabeth J. Rave, Carolyn C. Larsen.
    p.   cm.
    Includes bibliographical references and index.
    ISBN 0-89862-089-9
    1. Feminist therapy—Moral and ethical aspects. I. Rave,
Elizabeth J. II. Larsen, Carolyn C.
RC489.F45E86   1995
174'.2—dc20   95-18762
                                                     CIP

Book Editors

Elizabeth J. Rave, EdD, is Professor Emeritus of School Psychology and Women's Studies. While at the University of Northern Colorado, she developed courses in psychology of prejudice, psychology of women, violence against women and children, eating disorders, sexual abuse of children, and teen pregnancy. She served as coordinator of the School Psychology programs and was a member of the Women's Studies governing committee. Her research, presentations, and publications have been on antiracism, ethics, violence against women and children, play therapy, gender and ethnic effects on perceptions of behavior, and supervision ethics. As a founding member of the Feminist Therapy Institute (FTI) she has served on the Steering Committee and been Committee Coordinator and cochair of the Ethics and Accountability Committee, charged with developing the Feminist Therapy Code of Ethics. She is presently living in Seattle, learning about ageism, and developing a consultation practice.

Carolyn C. Larsen, PhD, is Senior Counsellor Emeritus and formerly Director, University Counselling Services and Adjunct Associate Professor, Department of Educational Psychology, The University of Calgary. She supervised graduate student practica, internships, and research. Carolyn has been in private practice as a partner with Alberta Psychological Resources, Ltd., for 13 years. She coauthored *A Woman's Choice: A Guide to Decision-Making*, which was developed from Contemporary Woman, a popular feminist esteem-building program for which she was a codesigner and consultant for 15 years, and is still being offered in Calgary. Carolyn collaborated with Jean Pettifor and Lorna Cammaert in developing the Ethical Guidelines for Counselling/Therapy with Women and *Therapy and Counselling with Women: A Handbook of Educational Materials* for the Canadian Psychological Association (CPA). She is a Fellow of CPA. A founding member of the Feminist Therapy Institute, she was on the Steering Committee for 10 years, serving as Committee Coordinator and cochair of the Ethics and Accountability Committee that facilitated the development of the Feminist Therapy Code of Ethics. Carolyn has contributed as author and section editor to two previous books sponsored by FTI.

Section Editors

Gail Anderson, MA, is a licensed psychologist working in private practice with Park Rapids Medical Clinic in rural Minnesota. Her generalist practice includes many children who survived abuse, and she specializes in feminist play therapy. This is Gail's first publishing venture.

Mary Ballou, PhD, is Associate Professor in Counseling Psychology at Northeastern University, Boston, and has a clinical practice in both Boston and Keene, NH. She has published extensively in both feminist psychology and crisis theory. Mary holds an ABPP Diplomate in Counseling Psychology, is a Fellow of the American Psychological Association, and a member of the Feminist Therapy Institute Steering Committee.

Maryka Biaggio, PhD, is Professor, School of Professional Psychology, Pacific University, Forest Grove, OR. She teaches a graduate level course in the Psychology of Women and supervises thesis and dissertation research. Maryka was Newsletter Editor and served on the Executive Board of the Association for Women in Psychology, 1990–1994. She is active in the Portland community, serving on the board of directors of both a large community mental health clinic and a transition program for recovering substance abusers. Maryka has published and presented research on sexual harassment, sexual victimization, anger arousal, and women in administration.

Jane Close Conoley, PhD, is a clinically certified psychologist, Professor, and Associate Dean for Research at the University of Nebraska–Lincoln Teachers College. Her areas of special interest are seriously disturbed children and family therapy. She is a past president of the Division of School Psychology of the American Psychological Association (APA) and is the editor of the Buros Mental Measurement Yearbook series. Jane is also the director of the Nebraska Internship Consortium in Professional

Psychology, an APA-approved predoctoral internship program specializing in child, family, and school-based approaches to treatment.

Susan Contratto, EdD, is Codirector of the Interdisciplinary Program in Feminist Practice, a Lecturer in Psychology at the University of Michigan, and in private practice. She teaches Advanced Feminist Therapy, Lesbian Psychology Development, and Feminist Pedagogy at the graduate level. Susan has published numerous articles and book chapters, including "The Fantasy of the Perfect Mother" with Nancy Chodorow, "Maternal Sexuality and Asexual Motherhood" in *Signs*, "Father Presence in Women's Psychological Development" in *Advances in Psychoanalytic Sociology*, "Psychology Views Mother and Mothering—1890–1990" in *In the Shadow of the Past*, and "A Too Hasty Marriage: Gilligan's Developmental Theory and Its Application to Feminist Clinical Practice" in *Psychology and Feminism*. She is currently chair of the Feminist Therapy Institute Steering Committee.

Kristin Glaser, PhD, completed her training at the University of Chicago in 1983. She has been in private practice in Montpelier, VT since the early 1970s. She has done both teaching and training. Currently helping to organize a practitioner-owned mental health provider network, Kristin is happy shaping a form of psychotherapist survival or going down in good company.

Beverly Greene, PhD, is Associate Professor of Psychology at St. John's University and a clinical psychologist in private practice in New York City. Beverly served as Director of Inpatient Child and Adolescent Psychology Services at Kings County Hospital, Brooklyn, NY. A Fellow of the American Psychological Association, she is coeditor of the series *Psychological Perspectives on Lesbian and Gay Issues* (Sage Publications), coeditor of *Women of Color: Integrating Ethnic and Gender Identities in Psychotherapy* (Guilford Press, 1994), and an author of *Abnormal Psychology in a Changing World* (Prentice Hall, 1994). Awards she has received include The Association for Women in Psychology first Women of Color Psychologist Publication Award, 1991, American Psychological Association Division 44 Award for Distinguished Professional Contributions to Ethnic Minority Issues, 1992, and the American Association of Applied and Preventive Psychology Distinguished Humanitarian Award, 1994, for exceptional outreach and advocacy efforts in the public interest.

Judy Harden, PhD, teaches at Goddard College in Plainfield, VT, where she is coordinator of the MA Counseling Psychology program, is an active participant in the undergraduate feminist studies program, and in a feminist research group of faculty and staff. Judy's current primary professional interest is in developing community-based research projects that benefit women and girls.

Jane Hassinger, MSW, ACSW, has been in psychotherapy practice with individuals and groups in Ann Arbor, MI since 1975. Her long-standing affiliation with the University of Michigan has included teaching courses on gender and group dynamics in Women's Studies and graduate and faculty seminars on Interdisciplinary Feminist Practice and Feminist Perspectives on the Treatment of Trauma. As an affiliate scholar with the Center for the Education of Women, Jane is coprincipal investigator for a study of women graduates about their methods of planning for and coping with work and family role and a founder with Susan Contratto and Marcy Plunkett, of the Interdisciplinary Program in Feminist Practice. Jane is a vocalist, specializing in the works of women jazz singers from the 1920s–1930s. Her publications include a chapter on women and jazz in Ellen Koskoff (Ed.), *Women and Music in Cross-Cultural Perspective* (Greenwood Press, 1987).

Marcia Hill, EdD, is a psychologist in private practice in Montpelier, VT. A feminist therapist for 20 years, she also teaches, writes, and consults in the area of feminist therapy theory and practice. Marcia is the new coeditor of *Women and Therapy*. She is past chair of the Feminist Therapy Institute Steering Committee.

Paula Larson, MS, is a certified school psychologist employed with Millard Public Schools in Omaha, NE, and a PhD candidate in school psychology at the University of Nebraska–Lincoln. Among her work responsibilities are conducting psychological evaluations, parent training and social skills groups, and consulting with staff, parents, and students to develop academic and behavioral interventions. Paula's special interests include educational programs and therapeutic interventions for youth with serious emotional and behavioral problems, improving home/school collaboration, and parent training.

Rosemary Liburd, PhD, is Professor of Educational Psychology and Women's Studies at The University of Alberta, Edmonton, Alberta. She trains psychologists and is a feminist therapist in private practice. Rosemary was affiliated with the Faculty of Extension Women's Program and Resource Centre for 12 years where she developed and conducted a variety of workshops and contributed to the development of the Counselling Women Certificate Program, teaching one of the core courses. Rosemary has published and presented at professional meetings in Canada and the United States.

Ruth Parvin, JD, PhD, has a private practice and law–psychology consulting business in Portland, OR. She has combined her legal and psychological background through work in the U.S. Senate, academic appointments at several colleges and universities, and administrative positions in outpatient therapy clinics. She is the editor of the Feminist Therapy Institute publication *Interchange*. Her other publishing has been in client-oriented, popular-press newspapers and journals.

Natalie Porter, PhD, is Associate Professor and Chief Psychologist in the Division of Child and Adolescent Psychiatry, University of New Mexico School of Medicine. She directs Programs for Children and Adolescents, an outpatient mental health program. Her writings have focused on training and ethical issues. She is coeditor of *Feminist Ethics in Psychotherapy*. Articles she has written include "A Feminist, Anti-Racist, and Cross-Cultural Model of Supervision," "Resistance in Family Therapy from a Cross-Cultural Perspective," and "Empowering Therapists to Empower Others: A Developmental Supervision Model." Natalie is past president of the Division on the Psychology of Women (Division 35) of the American Psychological Association.

Esther Rothblum, PhD, is Professor in the Department of Psychology at the University of Vermont and past chair of Women's Studies. She was the University Scholar at the University of Vermont for 1992–1993. Esther has chaired the Vermont Psychological Association's Committee on Women and Minorities, Women's Special Interest Group of the Association for Advancement of Behavior Therapy, and the Committee on Feminist Research of the Association for Women in Psychology. Esther was awarded a Kellogg Fellowship, which focused on travel to Africa to study women's mental health, and has received a grant to travel to the Antarctic to study women's stress and coping. Esther is coeditor of the journal *Women and Therapy* and has coedited 13 books, among them *Another Silenced Trauma: Twelve Feminist Therapists and Activists Respond to One Woman's Recovery from War*, which won a Distinguished Publication Award from the Association for Women in Psychology.

Rachel Josefowitz Siegel, MSW, BCSW, born in 1924, opened her private practice in Ithaca, NY, in 1976 after three years at the County Mental Health Clinic. She has been an active member of FTI since its inception, contributing to the process of creating the Ethics Code while serving six years on the Steering Committee. Rachel has written several articles about women in midlife and women over 60 and writes and lectures about Jewish women. She is coeditor of *Women Changing Therapy: New Assessments, Values and Strategies in Feminist Therapy*

(Haworth Press, 1983) and *Jewish Women in Therapy: Seen but Not Heard* (Haworth Press, 1991).

Theo B. Sonderegger, PhD, is a Professor of Psychology in the Department of Psychology, University of Nebraska–Lincoln and a Professor of Medical Psychology (courtesy appointment) at the University of Nebraska Medical Center, Omaha. Her graduate degrees from the University of Nebraska are in physical chemistry, experimental psychology, and clinical psychology. She is a licensed clinical psychologist in California and Nebraska. During 1992 Theo edited two books, *Perinatal Substance Abuse: Research Findings and Clinical Implications* (Johns Hopkins University Press) and *Psychology for Aging*, a volume in the Nebraska Symposium on Motivation series (University of Nebraska Press). She is also editor of *Psychology and Gender*, the 1984 volume in this series. She has published in numerous scientific journals and in 1994 assumed the editorship of a new series, *Agendas for Aging*, to be published by the Nebraska Press. Theo's recent honors include Outstanding Research Scientist Award, Sigma Xi–Nebraska Chapter (1991), Certificate of Appreciation for Service, National Institute of Drug Abuse (1993), and Outstanding Contribution to the Status of Women Award, University of Nebraska–Lincoln (1994). She has been an active member of the Feminist Therapy Institute since its inception and served as editor of the *Interchange*, its publication, for several years. Theo is a Fellow of the American Association for the Advancement of Science, the American Psychological Society, and the American Psychological Association, Divisions 28, 35, 37. Her research interests include perinatal substance abuse, psychology of women, and aging.

Denise C. Webster, PhD, is Associate Professor and Program Coordinator, School of Nursing, University of Colorado Health Sciences Center, Denver. She did her graduate work at the University of Illinois, Chicago, receiving a master's degree in psychiatric nursing and a PhD in nursing sciences. Denise holds certification as a Clinical Specialist in Adult Psychiatric/Mental Health Nursing, American Nurses Association. She has given many presentations to professional meetings and published extensively; among these are review articles on "Women and Mental Health" for Volumes I, II, and III in C. Leppa and C. Miller (Eds.), *Women's Health Perspectives: An Annual Review* (Oryx Press, 1988, 1989, 1990) and B. McElinurry and R. Sprengler (Eds.), *Annual Review of Women's Health*, (National League for Nursing, 1983).

Acknowledgments

We are grateful for the feminist women who contributed to this book by writing, editing, submitting ethical dilemmas, responding to ethical dilemmas, and providing feedback on particular issues about which they have special expertise. We are particularly appreciative of the many authors and editors who met deadlines, followed the format, and proofread carefully. All of us are indebted to the clients and students who have been our teachers. Their influence is evident throughout the book.

The Feminist Therapy Institute Steering Committee has provided interest and support for which we are grateful over the seven years since the idea for this book was first proposed. Barbara Watkins, Senior Editor at the Guilford Press, has a depth of knowledge about feminism, therapy, and ethics that allowed her to provide clear direction and encouragement to us and to the section editors. Her patience and understanding of the complexity of this project and her ability to communicate positively and directly are much appreciated. Doris DeHardt, Natalie Porter, and many other feminist therapists provided feedback in their special areas of expertise. Each section editor also relied on colleagues and other feminist therapists for feedback and support.

There have been many women who have contributed their organizational and clerical skills to the completion of the sections of the book. As one example, Pat Rand promptly and with care prepared the "Conflict in Care: Later Years" section. All the other women behind the scenes who helped bring this volume to reality also deserve our appreciation.

All of us involved in creating this book have special people in our lives who have sustained us through the long process. Donald Larsen, whose perspective, caring, advice, and humor have been invaluable, is one model of the countless others who have personally nurtured those of us named as contributors to the book.

ELIZABETH J. RAVE
CAROLYN C. LARSEN

Preface

The Feminist
Therapy Institute

The Feminist Therapy Institute (FTI) had its begin-
nings at a gathering of feminist therapists in Vail,
CO, in 1982. Forty women therapists who identi-
fied themselves as feminists and who had been in practice for at least
five years were present. Participants decided to form an ongoing international organization with annual meetings to develop feminist therapy
theory and practice. Annual meetings of advanced feminist therapists
have been held, several books about feminist therapy and feminist ethics
have been published (Brown & Root, 1990; Lerman & Porter,1990;
Rosewater & Walker, 1985), and a newsletter, *Interchange*, is distributed
to members.

At the 1983 meeting of the Advanced Feminist Therapy Institute
(AFTI), the annual conference for members of FTI, ethics quickly
emerged as a central issue. The need for ethical guidelines was acknowledged, and a committee with Carolyn Larsen and Elizabeth Rave as
cochairs was established to facilitate this task. Over the next four years,
the FTI Feminist Therapy Code of Ethics (1987) was developed (Rave
& Larsen, 1990). The process was deliberately collective and inclusive
with lengthy discussions and debates at AFTI meetings and feedback
from committee members at each stage as drafts were developed, reviewed, revised, and sent out again for the next round of feedback. The
Feminist Therapy Code of Ethics was approved in May, 1987, and it
continues to guide feminist therapists.

NEED FOR A FEMINIST ETHICAL CODE

Early in the development of the FTI and meetings of the organization it became clear that several ethical issues were important to the membership. The issue that was, and still is, most problematic to feminist therapists is that of dual or overlapping relationships between therapist and client. The major reason dual relationships posed difficult, often unique and sometimes agonizing, ethical questions for feminist therapists is the overlap of clients in the therapists' practice and in their social and political communities. Feminist therapists frequently live and work in the same communities as their clients. This overlap is highlighted in rural, lesbian, and ethnic communities. It is inevitable that therapists and clients will belong to the same social, political, and volunteer organizations or overlap at community, cultural, or recreational events. In the 1970s and early 1980s, professional codes of ethics did not address these relationship issues specifically, and the assumption seemed to be that overlapping relationships would not occur, or if they did, the therapist would simply avoid clients. Younger feminist therapists who received their training after the late 1980s may not realize how significant the issues surrounding overlapping relationships were in galvanizing activism and togetherness of feminist therapists in the first decade of feminist therapy.

Feminist therapists as women are more apt to be on the receiving end of the misuse of power through dual relationships with supervisors and therapists during their own training or therapy (Pope, Sonne, & Holroyd, 1993). Such personal experiences make feminist therapists more cognizant of these issues. Feminist philosophy also sensitizes therapists to the existence of and problems with dual/overlapping relationships. Feminist tenets of valuing and respecting all people and of helping people, especially women, develop and protect their personal physical and psychological boundaries contribute to this sensitivity.

Cultural diversity and concerns about the "sameness" of the FTI membership also were major topics at steering committee meetings as well as conferences. The organization took a major step with a one-year delay in admitting new white members while encouraging women of color to apply. Painful personal growth in individual members occurred around diversity issues probably more than within any other issue within the organization.

Power differentials between therapist and client and the importance of treating those differentials with care and respect were themes at an early AFTI conference and developed as ethical concerns for inclusion in the Code. Concerns for therapist accountability also played a role in developing the Feminist Therapy Code of Ethics as members thought back on their own experiences in therapy as well as remembered clients' concerns about lack of therapist accountability.

Perhaps it is not surprising that a decade ago there was a lack of attention to the ethical issues of dual/overlapping relationships and other issues crucial to feminist therapists. Not until the 1990s have these issues begun to be addressed in traditional professional codes of ethics.

CULTURAL DIVERSITY

A multicultural and anti-racist perspective has guided the organization, and members of the Feminist Therapy Institute have struggled with the complexity of multiculturalism and cultural diversity. The application form for membership in FTI includes an affirmative action policy statement: "Feminist therapy is by and for women of all colors and backgrounds. Its theory, practice, and research must be developed from and by a full diversity of women" (Feminist Therapy Institute, n.d.).

The Feminist Therapy Code of Ethics includes statements dealing with the integral significance of diversity (Preamble, I). The book *Diversity and Complexity in Feminist Therapy* (Brown & Root, 1990) developed from the 1988 conference theme. FTI's annual call for papers and presentations also includes a statement developed by FTI's Anti-Racism Committee (1989).

After observing that women-of-color presenters tend to be clear in identifying the people in their presentations, the statement points out that white presenters often proceed as if ethnicity needs to be identified only if the subjects are not white. The aim of the questions is to help minimize unexamined assumptions and dominant-culture biases.

1. If you offer a literature review, does it provide information about only one culture group, or is it diverse and accurately descriptive to the best of your knowledge?

2. Is your presentation based on a single ethnic group? If so, have you clearly identified the group and avoided even implicit generalizing to other groups of women? (The concept here is that studies based on a single ethnic group should be considered subcultural or monocultural studies, not as representing, e.g., "women.")

3. Has white privilege influenced your analysis? If so, in what ways? If not, how have you avoided it?

OMISSIONS IN THE ETHICS CODE

Because the Feminist Therapy Code of Ethics is intended to be additive to other codes, it does not include topics covered in most professional codes. Instead the focus is on those areas that are especially important to women therapists and clients.

In developing the Code, one topic, the issue of money, did not come up frequently, if at all. There was discussion of the need to make a living, as such, but not a discussion about how charging fees for service might raise ethical issues. In fact, the first book on ethics sponsored by FTI has only one article dealing with monetary issues (Brown, 1990). Issues surrounding charging fees for service were and are considered to be subsumed under power differentials. This book contains a section exploring the Code's implications for money-related issues.

Another decision made by the committee and the Institute membership was not to develop the Code according to work settings, that is, agencies, private practice, or academia. Instead, it was assumed that the feminist therapist could apply the ethical principles to the specific setting where she worked. Additionally, the Code was considered applicable to educators, researchers, and supervisors, among others, and ethical principles were not differentiated or written according to professional responsibility.

BOOK DEVELOPMENT

The topics included in this book emerged from discussions at AFTI conferences and mailings to FTI members. Over a period of three years and several revisions, the original list of 30 topics was combined into the final eight, which represented the list that came up most frequently. Several topics were combined into one. A few emerging topics, such as reproductive technology, service delivery, and managed care, are changing very rapidly. By focusing on ethical issues rather than specific topics, the section editors facilitate relevance regardless of technological or sociological advances occurring between writing and publication of the book.

Several requests were made for scenarios at conferences, through mailings, and through the organization's newsletter. Most general requests elicited only scenarios dealing with overlapping relationships, another indication of that topic's importance to feminist therapists. The majority of scenarios were developed after discussion with many therapists, came from therapists' experience as clients or with their clients, and were adapted to fit the format of the book.

ELIZABETH J. RAVE
CAROLYN C. LARSEN

REFERENCES

Brown, L. S. (1990). Ethical issues and the business of therapy. In H. Lerman & N. Porter (Eds.), *Feminist ethics in psychotherapy* (pp. 60–69). New York: Springer.

Brown, L. S., & Root, M. P. P. (Eds.). (1990). *Diversity and complexity in feminist therapy*. New York: Harrington Park Press.

Feminist Therapy Institute. (1987). *Feminist therapy code of ethics*. Denver: Author.

Feminist Therapy Institute. (n.d.). [Membership application]. Denver: Author.

Lerman, H., & Porter, N. (Eds.). (1990). *Feminist ethics in psychotherapy*. New York: Springer.

Pope, K. S., Sonne, J. L., & Holroyd, J. (1993). *Sexual feelings in psychotherapy: Explorations for therapists and therapists-in-training*. Washington, DC: American Psychological Association.

Rave, E. J., & Larsen, C. C. (1990). Development of the code: The feminist process. In H. Lerman & N. Porter (Eds.), *Feminist ethics in psychotherapy* (pp. 14–23). New York: Springer.

Rosewater, L. B., & Walker, L. E. A. (Eds.). (1985). *Handbook of feminist therapy*. New York: Springer.

Contents

ONE

Context of Feminist Therapy Ethics

Carolyn C. Larsen
Elizabeth J. Rave

Codes of ethics for the mental health professions protect the welfare of clients by requiring professional competency. They clarify the rights and responsibilities of mental health professionals and provide standards of conduct, common values, attitudes, and principles for using the knowledge and skills of the profession. An ethical code forms what is essentially a social contract between the profession and the public it serves.

That public consists primarily of women who continue to be the majority of clients in therapy regardless of its type or setting. Except for veterans and other military groups, women outnumber men in individual and group therapy, in private, public agency, outpatient, and inpatient settings. Self-help groups are also largely populated by women. Knowledge about the issues that women bring to therapy is essential for effective ethical treatment.

Guidelines for ethical therapy practice are vital. So much of therapeutic work occurs in the privacy of the practitioner's office that client(s) and the discipline rely on the individual therapist to manage the therapeutic relationship in a competent, caring way. Ethics focuses attention on providing for the welfare of the individual client and society more generally as a priority over the welfare of therapists or their profession.

Codes of ethics for mental health professionals vary in length, level of abstraction, and topics included. The Feminist Therapy Institute (FTI) Feminist Therapy Code of Ethics (1987) was developed to provide more guidance on issues not addressed in traditional professional ethics codes, particularly in areas relevant to women therapists and clients. It is intended to be additive to traditional codes. But neither the FTI Code nor traditional codes are exhaustive, and there is often a need to interpret the guidelines when applying them to a particular situation. The abstract principles of a code may appear clear and obvious, but the real world can be complex and confusing. What is the ethical course when two or more principles conflict? How best can ideal principles be applied in an imperfect world? This book grapples with these questions. Experienced feminist therapists, over 90 respondents, discuss ethical issues and comment on case scenarios that raise ethical dilemmas typical of everyday practice with women clients. A major goal of this volume is to sensitize therapists and therapists-in-training to ethical issues affecting women and girls in therapy.

Feminist therapists explain how they might respond to ethical situations, and readers can compare those responses to their own, possibly different, philosophical viewpoints or therapeutic approaches. The book is intended for therapists and students from psychology, social work, counseling, psychiatry, and nursing, and for therapists in private practice, agencies, and academic institutions. Until recently, ethics education has been minimal in many mental health training programs. But it is now increasingly recognized as an essential component of training and of continuing education.

This section offers a brief orientation to women's issues in psychology and to the main characteristics of feminist therapy ethics. Some questions to consider when reading the dilemmas and responses in the following sections are also offered.

WOMEN AND PSYCHOLOGY

The history of women in psychology is short. Significant efforts, mostly by women, to address psychology's neglect and misrepresentation of women began in earnest only in the early 1970s. These efforts included research on women, publication of books and journals devoted to the psychology of women, and the organization of professional associations to promote research on women, the status of women in the professions, and the rights of women clients to respectful treatment. A landmark study by Broverman, Broverman, Clarkson, Rosenkrantz, and Vogel (1970) illustrated that clinicians used different criteria for describing the mental health of women and men. This study was one of several developments that spurred on efforts to consider women equally in psychological research, in training opportunities, and within the mental health field as both professionals and as clients.

Texts on the psychology of women (Bardwick, 1971; Sherman, 1971) were published; topics of particular relevance to women, such as family violence, eating disorders, the female reproductive cycle, and math anxiety, were being discussed and researched. Review articles on women psychologists and the psychology of women began to appear (Astin, 1972; Greenglass, 1973a, 1973b), and for the first time, the *Annual Review of Psychology* published a chapter about women (Mednick & Weissman, 1975). The Association of Women in Psychology (AWP) was founded in 1970 to monitor and pressure the American Psychological Association (APA) regarding women's issues. Division 35 of APA, Psychology of Women, was founded in 1973 and began publication of the *Psychology of Women Quarterly* in 1976. APA established a Committee on Women in Psychology in 1978 and later a Women's Programs Office to promote the status of women in psychology.

The Canadian Psychological Association (CPA) was unresponsive to women's issues in the early 1970s, resulting in independent symposia at annual conventions. In 1975, the CPA Section on Women and Psychology (SWAP) was organized to monitor CPA, provide more programs relevant to and about women at the annual convention, and promote women within the profession. CPA finally took a comprehensive approach to women's concerns with the Task Force on the Status of Women in Canadian Psychology, which produced 90 recommendations (Wand, 1977), and led to establishing The Committee on the Status of Women, which has been active in implementing these recommendations. Pyke (1994) reviews progress in implementing these recommendations, particularly within CPA and academic institutions, and reports many achievements but continuing significant impediments to equality and equity for women within Canadian psychology.

Not until 1975 did sexual exploitation by therapists of clients become officially recognized and studied by the American Psychological Association (American Psychological Association, 1975). As more women became therapists and shared their experiences as survivors of therapist and professor abuse (Holroyd & Brodsky, 1977), momentum developed for inclusion of the issue in ethical guidelines. The APA Task Force on Sex Bias and Sex-Role Stereotyping in Psychotherapeutic Practice published guidelines for therapy with women (American Psychological Association, 1978). Division 17 of APA, Counseling Psychology, also adopted principles focusing on the need for therapists serving women clients to have specialized knowledge, attitudes, and skills (American Psychological Association, 1979). Sex between therapist and client was formalized as unethical behavior in the APA Code of Ethics in 1981 (American Psychological Association, 1981). In Canada a set of guidelines for counseling and therapy with women were adopted by CPA (Canadian Psychological Association, 1980), and educational materials were developed to assist in training professionals and consumers about feminist therapy (Pettifor, Larsen, & Cammaert, 1984).

Only in the latter part of the 1980s have other professional organizations seriously looked at and included in their codes more specific statements about therapists' sexual and personal relationships with clients. The unethical nature of any sexual relationship between client and therapist during therapy, and in many cases following termination of therapy, had been clearly stated in the ethical codes of most mental health professions by the late 1980s. Both the American and Canadian Psychological Associations included statements about sexual and other dual relationships in their revised codes of ethics (American Psychological Association, 1992; Canadian Psychological Association, 1991). With the most blatant sexual behaviors included in ethics codes and complaints being prosecuted by professional association disciplinary committees and in the courts, many of the more subtle ways in which therapists' and clients' lives overlap and create potential ethical problems are now being examined and studied (Adleman & Barrett, 1990; Brown, 1994; Herlihy & Corey, 1992; Kitchener, 1988; Peterson, 1992).

FEMINISM AND THERAPY

Not all feminist therapists define "feminism" or "therapy" in the same way. However, there are many values and behaviors feminist therapists have in common. Feminism is most popularly defined as a belief in the equal valuing of all people and in social, economic, and political equality for all. The emphasis is usually on equality for women, since historically women have played subordinate roles to men in patriarchal Western societies. Cammaert and Larsen (1988) identified many of the core values that underpin feminist therapy. First, the personal is political, with individual experiences and situations both reflecting and influencing the values of society. Second, women have a full range of choices about how to live their lives. Third, feminists work toward equalizing power in interpersonal relationships by recognizing that each person deserves respect and the right to have equal personal power in relationships. Fourth, therapists are role models as both women and therapists. Fifth, therapists help women move beyond sex role stereotypes to realize their fullest potential. Sixth, therapists engage in social action to change the system to benefit all women. Feminist therapists strive to behave in ways that reflect these values with clients, in other professional relationships, and in their daily lives. The philosophical bases of feminist therapy ensure that ethical issues are a primary part of the fabric of that therapy.

There is great diversity among feminist therapists in their feminist philosophical influences and preferences, training, background, and implementation in practice. Enns (1993), for example, differentiates four enduring feminist philosophies that represent a way to understand "the multifaceted nature of feminist therapy" (p. 45). They are liberal, cultural, radical, and socialist approaches that Enns elaborates to illustrate this diversity.

For the most part, feminist therapists have been trained in traditional professional programs. What they bring to their therapy are a philosophical lens and a set of values that influence how they work with their clients, students, trainees, and other colleagues. Starting in the late 1960s, feminists who were therapists began calling themselves feminist therapists, and anyone who called herself one was considered one! Slowly, through the 1970s and into the 1980s, feminist therapy became more defined and established (Enns, 1993; Gilbert & Osipow, 1991; Kaschak, 1981; Marecek & Hare-Mustin, 1991; Sturdivant, 1980). Workshops, conferences, and organizations emerged that allowed feminist therapists to share the growing research and grassroots knowledge about women, to examine societal and professional attitudes about women, and to teach what was and is being learned that would help move women toward economic, social, and political equality.

There are still few feminist therapy training programs per se, although many professional training programs now have feminist therapists on staff who contribute feminist principles and practice to the training of future therapists, consultants, teachers, and researchers. It remains for prospective students to seek out institutions and training programs where there are feminists who can transmit their knowledge, attitudes, and skills to the next generations of feminist therapists. There is no official credentialing of feminist therapists. But within psychiatry, psychology, social work, nursing, and other professions, feminist therapists have learned to utilize the full array of therapy theories, treatment strategies, and techniques. What aspects are unique about their approach are feminist analyses and modification of these theories and practices to bring them in line with feminist philosophies and values. The diversity of training, discipline, and theoretical orientations that feminists bring to their work has enriched feminist therapy theory and practice just as the feminist perspective has enriched the more traditional perspectives. Thus, feminism has been additive to many professional programs and allows feminists to utilize established, but adapted, techniques in their work. An example is the use of hypnosis as a therapeutic adjunct. Hypnosis is often seen as an authoritarian treatment approach, but many feminists have found creative methods to use hypnosis in an effective, cooperative way with clients (Laidlaw & Malmo, 1990).

TRADITIONAL CODES

In addition to the FTI Code, this book frequently refers to the American Psychological Association Ethical Principles of Psychologists and Code of Conduct (1992) and the Canadian Code of Ethics for Psychologists of the Canadian Psychological Association (1991). Both documents undergo continual revision and apply to psychologists as they carry out their many professional and scientific roles as therapist, teacher, supervisor, administrator, researcher, and consultant. Psychologists are not only expected to behave ethically in work-related activities but also to encourage ethical behavior in others with whom they work.

The APA code develops six ethical principles: (1) competence, (2) integrity, (3) professional and scientific responsibility, (4) respect for people's rights and dignity, (5) concern for others' welfare, and (6) social responsibility. These principles are followed by ethical standards that are rules for conduct. Some decision rules for resolving ethical dilemmas are also provided as part of the Code.

The CPA Code presents four ethical principles: (1) respect for the dignity of persons, (2) responsible caring, (3) integrity in relationships, and (4) responsibility to society. Each principle is followed by a statement of values and then a list of ethics standards that illustrates the application of the specific principle and values to the activities of psychologists. The CPA Code includes an ethical decision-making process.

Most feminist therapists have been trained in traditional professional programs and are guided by the ethical codes of their respective professions. Why, then, do feminist therapists need another code? How is the FTI Code different from other codes of ethics?

CHARACTERISTICS OF
FEMINIST THERAPY ETHICS

Feminist therapists wanted and needed a code that would go beyond their professional codes in acknowledging feminist tenets, deal more extensively and specifically with overlapping relationships, recognize the power differential between client and therapist, incorporate concerns about diversity, increase access by all to both knowledge and treatment, require therapist self-monitoring and self-care, and encourage therapist and client proactive behavior for social change. There was a significant need for clear ethical statements that would reflect feminist philosophy, provide positive proactive direction, and include issues that traditional codes had not yet addressed. This effort was motivated by the desire to provide direction to therapists and also to reduce the probability of any additional oppressions against women clients through the behavior, deliberate or inadvertent, of the therapist.

The exploration and understanding of power in people's lives continue to be a core issue for feminist therapists. The power inequities that women experience in other aspects of their lives should not recur in the therapeutic relationship. Feminist therapy seeks to help clients understand how power inequities contribute to their problems and to personally empower clients through understanding and action. Initially, feminist therapists denied that power differentials existed in the feminist therapeutic relationship. They then believed it possible to achieve the ideal of equality of power between client and therapist within the therapeutic relationship. That view has been modified to acknowledge that power differentials are inherent in therapy and other relationships. The tasks of the therapist, then, are to be sensitive to power issues, to use power responsibly in the service of clients, and to assist the clients in gaining perspective on how power affects them individually.

Feminist therapists are keenly aware of how both their personal and professional selves are present in the therapeutic relationship. The therapist is a powerful role model for the client, as well as for colleagues and supervisees. Feminist therapists seek to be responsible in conducting their personal and professional lives in an ongoing effort to function effectively. The imperative is to use and develop this awareness to take care of personal needs within their private lives, to be sensitive to their own values and biases and how they are expressed, and to seek needed support within their own community. These precautions ensure that the therapeutic relationship primarily serves the client's needs and not the therapist's needs. Therapists' own experiences have taught them how often and with what effect this ethic can be violated. Professionally, the feminist therapist is careful to work within her areas of competence, stay current, self-monitor as well as seek consultation, and engage in ongoing evaluation of integrating feminist principles into her theory and practice.

Many philosophical streams of therapy recognize the importance of social change. Additionally, many therapists adhere to the idea that individual change is not sufficient by itself. For feminist therapists, however, societal change and individual change are inherently intertwined. Feminists recognize that social conditions harmful to individual development must be alleviated as well as the personal dysfunction that results from those conditions. Facilitating change for one person at a time would not be sufficient for feminists. Feminist therapists believe in social as well as individual change.

Feminist therapists active in social change efforts may run more risk of interacting with their clients outside of the therapeutic experience. After two and a half decades of feminist therapy, overlapping relationships are still particularly problematic for feminist therapists. No one has systematically evaluated whether dual relationships are of more concern to feminist therapists than to other types of therapists. However, looking at convention topics covered by Division 35 of APA, Psychology of Women, as compared to other divisions over the years, one discovers a consistency of presentations on the topic in Division 35 that does not appear in the other Divisions.

Feminist therapists are more apt to meet colleagues in professional settings who are former clients, students, or supervisees. Additionally, feminist therapists recognize that it is not always possible or feasible to totally avoid clients in other settings. Therapists and clients may meet at or be members of the same social, volunteer, or political organizations, for example. An ethics code that stipulates there should be no overlapping relationships may be unrealistic in the majority of settings for feminist therapists. The Feminist Therapy Code of Ethics started with the assumption that there are some unavoidable overlapping relationships, and therapists need to develop strategies for dealing with these situations so that neither clients nor therapists are negatively affected.

The Preamble to the Feminist Therapy Code of Ethics is central to the Code, providing essential background and context for use of the guidelines that follow. The Preamble defines feminist therapy and sets out the role expectations of feminist therapists in all areas of their work. The Code has a unique and carefully specified relationship to other professional codes of ethics. The Preamble states very clearly, "Feminist therapists who are members of other professional organizations adhere to the ethical codes of those organizations" (Feminist Therapy Institute, 1987). Some feminist therapists do not belong to professional organizations, and the assumption is made that those women will be guided by the professional code of ethics "closest to their mode of practice" (Feminist Therapy Institute, 1987). The connotatively positive statements in the FTI Code provide more specific guidelines on the ethical issues of importance to feminist therapists than do most ethical codes. If a feminist therapist finds herself in conflict between the guidance of two codes, she is "accountable for how she prioritizes her choices" (Feminist Therapy Institute, 1987).

SIGNIFICANCE OF DIVERSITY

Members of the FTI continue to struggle with the complexity of multiculturalism and cultural diversity. A primary goal of the book editors then was to reflect the diversity of feminist therapists and feminist therapy. Therapists themselves come from a wide variety of training programs, including psychodynamic, behavioral, psychosocial, humanistic, and all the combinations and variations possible. Additionally, feminist therapists are trained as psychologists, psychiatrists, nurses, social workers, and counselors. Each of those professional or theoretical backgrounds may or may not affect the viewpoint of the feminist therapist.

The number of contributors alone implies a tremendous diversity in personal and sociohistorical characteristics whether these characteristics are obvious or not. For example, both heterosexual and lesbian writers are included, but that identity is not always stated. As a result, the reader should not assume that if a scenario character or respondent does not identify herself as a lesbian, she is automatically a heterosexual feminist or vice versa.

Additional issues surrounding diversity include class, age, sexual orientation, physical ability, religion, geographic location, race, and ethnicity. The editors were not explicit in asking for all characteristics. Contributors were given the opportunity to identify themselves, especially by ethnicity, if they chose to do so. Not all contributors did so choose.

The most problematic area of diversity is still ethnicity and color. Both book editors and section editors diligently sought out feminist therapists who represented a diverse population as respondents to ethical scenarios. Special attention was paid to a diversity of ethnic backgrounds. The final mix of contributors is not representative of the proportion of diversities in Canadian and U.S. cultures but is representative of the diversity of cultures in those two countries.

Although contributors were given the opportunity to identify themselves by ethnic background, editors needed to decide when and how to identify scenario personnel. Identifying all clients and therapists in scenarios by ethnicity was one possibility. The question then became how far to go in identification. For example, should Caucasian be the only reference used, or was more specificity called for, such as Irish-American, French-Canadian, Swedish-American–Canadian transplant, etc.? It is possible to trivialize the importance of ethnicity through overidentification and labeling. Individuals were identified in scenarios by ethnicity when ethnicity may have contributed to the ethical dilemmas involved.

In many ways the issues surrounding ethnicity become ones of privilege. For example, do representatives of one group experience more privileges on a daily basis than representatives of other groups? Do they have privilege of access? Do they feel safe and secure in their world on a daily basis? A full discussion of privilege and power is beyond the scope of this book. The reader is encouraged, however, to analyze scenarios and discussions with the implications of privilege in mind.

People of color in Canada and the United States clearly are the ones who feel the impact of racism more personally on a daily basis. Caucasians can more easily "blend in" whether they choose to or not. They also have the option of forgetting about racism if they choose and deciding not to deal with the effects for whatever length of time they wish. People of color typically do not have that option.

At the same time, in both the United States and Canada, the majority cultures are taught to "think white." In many ways, all people are taught to "think white." Because of that tendency, it seemed important to point out when someone is not of the majority cultures. "White" is not considered the norm by the authors, but whites may need the most reminders surrounding ethnicity issues. It is assumed that people of color learn to be bicultural. No reader should assume, however, that if ethnicity or color is not labeled it automatically means Caucasian. The same statement could also be made of all other physical, sociohistoric, and personal characteristics.

The meaning of ethnic characteristics is not necessarily the same for two people with the same ethnic background. Two Jewish women may come from considerably different backgrounds and experiences. Additionally, if both the therapist and client are Swiss-American, can the therapist assume she knows the significance of the client's background? The issue of Caucasian therapist and Caucasian client has not really been explored in the literature (Rave, 1990). Yet assumptions may be made by the therapist that interfere with therapy in ways similar to a different ethnicity interfering with understanding. The negative effects of assumptions by therapists of similar ethnic backgrounds will probably be less than by therapists of differing ethnic backgrounds than their clients.

The important point to remember is that the responsibility in determining significance of ethnicity to the client is the therapist's in conjunction with the client. It is, therefore, incumbent upon the therapist to be aware of her own biases and to continually work with a consultant when the therapist has any concern about her adequacies working with an ethnically different client. It also is possible for the client to be unaware of the impact of ethnicity on her own life. Even in such a case, it is the therapist's responsibility to facilitate the client's awareness.

Kanuha (1990), in discussing oppression, describes the components of ethical feminist therapy philosophy and practice. She lists four necessary components.

1. Discussion and development of the philosophy and practice of feminist therapy principles must directly address the concept of an integrated analysis of oppression.
2. All policies and position papers that describe the tenets of feminist therapy must include an integrated analysis of oppression.
3. All feminist therapists should have education and training in antiracism, homophobia, class issues, anti-Semitism, and all other forms of oppression that affect the lives of women not only in the United States, but internationally.
4. Specific strategies must be developed to actively recruit and support nonwhite, non-middle-class, nonheterosexual women into the feminist therapy profession. (pp. 30–33)

Overall, issues surrounding cultural diversity and oppression remain high among feminist therapist concerns. FTI's membership continues to struggle and learn in these areas. As overall populations in Western societies become more diverse and as therapy clientele reflect that diversity, it becomes even more important for therapists to increase their own knowledge about cultures and to continue exploring their own prejudices and racism for the purpose of increasing their effectiveness with a diverse population.

ORGANIZATION OF THE BOOK

The section by Hill, Glaser, and Harden, immediately following this introduction, gives practitioners a way to think about ethically problematic behaviors. Too often therapists' thinking about the ethical implications of their behaviors comes after the behaviors have occurred. "A Feminist Model for Ethical Decision Making" offers an innovative method to approach ethical decisions. Although other codes of ethics and authors have developed decision-making models (e.g., Canadian Psychological Association, 1991; Keith-Spiegel & Koocher, 1985; Schulz, 1994), this model is the first to acknowledge and use affect in making ethical decisions. Decisions regarding ethical therapist behavior are made in an emotional as well as rational context whether that context is acknowledged or not. To use the feelings of the therapist, consultant, or client as a factor in the decision-making process is a revolutionary step.

The Feminist Therapy Code of Ethics, the common denominator of all the discussions that follow, is reprinted on pages 37–41. Respondents' discussions through the book are referenced to its Preamble or to specific guidelines of the Code in parentheses.

The ethical issues and dilemmas presented are organized by topic. Ethics casebooks are often organized around the principles of the code of ethics being illustrated (American Psychological Association, 1987; Keith-Spiegel & Koocher, 1985; Schulz, 1994). That approach was considered but rejected. The FTI Code itself grew out of therapists' grassroots experiences with their clients. It is usually through specific content-laden situations, rather than through an ideal principle, that ethical dilemmas first arise. Few situations involve only one ethical principle. It seemed consistent and useful to organize the dilemmas around topics significant to women and then to reference responses back to the Code rather than vice versa. This organization also makes it easier for the reader to access topics and the ethical implications involved.

Each section focuses on a specific topic and follows a similar format. First, a brief introduction to the issue is offered including recent developments, importance to women clients, and approaches of ethical codes. Each section then presents three to nine ethical dilemmas, each followed by two or more responses by feminist therapists. Fictitious names are used for both therapists and clients in all the dilemmas, and every effort has been made to change them to protect confidentiality.

The respondents to each scenario explore the ethical dilemmas presented by the situation and apply the FTI Code to suggest ethical resolutions. The final part of each section is devoted to the implications raised by the respondents. The discussions within each section, however, are not comprehensive. The section editors have assumed that readers have some knowledge about ethics and the context of an issue. Most topics have had entire books written about them. At the end of each section, readers are provided with references for the topic together with brief descriptions of the backgrounds of the respondents.

OVERVIEW OF ETHICAL ISSUES

Each of the topics covered in the sections profoundly impacts therapists, clients, therapeutic strategies, and therapeutic process. The intent is to encourage thought and discussion among therapists and therapists-in-training. Some questions and ideas for readers to consider in approaching each of the issues are offered.

Naming the Issue

The diagnostic label given to clients affects how they think about themselves. Women have the added burden of being socialized into behaviors such as submissiveness, that may then be pathologized, such as masochistic personality disorder. Hopefully, readers will develop an increased sensitivity to labels and always question their impact. How does attaching a specific label affect treatment? How does it affect payment for services? How might the client be included in the labeling process?

Monetary Issues

In some ways monetary issues become more important as people further removed from the therapeutic process become involved. Therapists need to be even more concerned with the restrictions that money places on treatment of clients. What are the ethical implications when specific labels are required for a particular length or type of treatment? What are the practical and ethical implications when insurance companies have specific degree and training requirements for therapists? How much should insurance companies affect training programs? When should training program personnel take a more proactive stance in affecting insurance companies' decisions? How do fees and the different ways fees are paid impact the therapist–client relationship? What are the ethical ramifications of differing payment arrangements, such as direct payment by the client with insurance reimbursement or the insurer paying the therapist directly? What steps can therapists take to prepare themselves and the client for fee payment? How does a therapist who provides a range of fees or lower fees deal with complaints of undercutting the competition, considered unethical in some ethical codes?

Overlapping Relationships

Obviously overlapping relationships are still a contentious issue for therapists. Training programs would be an excellent place for professors and supervisors to model effective behaviors in this area. Too frequently, however, the professor and supervisor are not clear themselves about the dangers to a student of their becoming personally involved with that student. Because both individuals are "adults," it is often too easy for the professional to assume that the trainee has equal status and power in learning situations. Educators might ask themselves what the qualities of positive mentoring are and what the ethical issues are in this relationship. When is the professor mentoring and opening new horizons for the student, and when is the professor primarily meeting her or his own needs? How is the mentoring relationship modeling the therapist–client relationship? As therapists read the scenarios and think about their own dual experiences with clients, the main question may be whether the client had the real option of rejecting the experience. In other words, did the therapist misuse power with the client? Did the therapist fail to recognize the potential for conflict of interest in the situation?

Violence against Women

Violence against women continues to be a major social and health issue. Because there has been some publicity about the issues and considerable reading material is available, therapists may assume their knowledge about violence against women is sufficient. Therefore, an important question involves whether the therapist has the training to work with clients who have been abused. Training-program personnel need to question whether they offer sufficient background in this area. Does the therapist recognize whether the client is a survivor of interpersonal violence? Does the therapist have skills in understanding the symbolic content of violence, and is she also able to elicit that content without suggesting it? What ethical concerns may arise when a therapist coordinates community support for a victim of violence?

Reproductive Health

One of the most rapidly changing areas for women is reproduction technology. How can a therapist remain up to date with the new technologies? In the highly emotional area of choice, how does a therapist listen to a client objectively if the client has a different belief system? How might the client's socioeconomic status affect her choices in reproductive health care? In this section the reader might also keep in mind issues surrounding social activism and its impact on clients.

The Medical Model

The section dealing with the medical model raises other questions. What are the limits of the medical model in treating clients? How does the medicalization of clients impact treatment? Perhaps more subtly but equally as important, what are the effects of research from a patriarchal system on treatment? How can therapists who question research developed from a medical model perspective evaluate those results and inform clients of the significant applications of those results? How might training programs more effectively develop skills in research evaluation, especially in non-research-based programs? What is the ethical responsibility of therapists to influence the medical system when information, labeling, research strategies, or results are detrimental to women? How would action dealing with such issues be ethically implemented?

Conflicts in Care

Children and older adults share a common problem. Others, usually caring family members, make decisions for them. The question then becomes when a child can make decisions for herself or himself. For older adults, it becomes when they can no longer make decisions for themselves. Unfortunately the caring family member frequently does not include the child or the older adult in this basic and all-important decision about self-decision-making. To what extent and how can the therapist intervene on behalf of a child or older adult who is being given limited decision-making power? While reading the scenarios, readers may want to ask themselves whether the client was given as large a range as possible in decision making.

Self-Care

Therapist self-care is still an issue not addressed at much length in the literature. Its importance is acknowledged, but the specifics of self-care are not really discussed. Therapists may have difficulty acknowledging they are in psychological distress themselves. How does the therapist know when she is too stressed and needs help herself? How does a colleague facilitate a therapist's getting the help she needs? How can training programs model and alert therapists in training about self-care issues? What policies can institutions and agencies adopt to assist staff in taking care of themselves so they can function effectively in their roles? What assumptions need to be challenged that encourage therapists to overextend themselves at the expense of their own health?

Looking toward the Future

The final section of the book includes thoughts by the book editors developed while editing the volume. The editors react to the topics and ethical dilemmas presented and also suggest some concerns about future ethics' code development. They also discuss some impacts of societal trends on therapy and ethics.

REFERENCES

Adleman, J., & Barrett, S. E. (1990). Overlapping relationships: The importance of the feminist ethical perspective. In H. Lerman & N. Porter (Eds.), *Feminist ethics in psychotherapy* (pp. 87–91). New York: Springer.

American Psychological Association. (1975). Report of the task force on sex bias and sex-role stereotyping in psychotherapeutic practice. *American Psychologist, 30*(1), 1169–1175.

American Psychological Association. (1978). Task force on sex bias and sex-role stereotyping in psychotherapeutic practice: Guidelines for therapy with women. *American Psychologist, 13*, 1122–1123.

American Psychological Association, Division 17, Counseling Psychology. (1979). Principles concerning the counseling and therapy of women. *Counseling Psychologist, 8*(1), 21.

American Psychological Association. (1981). *Ethical principles of psychologists.* Washington, DC: Author.

American Psychological Association. (1987). *Casebook on ethical principles of psychologists.* Washington, DC: Author.

American Psychological Association. (1992). Ethical principles of psychologists (revised). *American Psychologist, 47,* 1597–1611.

Astin, H. S. (1972). Employment and career status of women psychologists. *American Psychologist, 27,* 371–381.

Bardwick, J. M. (1971). *Psychology of women: A study of bio-cultural conflicts.* New York: Harper & Row.

Broverman, I. K., Broverman, D. M., Clarkson, F. E., Rosenkrantz, P. S., & Vogel, S. R., (1970). Sex role stereotypes and clinical judgments of mental health. *Journal of Consulting and Clinical Psychology, 34,* 1–7.

Brown, L. S. (1994). Boundaries in feminist therapy: A conceptual formulation. *Women and Therapy, 15*(1), 29–38.

Cammaert, L. P., & Larsen, C. C. (1988). Feminist frameworks of psychotherapy. In M. A. Dutton-Douglas & L. E. Walker (Eds.), *Feminist psychotherapies: Integration of therapeutic and feminist systems* (pp. 12–36). Norwood, NJ: Ablex.

Canadian Psychological Association. (1980). *Guidelines for therapy and counselling with women.* Ottawa: Author.

Canadian Psychological Association. (1991). *Canadian code of ethics for psychologists* (rev.). Old Chelsea, PQ: Author.

Enns, C. Z. (1993). Twenty years of feminist counseling and therapy: From naming biases to implementing multifaceted practice. *Counseling Psychologist, 21*(1), 3–87.

Feminist Therapy Institute. (1987). *Feminist therapy code of ethics.* Denver: Author.

Gilbert, L. A., & Osipow, S. H. (1991). Feminist contributions to counseling psychology. *Psychology of Women Quarterly, 15,* 537–547.

Greenglass, E. (1973a). Women: A new psychological view. *Ontario Psychologist, 5,* 7–15.

Greenglass, E. (1973b). The psychology of women: Or the high cost of achievement. In M. Stephenson (Ed.), *Women in Canada* (pp. 108–118). Toronto: New Press.

Herlihy, B., & Corey, G. (1992). *Dual relationships in counseling.* Alexandria, VA: American Association for Counseling and Development.

Holroyd, J. C., & Brodsky, A. M. (1977). Psychologists' attitudes and practices regarding erotic and nonerotic physical contact with clients. *American Psychologist, 32,* 843–849.

Kanuha, V. (1990). The need for an integrated analysis of oppression in feminist therapy ethics. In H. Lerman & N. Porter (Eds.), *Feminist ethics in psychotherapy* (pp. 24–35). New York: Springer.

Kaschak, E. (1981). Feminist psychotherapy: The first decade. In S. Cox (Ed.), *Female psychology: The emerging self* (pp. 387–400). New York: St. Martin's.

Keith-Spiegel, P., & Koocher, G. P. (1985). *Ethics in psychology: Professional standards and cases.* New York: Random House.

Kitchener, K. S. (1988). Dual role relationships: What makes them so problematic? *Journal of Counseling and Development, 67*(4), 217–221.

Laidlaw, T. A., & Malmo, C. (1990). *Healing voices: Feminist approaches to therapy with women.* San Francisco: Jossey-Bass.

Marecek, J., & Hare-Mustin, R. T. (1991). A short history of the future:

Feminism and clinical psychology. *Psychology of Women Quarterly, 15,* 521–536.

Mednick, M. T. S., & Weissman, H. J. (1975). The psychology of women: Selected topics. *Annual Review of Psychology, 26,* 1–18.

Peterson, M. R. (1992). *At personal risk: Boundary violations in professional–client relationships.* New York: W. W. Norton.

Pettifor, J. L., Larsen, C. C., & Cammaert, L. P. (1984). *Therapy and counselling with women: A handbook of educational materials.* Ottawa: Canadian Psychological Association.

Pyke, S. (1994). CPA achievements and weather trends in academe. *Newsletter of the CPA Section on Women in Psychology, 21*(1), 12–15.

Rave, E. J. (1990). White feminist therapists and anti-racism. *Women and Therapy, 9*(3), 313–326.

Schulz, W. E. (1994). *Counselling ethics casebook.* Ottawa: Canadian Guidance and Counselling Association.

Sherman, J. A. (1971). *On the psychology of women: A survey of empirical studies.* Springfield, IL: Charles C. Thomas.

Sturdivant, S. (1980). *Therapy with women: A feminist philosophy of treatment.* New York: Springer.

Wand, B. (1977). Report of the task force on the status of women in Canadian psychology. *Canadian Psychological Review, 18,* pp. 3–18.

TWO

A Feminist Model for Ethical Decision Making

Marcia Hill
Kristin Glaser
Judy Harden

What is an ethical dilemma? By definition, a dilemma implies a conflict. Therapists make any number of ethical decisions over the course of a week, or even a day: to avoid revealing information about clients to colleagues or friends, to take a client's background into account in a therapy session, or to attend a workshop as a way of staying current in the field. Generally, these decisions are not experienced as dilemmas. Ethical codes as well as the therapist's moral principles serve as guidelines for behaviors that are well integrated into the therapist's professional identity.

A dilemma arises when the clinician experiences conflict, especially conflict that is not clearly addressed by one's principles or ethical code. Kitchener (1984) describes an ethical dilemma as "a problem for which no course of action seems satisfactory" and goes on to note that "the dilemma exists because there are good, but contradictory ethical reasons to take conflicting and incompatible courses of action" (p. 43). Any combination of one's values, ethical codes, the law, one's personal or professional loyalties, clinical knowledge, or personal feelings may come into conflict in a particular situation. For example, a therapist may have to choose whether to adhere to a legal requirement to report child abuse, knowing that doing so will destroy the therapeutic relationship and may not ultimately protect the child. In such cases, the therapist must find a way to sort through the variables involved, weighing consequences and prioritizing values, in an effort to come to the best possible decision.

Ethical dilemmas are situations in which there is no "right" decision, only a decision that is thoughtfully made and perhaps "more right" than the alternatives. And, as every clinician knows, often the wisdom of a particular course is not evident until long after the choice itself. For clinicians, an ethical decision is a particular subset of treatment decisions, choices that affect one or more clients in the context of the therapist's professional relationship with that person. Ethical decisions are treatment decisions that in some way engage concerns about right and wrong, rather than (or in addition to) other treatment issues such as effectiveness, timing, or appropriateness of particular interventions.

When confronted with an ethical dilemma, a clinician needs more than a code of ethics for guidance. She or he also needs some understanding of how to use that code, as well as other resources, in order to come to a decision that is "more right." As Welfel and Lipsitz (1984) state:

> Just as morality is more than a behavior that ends up helping or hurting someone else, ethics is more than the outcome behavior that conforms to or violates a code. The internal processes (intentions, motivations, way of cognitively structuring the ethically sensitive situation) are equally important. (p. 38)

This section reviews the literature on ethical decision-making processes, which covers intuitive and cognitive levels of reasoning and concrete models for ethical decision making, and comments on the limitations of these guidelines and models from a feminist perspective. The second section offers a more inclusive model for making ethical choices and concludes with an application of the model to an example of an ethical dilemma. This model for decision making is feminist in that the process takes into account the emotional–intuitive responses of the therapist, as well as the location of the therapist, client, and consultant in the social context. Values, beliefs, and factors such as gender, race, class, and sexual/affectional preferences of the people involved are assumed to affect the various aspects of the ethical dilemma. In addition, this model includes the client in the decision-making process whenever possible, which is compatible with the feminist principle that power should be made more equal between the therapist and client when appropriate.

COMPONENTS OF AN ETHICAL
DECISION-MAKING PROCESS

Moral Reasoning

Hare (in Kitchener, 1984) suggests two levels of moral reasoning when one is confronting an ethical situation: the intuitive level and the level of critical evaluation. The intuitive level is the way one first responds to the facts of a situation, the "ordinary moral sense" or the immediate sense of what to do, prior to reflection, and is based on beliefs and assumptions, including knowledge of relevant professional codes. There are some difficulties inherent in primary and exclusive reliance upon an intuitive level of moral reasoning, even though many ethical situations are simple and straightforward enough to resolve themselves quickly and without further deliberation. One concern is that intuitive thinking is permeated with cultural values, including values detrimental to women and other historically undervalued groups. In addition, reliance upon even an informed intuition can lead to a moral relativism that does not always result in sound ethical choices and that can be destructive to clients. The number of therapists who have defended sexual relationships with their clients as in the client's best interests (Rutter, 1989) provides one example of this concern. The limitations of intuitive moral reasoning make critical–evaluative reasoning, described by Hare (in Kitchener, 1984), necessary "to guide, refine, and evaluate our ordinary moral judgment" (p. 44). There are two aspects of critical–evaluative moral reasoning. First is the consideration of the basic and specific ethical rules, such as the Ethical Principles of Psychologists (American Psychological Association, 1992), or the Canadian Code of Ethics for Psychologists (Canadian Psychological Association, 1991). Second is consideration of the more general and fundamental ethical principles or higher-level norms (Beauchamp & Childress; Drane; both described in Kitchener, 1984) to which one can refer when the concrete codes are ambiguous, incomplete, or conflicting.

The basic and specific ethical rules consist of the appropriate professional code, laws, and case law. Thus, if a psychologist had a question about the appropriateness of barter, she or he would look at the new Canadian Psychological Association (1991) or American Psychological Association (1992) code of ethics and relevant casebooks, and a social worker would consider her or his own standards. One also needs to be aware of the state or provincial rules that govern the practice of one's profession and relevant provincial or state laws such as those that legislate mandatory reporting if child abuse is suspected. In some instances, federal legislation must also be considered, such as the U.S. law that mandates equal educational opportunities for differently abled children. Finally, case law such as the *Tarasoff* (1976) decision concerning "duty to warn" have become part of the standards that professionals must consider. One needs to renew continually one's knowledge of standards, since they evolve over time and reflect changing professional values. For example, the new APA Code of Ethics adds rules about barter and reflects much greater concern with the rights of and protection of the consumer of psychology than the previous Code.

The more general and fundamental ethical principles described in Kitchener (1984) that form the foundation of this cognitive level of ethical reasoning in psychology include autonomy (the right to act as an autonomous agent, including the right to choice and privacy about that choice), nonmaleficence ("above all, do no harm"), and beneficence (promoting the welfare of others), justice, and fidelity (promise keeping). Nonmaleficence is considered by many ethicists (Kitchener, 1984) to be the strongest ethical obligation, to be given priority when two principles conflict, such as when a situation calls for both confidentiality and doing no harm, and doing both is not possible. Kitchener describes some problems and limitations associated with this level of reasoning, many of which she and the authors she reviews have addressed. One issue concerns the validity of the principles, whether they should be considered valid absolutely, only relatively, or in a prima facie way. Kitchener's review (1984) led her to conclude that ethical principles are "'conditional' duties. . . . The conditions under which they may be overturned must, however, be morally relevant ones (i.e., when there are stronger moral obligations)" (p. 52). A second issue is the dilemma one faces when two or more of these principles conflict in a given situation.

Another problem inherent in the critical–evaluative level of moral reasoning that has not been addressed or resolved by the literature so far is that one's interpretation of the ethical codes, and the principles on which they are based, varies according to where one is located within a context of power (race, gender, class, etc.). Since the ethical principles are seen as fundamental to the more specific ethical codes of conduct, a look at some of these in terms of feminist principles will illustrate the nature of the problem.

All of the ethical principles reviewed here rest upon certain assumptions about those professionals making the decisions; one is that there is some common and agreed-upon sense of what constitutes harm and human welfare, and more significantly, that one's judgment about these principles is unaffected by one's personal and social context. The authors would argue that one's position in the culture, particularly in relation to power, deeply affects how one defines each of these principles and thus is at the very heart of one's ethical decision making.

Nonmaleficence, or "above all, do no harm," is ambiguous at its core in that what constitutes "harm to clients" is never defined. The authors argue that much harm has been done to female clients through the very nature of many theoretical models of psychotherapy that rely solely upon intrapsychic explanations of behavior and thus define human problems and their solutions in ways that blame the victim. Just a few years ago, women were frequently counseled to calm down and return to abusive situations, and they, rather than the perpetrator, were often defined as the problem. Such practices were considered not only professional, but well within specific ethical guidelines as well, and they have been harmful to women.

Similar concerns are associated with the principle of beneficence, since what promotes human welfare is equally ambiguous, and thus subject to influence by factors of culture and power. To the extent that women are viewed as "irrational" or otherwise "incompetent" by virtue of being women, to that extent can many acts of paternalism be committed "for her own good." For example, to the extent that marriage and heterosexual relationships are assumed to be the healthy norm, clients with other affectional preferences can be encouraged in a direction not in their best interests.

Kitchener also does not distinguish among different effects of ethical decision making depending on the particular characteristics of the client in terms of power. For example, in her acknowledgment of the lack of a clear definition of what constitutes harm, she describes the difficulty in determining "how much discomfort is justifiable in therapy" (1984, p. 48); she does not acknowledge that one's sense of discomfort can be exacerbated by one's relative power in the therapy situation. Exploration of an incestuous relationship by a young woman client with an older male therapist may have added layers of discomfort compared to exploration with a female therapist, where the power differential is not as great. Similarly, although Kitchener acknowledges the potential harmful consequences of diagnostic labeling associated with the medical model of mental illness, she does not address the differential impact of this labeling depending on one's racial or gender identification.

Models for Decision Making

The intuitive and the critical–evaluative levels of moral reasoning described by Kitchener (1984) provide a general background for the more concrete models of decision making, such as the ones offered by the Canadian Psychological Association (1991), Haas and Malouf (1989), Jacob and Hartshorne (1991), Lafer and Lee (1990), and Tymchuk (1989). Haas and Malouf, in a very accessible general ethical guide, offer a flow chart for decision making. They illustrate the model, chapter by chapter, as they present ethical issues such as dual relationships, confidentiality, and so forth. The first step in the model is information gathering. The clinician first identifies whether there are one or more ethical problems. One must clarify who the "legitimate stake holders" are, particularly if insurance companies, hospitals, or guardians are involved. A decision must be made about who is the primary client and who has ultimate say. Finally, one must identify the applicable standards such as ethical codes, principles, and laws.

One enters the Haas and Malouf flow chart by asking if a single relevant professional, legal, or social standard exists for the question. If yes, and there is no reason to deviate from it, there is no dilemma, and one simply implements the recommended action. If no single standard seems apparent, one tries to identify the competing ethical principles and decide whether one principle is primary. If so, one seeks an appropriate course of action and implements it. If there is no clarity, one consults with others, researches the literature, and attempts to prioritize the principles. Where no ethical characteristic is primary, a variety of actions could be appropriate. The clinician brainstorms solutions, looking for answers that reconcile the competing principles or achieve a balance between doing the least harm and accomplishing the most benefit. The cost–benefit analysis is then applied to the various affected parties to see if the solution works for everyone. One also asks if the decision would cause any new ethical problems and whether the decision is both practical to implement and prudent for the practitioner. One then initiates the action and evaluates the outcome. Review and consultation are again recommended.

Haas and Malouf point out that the weakness of this model is that it is based on rationality and could therefore be used in a self-serving manner to rationalize poor decisions. The authors suggest that the assumption that this complex process ever could be strictly rational is erroneous. Most complex issues stir up feelings in the protagonists, and not to account for the practitioner's psychology is to leave out critical factors. The authors suggest a more complete model that is based on acknowledging both the rational and emotional components of an ethical decision-making process.

Additional Aspects of Ethical Decision Making

The literature about the ethical decision-making process, then, describes ethical codes, the general moral principles underlying those codes, and various models based on one or both of these guidelines. However, these approaches consider ethical dilemmas from a perspective that is almost exclusively cognitive and that gives minimal attention to the person of the therapist as a factor in the decision-making process. Ethical guidelines, as well as ethical decision-making models, look at ethical dilemmas objectively and from an intellectual distance. In actual practice, clinicians experience ethical dilemmas with an immediacy and personal involvement that cannot be completely separated out from their decision-making process. According to feminist principles, one's personal experience and involvement are legitimate and necessary factors to take into account in any analysis. In addition, ethical guidelines are of necessity generalizations and will therefore lack the complexity and specificity of any given ethical dilemma. As a consequence, it is understandable that most clinicians believe that they are not well enough informed to make ethical decisions (Tymchuk, 1986).

Situational or contextual elements in the particular ethical dilemma are missing from most ethical guidelines as well as from most research about ethical decision making; these elements are also a necessary aspect of a feminist analysis. Exceptions to this omission are Brosig and Kalichman (1992) who review the literature on child-abuse reporting. They suggest that someone can only understand whether or not a clinician will report by looking at all the situational variables. They examine legal factors such as clinician's knowledge of the law and the specific requirements and language of the law; clinician characteristics such as years of experience, training, and attitudes; and situational factors such as victim attributes, type and severity of abuse, and available evidence. Similarly Lafer and Lee (1990) discuss the making of ethical treatment decisions with dying patients. In their examples they illustrate how the correct choice is unique for each patient based on her or his understanding of the illness, the characteristics of the staff, and the family context.

A book such as this one is also an effort to integrate the context into ethical guidelines. Although it is obvious that not all situations related to a given ethical issue can be addressed, specific examples may help the therapist better understand how the context influences the way in which ethical guidelines are prioritized and applied.

The person of the therapist has been strikingly absent from the public discourse on ethical decision making. It is perhaps this omission, more than any other factor, that has left clinicians feeling so inadequately advised about making ethical decisions. The omission itself is significant; what is not said often has as much meaning as what is said. In this case, what is implied by the failure to include the therapist in discourse about ethics? Does discussing ethics without discussing the therapist mean that the personal characteristics of the therapist (experience, culture, style, etc.) are or should be irrelevant to one's ethical decisions? Does it imply that the therapist's feelings about the ethical dilemma (intuition, countertransference, etc.) are or should be irrelevant as well? If guidelines are developed that do not include the therapist as a factor in decision making, then therapists who try to make ethical choices have guidance in certain aspects of the decision but no help in other aspects. By omission, therapists are implicitly instructed that certain factors should be ignored.

Some authors have looked at therapist characteristics as they relate to ethical choices without offering suggestions to therapists about how to take these factors into consideration. Kimmel (1991), for example, notes that "ethical decisions and moral judgments may be affected by the investigator's cultural and personal characteristics" (p. 786). His research indicated that clinician characteristics such as gender, years of experience, area of training, and employment setting were related to whether the clinician emphasized the benefits of research or the costs to the research participants in making ethical decisions about research. His study showed that clinicians who had held a degree longer, those with degrees in basic rather than applied psychology, those employed in research rather than service contexts, and male clinicians emphasized the benefits over the costs of research. Haas, Malouf, and Mayerson (1988), using a variety of clinical vignettes, showed that for some situations, therapists' ethical decisions differed by gender and years of experience. Brosig and Kalichman (1992) also show years of experience as being a factor in therapists' decisions to report child abuse. Welfel and Lipsitz (1984) state that a review of the literature finds conflicting results as to the effect of various therapist characteristics on their ethical judgments.

What is perhaps most useful to draw from the literature on clinician characteristics is the knowledge that it is likely that a therapist's personal characteristics (e.g., training, gender) will influence her or his priorities and values. Values are inherent in every work or training setting, as well as in every theoretical orientation, whether they are made explicit or not.

Time in a particular setting or working from a certain theoretical base represents at least a certain amount of exposure to specific values and often a personal investment in those values. Factors such as gender, ethnicity or race, religious background, geographic location, and so forth, are even more obviously related to values. The therapist's personal experiences of oppression and the uses of power, (e.g., through race, sexual orientation, gender, size, disability, class, and age) will sensitize that individual in certain ways. Those same factors and others (such as religious background, family or living situation, or geographic location) will influence the therapist's priorities and assumptions. In order to make a feminist model for decision making, these aspects of who the therapist is cannot be separated from the decisions that she or he makes. If therapists turn to ethical decision-making models that do not address these factors, they then run the risk of making these factors invisible and thus not open to scrutiny.

The other general aspect of the person of the therapist that has not been included in models for making ethical choices is the psychological, a curious lacuna for a group of professions that claim expertise regarding the influence of the psychological on human behavior. Psychological characteristics of the therapist include those that might loosely be designated as countertransference, such as feelings about the client, the ethical situation itself, the process of consulting, and so forth, as well as personal characteristics that might best be ascribed to temperament or style.

Countertransference can include a range of feelings that influence the clinician's judgment in a given ethical dilemma. In the most traditional use of the term, the therapist might have feelings about the client or responses related to how closely the ethical dilemma touches her or his personal life. The therapist may also have feelings about her or his supervisor or consultant. More generally, there are the therapist's feelings about her or his competence, about the way in which she or he may have contributed to the ethical dilemma, feelings of responsibility or self-blame, or shame associated with the situation itself or with sharing it with a colleague. In examining an ethical dilemma, it is important that these responses be taken into account not only because they can get in the way of making a good decision, but also because they may be subtle indicators of aspects of the ethical dilemma that have not been fully considered. For example, a therapist may respond to a client's request for some special consideration by withholding and feeling guilty. Those feelings might be strictly personal, but they could also indicate that the request is inappropriate.

A therapist's temperament or style does not so much change an ethical decision as it shapes the form in which the decision will be carried out or fine tunes matters like timing or detail. A therapist with relatively high tolerance for anxiety may choose to wait and watch with an angry and potentially destructive client in a situation where another therapist might intervene more actively. A clinician with a more formal persona might be more inclined to avoid social settings in which clients are present, while a less formal clinician might address the boundary issues through negotiation and discussion with the clients involved. In any ethical decision, the therapist will find the most personally authentic solution if she or he is able to take these kinds of personal characteristics into account.

Another dimension not adequately addressed in the literature is the role of the consultant in the decision-making process. In the authors' experience, seeking consultation about ethical issues is quite common, even among very experienced practitioners. The consultant's values, conceptualization of therapy, and relationship to the questioner are likely to have significant impact. For example, depending on training and personal experience, one advisor is likely to have a more rigid or loose definition of boundary issues than another. In a different situation, an advisor would have a more distanced or impassioned reaction to the issue of reporting child abuse based on her or his personal experience with both abuse and reporting. Given that the therapist is seeking advice, or at least validation and reassurance about a dilemma, the characteristics of the advisor and the consulting relationship should also be scrutinized.

Finally, it is essential that the client be explicitly included in the ethical decision-making process as fully as is possible and appropriate. This position is informed by the feminist principle that power should be equalized between therapist and client to the extent compatible with good treatment principles. But perhaps more than that, inclusion of the client in the decision-making process is simply a matter of making the best possible decision. The client's perspective and reactions are valuable information that the clinician cannot afford to ignore. Sometimes, of course, not all those affected by a decision are available for discussion about the dilemma; occasionally, a client may not be competent to participate in such a discussion. In addition many aspects of any given situation are not appropriate to share with a client (most commonly, certain of the therapist's feelings, such as insecurity or shame or erotic feelings toward the client). Nonetheless, in most cases, the therapist can reasonably seek some form of collaboration with the client. Although clients may not be aware of the specific codes of ethics by which therapists are governed, they certainly are usually capable of understanding the general moral principles involved. The client's responses may well suggest factors or emphases in the dilemma that the therapist may not have considered. For example, a clinician might be trying to decide whether to accept for therapy someone who has difficulties that are outside the therapist's area of expertise. In this case, the therapist might be reassured to know that the client has other resources in that area or wishes to focus on concerns other than the area in question. In addition, even though the therapist carries sole responsibility for the ultimate decision, the perspective of the client should always be taken into account.

A FEMINIST MODEL FOR ETHICAL DECISION MAKING

A feminist model for ethical decision making combines the rational–evaluative model found in the literature (Canadian Psychological Association, 1991; Haas & Malouf, 1989; Jacob & Hartshorne, 1991; Lafer & Lee, 1990; Tymchuk, 1986), the emotional and intuitive aspects of the clinician's responses to the situation, awareness of the power difference between the therapist and client, and a recognition of possible cultural biases inherent in making value-based decisions. As feminists, the authors consider the inclusion of the person of the therapist in the description of the decision-making process crucial to making a decision that is more fully informed and less likely to be based on unexamined biases. Thus, the question "How does who I am affect this process?" is asked both emotionally and analytically throughout the course of making the decision. Although this model will be presented in a linear way, the steps may not always occur in this order, and certain steps may be repeated depending on the nature of the ethical dilemma. The actual process of decision making will weave back and forth between a more cognitive evaluation of the dilemma and attention to the clinician's experiential or feeling sense of the situation.

Recognizing a Problem

Recognition of a problem may come in any of several ways. Clinicians may simply recognize ethical problems from their experience and understanding of the therapy process or the ethical codes. Less experienced therapists may be informed by supervisors, colleagues, or clients. Frequently, the first indication that there is an ethical dilemma is the therapist's feeling of discomfort. It may be as simple as uncertainty concerning how to proceed in a given situation or may be complicated by other feelings. The initial task of the therapist is to identify any aspects of her or his feelings that stand in the way of understanding and sorting through the problem. One possibility is that the clinician has reactions to the nature of the situation that are not particular to the client involved. An example would be a therapist who knows that she or he is always a bit confused by difficult boundary dilemmas and tends to have trouble standing her ground when a client asks for special treatment in some way. Another general area of initial reactions that may be separate from the specific dilemma includes feelings that one may have about asking for help in examining an ethical decision. The clinician may feel that she or he should not have this problem, may feel exposed or ashamed for being in the situation at all, or may have feelings about her or his consultant. In any of these cases, the therapist may be able to resolve the difficulty before attempting to make the ethical decision. Alternatively, it may be enough simply to recognize that the particular feeling is an element of what she or he brings to the issue at hand and to mark it as something to stay aware of while going through the decision-making process. The decision to ask for consultation may occur at this point.

Defining the Problem

Now the therapist goes on to define the nature of the conflict. As previously described, a dilemma implies that there is more than one potentially right course of action. The therapist now asks, "What is the conflict?" in an attempt to identify what ethical principles, obligations, laws, or treatment imperatives may be at odds. The therapist identifies the people or institutions whose needs must be considered in the decision. Relevant standards, which might be formal ethical codes, general ethical principles, or laws, are also identified at this point.

Collaboration with the client is perhaps most critical during this stage of the decision-making process. The first step is for the therapist to determine the extent to which, consistent with good treatment principles, the client can be included in the process of sorting through the ethical dilemma. What perspective does the client bring to the therapist's understanding of the dilemma? How does the client define the problem? Both the rational and emotional dimensions of the client's responses may be explored.

In the emotional arena, the clinician can begin to use her or his felt experience as additional information about the ethical dilemma. Questions might include, "What else is my discomfort about? What do my feelings tell me about the situation? What am I worried about?" For example, a clinician knows that she should report child abuse that a client has revealed yet finds herself feeling very reluctant to do so. On reflection, she realizes that she does not trust the client's report and begins to consider her recent experiences with the client in this light, eventually wondering if the confession of child abuse were exaggerated in order to elicit a particular response from her.

Returning to the more rational aspect of defining the problem, the clinician at this stage would also take an initial look at the personal characteristics and values that she or he brings to the definition of the problem. This evaluation is particularly necessary if the clinician differs in any significant cultural way (gender, race, class, etc.) from the other players in the situation. It is important to ask oneself whether the client, for example, would define the problem differently based on cultural characteristics. For instance, the client may feel bound by cultural norms that the therapist cannot support, such as a particular attitude toward lesbians and gays or attitudes that significantly restrict options for women. These differences may lead the clinician into therapeutic, legal, or ethical conflicts. The therapist may feel that honoring the client's religious, ethnic, or other cultural expectations will ultimately harm the client. As with other conflicts, open discussion with the client and professional consultation are called for.

The decision to seek consultation may also occur at this point in the decision-making process. The therapist needs to be conscious and thoughtful about the consultant's personal characteristics and values and how they will influence the process. Under ideal circumstances, there would be open discussion between the two people about their influences on one another.

Developing Solutions

Now the therapist begins to generate possible options for responding to the situation. She or he will brainstorm possibilities and engage in a cost–benefit analysis of each option. Such an analysis is, in effect, an effort to address explicitly the primary ethical principles of nonmaleficence ("do no harm") and beneficence (do "the greatest good"). In addition, the therapist will consider whether the solution being considered is both practical and prudent (Haas & Malouf, 1989). Although the clinician may have already determined what factor in the decision is most important, in many cases the order of priority will emerge in this weighing-out process.

As she or he engages in a cost–benefit analysis, the therapist will also have intuitive or feeling responses to each of the alternatives generated. As described in the previous step, those responses are valuable information that can be used to refine further one's understanding of the nature of the dilemma and problems or benefits that may be associated with each possible response. Again, in many cases, the client can be appropriately included in the development of solutions. A fairly common example in small communities is the discovery that both the therapist and the client plan to attend the same social event. In discussing the dilemma, one or the other may offer not to attend or may suggest a way to interact that feels comfortable to both.

Choosing a Solution

The authors do not separate cognitive and emotional components in this step because the best decisions are made when both of these sources of information are included in an integrated way. The therapist asks, "Is this solution the best fit both emotionally and rationally? Does this meet everyone's needs, including mine? Can I implement and live with this?"

Reviewing Process

At this point, it is again critical for the clinician to ask how her or his values and personal characteristics might be influencing the choice of a solution. Once more, this questioning is especially important if the therapist differs from the client in some significant way. Would another clinician who is similar to the client in these dimensions make a different choice? Being in a position to make an ethical decision that involves the welfare of another person implies that one is in a position of power, and it is incumbent upon the therapist to look at how she or he is using that power. The "golden rule," which asks whether you would wish to be treated in this way, is a time-honored method to consider the rightness of a decision. The clinician might also ask her or himself whether the decision is universalizable (Haas & Malouf, 1989). Although every situation is unique, a decision that is too much of a special case may be a decision that is based too much on personal bias in some way. Haas and Malouf suggest that the decision be examined using the criterion of a "well-lit room." Does the clinician feel comfortable subjecting her or his choice to the scrutiny of others?

In a more intuitive frame, the therapist asks simply, "Does this feel right?" At this point, the clinician may wish to consider whether the specific form in which the decision will be enacted feels like a reasonably good match with her or his temperament or style. When time permits, it is often a good idea to sleep on a decision, to give oneself time to let any buried uncertainties or reservations emerge.

The therapist at this point generally communicates the decision to the client. When appropriate and realistic, the client can be asked to consider her or his reactions to the decision.

Implementing and Evaluating the Decision

Implementing the decision and evaluating the results are a unitary step in the decision-making process. The therapist carries out the decision while observing the consequences of this choice. Such action involves an ongoing reassessment of the ethical dilemma and the effectiveness of the chosen response. The clinician asks, "Is this the best I can do in this situation? Does my decision continue to feel right?" It is not uncommon for the therapist's intervention to throw more light on the situation, which might then lead to a redefinition of the problem, development of further solutions, and so forth.

The client's responses to the ethical decision are, of course, a primary consideration. When feasible and appropriate in terms of treatment considerations, the therapist may choose to include the client in the ongoing process of evaluating whether the decision continues to feel right or needs to be rethought.

Continuing Reflection

Every experience changes the people involved. After the ethical dilemma is resolved, the clinician integrates the experience in some way. Experience is valuable to the extent that it can be used to inform and enrich future understanding and choices. Cognitively, the therapist might consider what she or he learned from this situation. Are there things that she or he would do differently if faced with a similar dilemma in the future? More globally, the therapist asks, "How have I changed as a result of this decision?" For example, has this experience had the long-range impact of making the therapist more cautious about a particular issue or more sensitive in some area? This kind of self-knowledge may be part of what one brings to the next ethical dilemma.

Table 1 summarizes the steps of the decision-making process. The interaction between the rational–evaluative and the feeling–intuitive aspects of the model are also illustrated.

The following example illustrates how this model might be implemented in a clinical situation. Note that in actual practice one or several of the steps may need to be repeated as the clinician's understanding of the ethical dilemma unfolds.

AN EXAMPLE OF IMPLEMENTING THE MODEL

Recognizing a Problem

An experienced therapist had been seeing a quite troubled man in his early 20s for about six weeks. The young man described a history of difficult relationships, most often with himself in the victim's role. He was having an affair with a significantly older, married woman. The client seemed satisfied with the relationship, feeling that he was finally safe. He had few concerns about his lover's married status because he spent as much time with his lover as he wished. The therapist had mixed feelings but was biding her time, since the client was focused on other issues.

The young man then reported that his lover, as a necessary part of her training, wanted to participate in an upcoming certification workshop conducted by the therapist. The lover had asked the young man to check it out with the therapist. The client volunteered that he had no problem about it, and the therapist agreed to think it over.

The therapist's immediate response was mild discomfort and a sense of confusion. After the session, she realized that there were several conflicting ethical issues. Because of the conflicting issues and her sense of discomfort, she sought a consultation with a colleague who had strong feelings about boundary issues.

Defining the Problem

The therapist outlined the conflicting ethical guidelines to her colleague. She was enjoined by her professional ethical code to avoid overlapping relationships whenever possible. However, she also was the only available certifying practitioner in her rural area and to refuse might mean harm to the lover. The consultant was concerned about the implications of developing a dual relationship with the lover and immediately argued that the lover be turned down. The therapist also

Table 1. Feminist Ethical Decision-Making Model

Rational–evaluative process	Feeling–intuitive process

Recognizing a problem

Information from therapist's knowledge; advice from supervisor or colleague	Uncertainty about how to proceed in situation
	Identify what stands in the way of working through the problem: feelings about the nature of the issue, feelings about the consultant or about asking for help

(Decision to consult may occur here)

Defining the problem

What is the conflict? Who are the players? What are the relevant standards? (rules, codes, principles)	What else is my discomfort about? What do my feelings tell me about the situation? What am I worried about?
What personal characteristics and cultural values do I bring to this decision? How do these factors influence my definition of the problem?	
How does the client define the problem?	What are the client's feelings about the dilemma?

(Decision to consult may occur here)

What personal characteristics, values does the consultant bring to this process?	How do the consultant's characteristics affect me?

Developing solutions

Brainstorm possibilities Cost–benefit analysis Prioritize values	What do my reactions to each choice tell me?

Choosing a solution

What is the best fit both emotionally and rationally? Does this solution meet everyone's needs, including mine? Can I implement and live with the effects?

Reviewing process

Would I want to be treated in this way?	Does the decision feel right?
Is the decision universalizable? Would this decision withstand the scrutiny of others?	Have I given myself time to let reservations emerge?
How are my values, personal characteristics influencing my choice? How am I using my power?	Does the manner in which I carry out this decision fit my style?
Have I taken the client's perspective into account?	

(cont.)

Table 1. *(cont.)*

Rational–evaluative process	Feeling–intuitive process
Implementing and evaluating the decision	
Carry out the decision	Is this solution the best I can do?
Observe consequences	
Reassess the decision	Does the outcome continue to feel right?
How has this decision affected the therapeutic process?	
Continuing reflection	
What did I learn?	Have I changed as a result of this process? How?
What would I do differently?	How might this experience affect me in the future?

Note. From "A Feminist Model for Ethical Decision Making" by M. Hill, K. Glaser, and J. Harden (1995). In E. J. Rave and C. C. Larsen (Eds.), *Ethical Decision Making in Therapy: Feminist Perspectives.* New York: Guilford Press.

became concerned about treatment implications. Would her acceptance of the lover make it seem as if she were condoning the affair? Would it replicate the conditions of the triangle? Would her power position as giver of certification create transferential feelings in either client or lover? How else would getting to know the lover (or refusing her) affect her therapeutic work?

Developing Solutions and Choosing a Solution

The therapist and consultant first brainstormed to see if there were other options than acceptance/refusal. They could not find other alternatives. They then considered the primary choices: (1) Accept the lover and work through the consequences as they evolve. The consultant did not care for this solution. (2) Refuse the lover and work through the consequences with the client. The therapist would clearly avoid the overlapping relationship but might engage the client in a deeper level of transference than appropriate for the current stage of therapy. The therapist was not very comfortable with this solution, but it seemed the better choice.

Reviewing Process

The therapist continued to think the situation over for a few days, remaining unsettled about the choice. Partially she realized she felt pushed by the consultant, but there was another source of yet unidentified disquiet.

To gather further data, she discussed the issue again with her client. He gave the issue more thoughtful consideration but said that he did not feel any danger to himself. He trusted both his lover and the therapist. The workshop was brief, and he did not understand what the "big deal" was. His reaction led the therapist to examine her own sense of caution and wonder if she were reacting differently than the client because of gender. Perhaps for some men these kinds of overlaps simply were not "such a big deal." She also considered, and then discarded as not important here, the substantial class-of-origin difference between her and her client.

Rechoosing a Solution

The therapist sought a second consultation from her colleague. As they reexamined the material, they realized that another treatment principle was at stake. Not to honor the client's choice without compelling reasons would constitute a paternalistic response from the therapist. At this stage of treatment the therapist did not feel as though she knew more than the client did about what was best for him. The risk of harm was less than the risk of refusing to work collaboratively with him about treatment decisions and of refusing to let him have as much power as possible in the therapeutic relationship.

When the therapist considered the possible negative consequences of accepting the lover, she realized that at the worst it would stir up transferential responses that she believed she could handle. The consultant agreed with the choice.

Implementing and Evaluating the Decision

The "most benefit, least harm" choice was made to accept the partner in the workshop. The therapist had opened discussion with the client, and they would continue to discuss his feelings as the situation unfolded. The therapist also realized that the choice also suited her character. Even though she has no trouble holding her ground with clients, she did not relish taking a paternalistic stance unless absolutely necessary.

Continuing Reflection

Several months later, the therapist reported that the decision seemed to have worked well. The lover had maintained a professional stance in the workshop, and the client had been so deeply absorbed in other work that he seemed to have no further reactions. Given that the outcome seemed so benign, the therapist had been wondering why it had become such a "big deal." She decided that she must have been more stirred up about the client's affair than she had realized and had displaced that concern onto the request about the workshop. She was glad she had not settled for her first decision. She also thought she had learned a lot about the ethical decision-making process in general. Of particular interest to her were the facts that the obvious decision is not necessarily the best; that frequently ethical decisions have an evolving, unfolding quality; that supervision is not an unbiased process; and that when possible, consultation with the client should be central.

In considering this case, it is important to realize that were the situational factors different, the choice and outcome could also have been different. If the therapist thought the affair were damaging or she had recently experienced troublesome boundary issues, she might have kept her original decision. If the consultant had been in a more powerful supervisory position with a less experienced therapist, the original choice might have prevailed. If the lover turned out to be a difficult person or a poor student, the outcome might not have been so successful. Most ethical decision-making processes are relative to the people and the conditions of that situation. Assessing the situational correctness is as important as the reconciliation of underlying principles and rules. Full consciousness of all the variables allows a fully informed decision.

CONCLUSION

The focus in this section has emphasized aspects of ethical decision making that the authors have experienced clinically and that are consistent with feminist principles of analysis but have been missing from the literature. As a feminist, one must consider the emotional–intuitive responses of the therapist; the sociocultural context of the therapist, client, and consultant, particularly as it relates to issues of power; and the client's participation in the decision-making process. More work needs to be done regarding how factors of ethnic identification, affectional preference, gender, class, and so forth affect the prioritization of values. Guidelines about the extent to which the client could be included in solving ethical dilemmas would also be valuable.

ACKNOWLEDGMENT

The authors gratefully acknowledge the assistance and support of Michele Clark in the preparation of this section.

REFERENCES

American Psychological Association. (1992). Ethical principles of psychologists and code of conduct. *American Psychologist, 47*, 1597–1611.

Brosig, C. L., & Kalichman, S. C. (1992). Clinicians' reporting of suspected child abuse: A review of the empirical literature. *Clinical Psychology Review, 12*, 155–168.

Canadian Psychological Association. (1991). *Canadian code of ethics for psychologists* (rev.). Old Chelsea, PQ: Author.

Haas, L. J., & Malouf, J. L. (1989). *Keeping up the good work: A practitioners's guide to mental health ethics.* Sarasota, FL: Professional Resource Exchange.

Haas, L. J., Malouf, J. L., & Mayerson, N. H. (1988). Personal and professional characteristics as factors in psychologists' ethical decision making. *Professional Psychology, 19*, 35–42.

Jacob, S., & Hartshorne, T. S. (1991). *Ethics and law for school psychologists.* Brandon, VT: Clinical Psychology Publishing Co.

Kimmel, A. J. (1991). Predictable biases in the ethical decision making of American psychologists. *American Psychologist, 46*, 786–788.

Kitchener, K. S. (1984). Intuition, critical evaluation and ethical principles: The foundation for ethical decisions in counseling psychology. *Counseling Psychologist, 12*, 43–55.

Lafer, B. H., & Lee, S. S. (1990). A framework for ethical decision making with dying patients. *Psychotherapy in Private Practice, 8*, 69–82.

Rutter, P. (1989). *Sex in the forbidden zone.* Los Angeles: Jeremy Tarcher.

Tarasoff v. Regents of University of California, 529 P.2d 533 (Cal. 1974); 551 P.2d 334, 331 (Cal. 1976).

Tymchuk, A. (1986). Guidelines for ethical decision making. *Canadian Psychology, 27*, 36–43.

Welfel, E. R., & Lipsitz, N. E. (1984). The ethical behavior of professional psychologists: A critical analysis of the research. *Counseling Psychologist, 12*, 31–42.

THREE

Feminist Therapy Code of Ethics

PREAMBLE

Feminist therapy evolved from feminist philosophy, psychological theory and practice, and political theory. In particular feminists recognize the impact of society in creating and maintaining the problems and issues brought into therapy. Briefly, feminists believe the personal is political. Basic tenets of feminism include a belief in the equal worth of all human beings, a recognition that each individual's personal experiences and situations are reflective of and an influence on society's institutionalized attitudes and values, and a commitment to political and social change that equalizes power among people by recognizing and reducing the pervasive influences and insidious effects of patriarchy on people's lives. Thus, a feminist analysis addresses the effects of sexism on the development of females and males and the relationship of sexism to other forms of oppression, including, but not limited to, racism, classism, homophobia, ageism, and anti-Semitism. Feminists also live in and are subject to those same influences and effects and continually monitor their beliefs and behaviors as a result of these influences.

Feminist therapists adhere to and integrate feminist analysis into all spheres of their work as therapists, educators, consultants, administrators, and/or researchers. Feminist therapists are accountable for the management of the power differential within the therapist/client relationship. Because of the limitations of a purely intrapsychic model of human functioning, feminist therapists facilitate the understanding of interactive effects of the client's internal and external worlds. Feminist therapists possess knowledge about the psychology of women and utilize feminist scholarship to revise theories and practices, incorporating new knowledge as it is generated.

Feminist therapists assume a proactive stance toward the eradication of oppression in their lives and work toward empowering women. They are respectful of individual differences, challenging oppressive aspects of both their own and clients' value systems. Feminist therapists engage in social change activities, broadly defined, outside of and apart from their work in their professions. Such activities may vary in scope and content but are an essential aspect of a feminist perspective.

Feminist therapists are trained in a variety of disciplines, theoretical orientations, and degrees of structure. They come from different cultural, ethnic, and racial backgrounds. They work in many types of settings with a diversity of clients and practice different modalities of therapy, training, and research. Amid this diversity, feminist therapists are joined together by their feminist analyses and perspectives.

Feminist therapy theory integrates feminist principles into other theories of human development and change. As a result, the following ethical principles are additive to, rather than a replacement for, the ethical principles of the profession in which a feminist therapist practices. Feminist therapists also will work toward incorporating feminist principles into existing standards when appropriate.

The code is a series of positive statements which provide guidelines for feminist therapy practice, training, and research. Feminist therapists who are members of other professional organizations adhere to the ethical codes of those organizations. Feminist therapists who are not members of such organizations are guided by the ethical standards of the organization closest to their mode of practice. These statements provide more specific guidelines within the context of and as an extension of most ethical codes. When ethical guidelines are in conflict, the feminist therapist is accountable for how she prioritizes her choices.

These ethical guidelines, then, are focused on the issues feminist therapists, educators, and researchers have found especially important in their professional settings. As with any code of therapy ethics, the well-being of the clients is the guiding principle underlying this code. The feminist therapy issues which relate directly to the client's well-being include cultural diversities and oppressions, power differentials, overlapping relationships, therapist accountability, and social change. Even though the principles are stated separately, each interfaces with the others to form an interdependent whole. In addition, the code is a living document and thus is continually in the process of change.

ETHICAL GUIDELINES FOR FEMINIST THERAPISTS

I. Cultural Diversities and Oppressions

A. A feminist therapist increases her accessibility to and for a wide range of clients from her own and other identified groups through flexible delivery of services. When appropriate, the feminist therapist assists clients in accessing other services.
B. A feminist therapist is aware of the meaning and impact of her own ethnic and cultural background, gender, class, and sexual orientation and actively attempts to become more knowledgeable about alternatives from sources other than her clients. The therapist's goal is to uncover and respect cultural and experiential differences.
C. A feminist therapist evaluates her ongoing interactions with her clientele for any evidence of the therapist's biases or discriminatory attitudes and practice. The feminist therapist accepts responsibility for taking action to confront and change any interfering or oppressing biases she has.

II. Power Differentials

A. A feminist therapist acknowledges the inherent power differentials between client and therapist and models effective use of personal power. In using the power differential to the benefit of the client, she does not take control or power which rightfully belongs to her client.
B. A feminist therapist discloses information to the client which facilitates the therapeutic process. The therapist is responsible for using self-disclosure with purpose and discretion in the interests of the client.
C. A feminist therapist negotiates and renegotiates formal and/or informal contracts with clients in an ongoing mutual process.
D. A feminist therapist educates her clients regarding their rights as consumers of therapy, including procedures for resolving differences and filing grievances.

III. Overlapping Relationships

A. A feminist therapist recognizes the complexity and conflicting priorities inherent in multiple or overlapping relationships. The therapist accepts responsibility for monitoring such relationships to prevent potential abuse of or harm to the client.

B. A feminist therapist is actively involved in her community. As a result, she is especially sensitive about confidentiality. Recognizing that her clients' concerns and general well-being are primary, she self-monitors both public and private statements and comments.

C. A feminist therapist does not engage in sexual intimacies nor overtly or covertly sexualized behaviors with a client or former client.

IV. Therapist Accountability

A. A feminist therapist works only with those issues and clients within the realm of her competencies.

B. A feminist therapist recognizes her personal and professional needs, and utilizes ongoing self-evaluation, peer support, consultation, supervision, continuing education, and/or personal therapy to evaluate, maintain, and improve her work with clients, her competencies, and her emotional well-being.

C. A feminist therapist continually reevaluates her training, theoretical background, and research to include developments in feminist knowledge. She integrates feminism into psychological theory, receives ongoing therapy training, and acknowledges the limits of her competencies.

D. A feminist therapist engages in self-care activities in an ongoing manner. She acknowledges her own vulnerabilities and seeks to care for herself outside the therapy setting. She models the ability and willingness to self-nurture in appropriate and self-empowering ways.

V. Social Change

A. A feminist therapist actively questions other therapeutic practices in her community that appear abusive to clients or therapists and, when possible, intervenes as early as appropriate or feasible or assists clients in intervening when it is facilitative to their growth.

B. A feminist therapist seeks multiple avenues for impacting change, including public education and advocacy within professional organizations, lobbying for legislative actions, and other appropriate activities.

FOUR

Naming the Issue

Mary Ballou

A rose may be a rose, but it could also be a tulip or perhaps even a daffodil. Naming and norming are central issues in feminist therapy theory in general and in feminist ethics in particular. Although naming and norming seem simple enough, they are in fact quite subtle and complex concepts. How a thing is called and the standard against which it is evaluated are important aspects of ethics that often go undiscussed. This section discusses and analyzes the power and influence at this less obvious and more subtle level of naming and norming. For far from simple, they are acts through which power is brokered. The section discusses the concepts, looks at some ethical cases and differing responses to them, and concludes with analysis.

NAMING AND NORMING

Naming is a powerful act. In naming, clinicians define and direct attention to certain things and away from other things. On the positive side, naming makes clear what is meant allowing effective and efficient communication. On the negative side, naming controls the way a subject will be perceived, establishes a cognitive set, and may cover particular values and views.

What a thing is called influences how it will be perceived, evaluated, processed, understood, and remembered. To illustrate, a group that (1) sets certain rules for its members, (2) offers identity, protection, and reward, and (3) asserts and fights for status and dominance could be named several things. Inner-city gang, law firm, religious group, or professional organization each fit the characterization. It is the naming that shapes reactions to each entity as much as the description of the activities and goals. The name "gang" makes listeners think: dangerous, illegal, drugs and violence, antisocial individuals, a social problem. To name "professional organization" makes listeners think beneficial, legitimate, status and influence, a social necessity.

Norming is often less overt than naming, but the two function together. Basically, a norm is an evaluative comparison. A norm is a standard to which other things are compared. Although orginally norms meant only averages or described a measured consensus, they have come to take on qualities of "rightness" or expectation. Normative criteria function then as the way something should be. At best a norm is a measured consensus or usual performance. However more commonly, and often without conscious intent, norms become standards of correctness with deviations evaluated as less than standard or wrong. In feminist ethics, when a behavior does not match a norm, questions are raised about hidden assumptions and views within the norm, rather than the judgment of deviance automatically being made.

Norming is also a part of naming. For example, criminal, psychotic, revolutionary, genius, or prophet are all names for one who violates normative standards. Yet each is understood and reacted to quite differently. The criminal has violated a law, the psychotic a thought or behavior standard, the revolutionary a political structure, the genius an intellectual pattern, and the prophet a secularization of a sacred rule. The argument is not that these are the same, but rather, that naming has implicit norms. Calling a thing a particular name invokes certain standards by which the named is evaluated. The result is implicit judgment of right–wrong, good–bad, normal–abnormal. Naming and norming, then, are much more involved than application of words that merely identify. They act in ways that shape thinking, inform evaluation, and set rules governing actions. The identified (named) is positioned in an evaluative manner (norming), according to a particular value structure.

Over the last four decades, traditional mental health naming and norming have been challenged in the United States. The radical therapy movement, behavorial and humanistic movements in the 1960s, feminist therapy in the 1970s and 1980s (Lerman, 1976), the multicultural movement in the 1980s (Brown & Root, 1990; Sue, 1981), and contextual nondominant perspectives of the 1990s (Brown & Ballou, 1992) have each reacted against the power and kind of naming and norming done in mainstream mental health. Each of these movements began with criticisms of mainstream mental health. Essentially, they all moved rather quickly (with either more or less political awareness) to question the power of mainstream mental health to control (name and norm) perspectives, function, and personnel.

Examples abound from the questioning of whether there is individual disease or social dis-ease to maladaptive learning or blockage of the potential for growth, to the move for patient rights, to the repression of the diagnostic system, to the inclusion of others in conceptualization and treatment and policy/payment, to the call for broader and more interactive theory, to reform of training and personnel in professional groups, and of course to standards of practice and ethics. There is a history and tradition of reaction against the particular naming and norming done in mainstream mental health, starting but not ending with community psychology. Although mapping that route and intersection would be fascinating, it is the subject of a different discussion.

Feminist theory as applied to mental health has accomplished a rather impressive disciplinary/professional development (Enns, 1993), including a consistent set of principles applied to theory, practice, organizational structure, and professional/social change. These principles require a different language and purpose for naming and norming and are central to feminist therapy. They direct analysis, theory building, practice, and ethics. Naming and norming are important to feminism; they are the central politic, for they reveal its different world view and value stance.

FEMINIST PRINCIPLES

The principles of feminist therapy are *valuing women's experience, pluralism, egalitarian relationships*, acknowledging the existence of *harmful environments* (monocultural, sexist, classist, racist, material), the *influence of external forces* on psychological causation, and a *questioning stance toward traditional mental health* theory, policy, and practice (Ballou & Gabalac, 1985). These principles lead to a very different position when used in naming and norming. Taken together they call for looking to actual *women's experience* as the criteria (essential norm) rather than a standard based unreflectively on traditional mental health assumptions. They call for truly realizing equally valid differences: *pluralism*, meaning that no single experience is universal or more right. Instead experiences exist and need to be fully understood in their particular and differing contexts. So *pluralism* and *experience* require conceptions that see diversity not only in colors and language but in social organization, world views, and values. With this diversity naming, or accurate calling, is extremely difficult and often mistaken.

This diversity is added to complexity (Brown & Root, 1990) with multiple influencing factors. The feminist principles of *harmful external environment* and *causative influences of external forces* (Ballou & Gabalac, 1985) call attention to the many influences on human growth and development. Internal psychological variables and family dynamics are simply not "good enough" to understand the multiple and interacting factors affecting people. Diversity also implies that many lived experiences for nondominant peoples are harmful. Sexism, classism, racism, monoculturalism, heterosexism, colonialism, and hierarchical control of authority, power, and resources are noxious and damaging to human beings. These factors influence the causation of pathology and development of personality (Brown & Ballou, 1992). With this complexity, norming or setting standards for mental health becomes at worst a political and at best a reductionist act.

When an *egalitarian relationship* (Sturdivant, 1980) is added to the mix, major shifts occur. No longer is the professional the knowing authority in defining the problem or recommending treatment that aims to restore normalcy. Instead the naming is shared or efforts are made to work power flexibly within the relationship. Power becomes seen as state specific rather than role dependent. The power to name and the right to bargain (Ballou, 1990) are extended into the relationship, the problem definition, and negotiating the outcome. If extended to the conceptual level, then egalitarian means that both diagnosis (naming) and setting treatment goals (norming) become shared, negotiated, and bargained.

The principle of *a questioning stance toward traditional mental health theory, practice, and policy* is quite obvious given the prior discussion. Traditional mental health needs to be questioned in its stance toward diagnosis, models of human personality and development, and psychopathology. It also needs to reexamine the American Psychiatric Association's *Diagnostic and Statistical Manual of Mental Disorders* (DSM) nosology, treatment models, and outcomes for adjustment to dominant social norms. Blaming the victim, noncontextualized individualistic views, professional collusion, and status grabbing are all too frequent consequences of traditional practice. Feminist principles direct naming and norming in mental health differently.

ETHICAL ISSUES

Naming the issues, then, is no easy feat. The discussion about it is actually quite intimidating. To name accurately with articulated norms and unearthed values is to be ethical in naming and norming. Labeling and evaluating are centrally important and appropriately difficult. They are difficult because there is no diverse, complex, interactive, and externally integrating comprehensive framework.

Yet the accuracy and ethicality of traditional diagnosis and treatment goals are severely compromised for nondominant peoples, who often fare the worst by the exclusion of consideration of external and structural factors as causative. Social myth, narrow individualistic perspectives, and conservative politics have all breached ethical diagnosis (naming) and treatment aims (norming). In the end, naming and norming are socially constructed and political, and hence ethical acts.

Both formal traditional mental health DSM diagnosis and pop psychology concepts from grassroot movements offer attempts at naming and norming. Although both have some real strengths, both clearly fall short of ethical naming and norming. The controversy about the DSM is detailed by the American Psychological Association's task force on misdiagnosis. Many of the feminist therapy theory writers have written compellingly about the myriad of issues composing the literature/struggle.

The power to name mental health difficulties and describe the normative standards for adjusted human behavior is of enormous import. Yet an inaccurate and perhaps unethical DSM system continues to be the gold standard of North American mental health. The DSM has been revealed to be narrowly socially constructed by a few conservative power holders in the psychiatric wing of the medical establishment. Although the DSM does have clarity in communication among initiates, its problems for nondominant people and especially women are legion. So mental health has a nosology—naming and norming—that does not fit. It is dominant-group normed and is at best a two-dimensional figure. Needed is a nosology that is either purely descriptive or multiple and differentially normed.

Naming and norming in pop psychology are also ethically problematic. Notions such as Adult Children of Alcoholics (ACOA), sex or love addict, codependent, incest survivor, and the inner child are troublesome in a different way. These industries are quite appealing in offering a phrase that summarizes a set of behaviors and attitudes. They also frame the problem in a straightforward, simple way and offer hope of understanding, clear actions for change, and community with others.

Separating the grassroots notions from the later ecomomic thrust also allows appreciation of ordinary people coming together for help and to help others in areas of real need that medical and legal systems in the culture do not address competently. To the extent that the professions now do help, it is through the grassroots influence. The notions of pop psychology contrasted with DSM diagnosis offer an alternative naming if not norming and are in accord with the principle of egalitarian relationship. Yet these pop notions are no more reflective of pluralism, complexity, respect for diverse experience, external causation, and harmful environments than most of professional psychology. Context and confoundedness and mutuality and differences are no better realized in these labels. The naming and norming may be more accessible, but they are no less socially constructed and used to hold folks individually accountable for gender, culture, class, and economic/material causative influences.

Within the feminist literature there are also problems of naming and norming. Concepts and labels do not always reflect feminist principles, that is, dominant free, externally caused, and structural ways. Learned helplessness, for example, runs the risk of ignoring the forceful and harmful environment. Instrumental versus expressive assumes dichotomy and does not acknowledge the social reward for instrumental and against expressive. Bem's (1983) androgyny and Chodorow's (1978) prescription for coparenting do not respond to cultural differences and the economic/power elements in social arrangements. The Harvard project notions of "ethics of care" and "self in relation" of the Stone Center are not cognizant of the narrow class/race/culture norms imbedded within the theories.

The use of any of these—DSM, pop psychology, or nonsexist namings and normings without thought, context, and structural analyses—is not in the welfare of the client or competent practice. In short, it is unethical.

The dilemmas that follow are discussed using the Feminist Therapy Code of Ethics, a guide for ethical decision making based on feminist principles. It is a code that attempts to name supported by clear norms and values.

DILEMMA A

Rhonda has an MA in counseling and has established a private practice. She recently took a two-day workshop on codependency and has read three or four books on the issue. Sue is Rhonda's fourth client and has been discussing her difficulties with relationships. She is having particular trouble with her employer. During the third session, Sue mentions that her husband drinks heavily but only on weekends. Sue is pleased that his drinking is "contained" and that her husband is not abusive. Sue insists she wants to deal with the issues involving her employer, but Rhonda focuses on Sue's reactions to her husband's drinking.

RESPONDENT 1

This is a difficult case because Sue's issues involving her husband's drinking may indeed be important and relevant to her relationships in other areas. The implication is that Rhonda does not have much experience and that her response to Sue is based on her recent workshop and readings rather than Sue's specific issues. An important question would be Rhonda's access to and use of supervision to make sure she is reacting to Sue appropriately.

Three possible areas of concern include power differentials (II) and therapist bias (I), therapist accountability (IV), and the concept of codependency. Rhonda is not actively negotiating with Sue to determine the therapeutic issue(s). She rather unilaterally decided what Sue should focus on rather than addressing Sue's expressed concerns.

Although Rhonda should raise the issues with Sue's husband with her, nonetheless, Sue has the right to decide how she wants to use therapy. The orginal contract is not being attended to, and Rhonda is not listening to Sue's readiness/willingness to deal with the issues but is saying, "I am the therapist. I know what you need." Rhonda's actions certainly do not empower Sue or facilitate therapy.

One would wonder if Rhonda has had enough training and experience to make an appropriate diagnosis or enough supervision to determine the main issues. It is easy enough for a therapist to see every client as having the particular problems that relate to the therapist's latest training, unless someone is available to call the therapist on it.

The last concern is the concept of codependency. What does this mean? Women are labelled and blamed when this term is used. It takes away power and is largely blaming and unhelpful. Is this not a feminist issue, one involving backgrounds in terms of feminism and psychological theory? Even though codependency seems to be widely used in the psychological community, it becomes a labeling tool and, as such, denigrates the woman and cuts off further investigation into her personal issues and means of coping. (Lee Fogarty)

RESPONDENT 2

One issue raised here is the general competence of Rhonda, the therapist (IV). The fact that she is in private practice with an MA degree may automatically imply to some that she possesses limited competence, but in itself, the degree is not sufficient information for that assumption. That Sue is her fourth client implies that Rhonda is relatively inexperienced. If Rhonda were a feminist therapist, she should receive consultation about her proposed use of codependency therapy in order to ensure that she is applying it appropriately (IV). If the general theme of the sessions is relationship issues, all relationships are grist for the mill. Despite the client's initial perception, there may or may not be issues related to the husband's drinking. Certainly, the client's feelings about that are worth exploring. It is necessary to keep in mind that the client wishes to focus on her relationship with her employer. This is apparently the most immediate issue for her and the one that seems to cause her the most overt distress at the moment. Her wishes need to be respected, although doing so does not contradict the idea that it would be appropriate to explore her feelings about her husband's drinking, at least to some degree. It would not be appropriate, however, at the present stage of therapy to focus exclusively or predominantly on the husband's drinking to the exclusion of the client's employer. Topics discussed are subject to the negotiation between therapist and client that consistently goes on in feminist therapy.

Another issue implied here is the degree of the therapist's knowledge of and degree of adherence to the model of codependency. Although this model may indict the client and blame her for her husband's actions, feminist therapists use a variety of theoretical models. It behooves a feminist therapist to make herself aware of the patriarchical aspects of any theoretical model she wishes to use. Having said that, it must also be said that clients have been helped by the use of nonfeminist approaches or feminist adaptations of traditional approaches. (Hannah Lerman)

DILEMMA B

Elsie is a therapist in a private clinic. A new client, Carol, has come to see her for the first session. Previously, Carol has taken several psychological assessments on intake, which indicate no severe psychological problems and only two indicators for depression. Carol maintains she needs to use insurance money to cover the cost of treatment and that she really needs to talk to a therapist because her life seems to be "falling apart." Elsie explains that she does not fit any categories for treatment, but Carol is insistent that if Elsie does not work with her she will find someone willing to fill out the necessary forms for insurance.

RESPONDENT 1

The ethical issue here is therapist accountablity (IV). In this situation, should the therapist think that she cannot in good conscience provide service to the client, she should refer Carol. On the other hand, if Elsie sees the issue as providing accessible services, she will utilize the client's insurance by providing a reimbursable diagnosis. Elsie and Carol must clarify limits regarding time and insurance usage.

In fact the issue here might well be one of class background or personal issues on how one deals with authority and bureaucracies. It would be important for the therapist to explore with Carol her justification for lying to the insurance company and in "playing" a system. Some therapists are amenable to stretching the system on the client's behalf and are willing to access services for people who otherwise might not be able to get help. Elsie might want to explore with her supervisor both the decision and its implications. (Elaine Leeder)

RESPONDENT 2

One issue here is the basis the therapist uses for assessment and evaluation of the client (I, IV). If the therapist bases her assessment wholly on psychological tests, she will probably be wrong. If she ignores such information, she is also subject to error. The most significant point is that if the client thinks her life is "falling apart," she is experiencing psychological distress for which she is seeking help and to which the therapist should be responding. Elsie's failure to respond is a more serious error because it violates the idea of ongoing interplay and negotiation between therapist and client (IV).

The issue of how to diagnose in order for insurance to pay for treatment is a difficult one. It is implied here that insurance companies require objective (i.e., psychological assessment) evidence to support a diagnosis. Such a belief is not correct. There are also many levels of diagnosis available in the DSM, for which insurance will reimburse, ranging from major depression to adjustment reaction with depression. If the client is experiencing distress, it is usually possible to arrive at some reimbursable diagnosis. If it is not possible, it is important for the therapist to adhere to her own value system. If Carol chooses to go elsewhere on that basis, that is her decision. Although feminist therapists recognize that the offical diagnostic schema are limited and highly subject to patriarchal assumptions, in the real world, they are the currency by which therapists communicate with insurance companies.

Clients are often not aware that when they use insurance, they are waiving confidentiality to the insurance company. The company may (although it usually does not) require detailed information about session content. In addition, once an insurance form or other information is sent to an insurance company, the therapist has no further control as to how and to whom this information, including the diagnosis, is made available. Feminist therapists would be more likely perhaps than other therapists to inform clients of this practice (IID). (Hannah Lerman)

RESPONDENT 3

Psychological tests are normed on the dominant group, and therefore the interpretations are to be questioned for women (I, II, IV). Allowing the results of psychological tests to determine the identification and naming of a presented problem ignores the important feminist principle of valuing women's experience as an essential norm.

The ethical guidelines for feminist therapists clearly indicate their responsiblity to continually "[integrate] feminism into psychological theory" (IVC). The feminist principle of pluralism, if understood by Elsie and integrated into her work, would afford her the insight that a client's experience needs to be understood in a larger context than that which is simply offered through psychological assessments.

Elsie, in determining that her client Carol does not fit any predetermined category for treatment, is creating a harmful environment by invalidating her personal experience. In doing so, Elsie abuses the power differential (II) inherent in the therapist/client relationship and denies Carol the right to define and name her problem for herself.

As a feminist therapist, Elsie is responsible for "[questioning] other therapeutic practices in her community that appear abusive to clients" (VA). Insurance practices that determine the course of treatment based upon psychological tests too narrowly normed to incorporate a woman's total experience could be considered abusive. A feminist therapist's most basic duty would be to maintain a questioning stance toward this practice and in addition to participate in actions leading to changes in such practice (VB). (Beth Lewis)

DILEMMA C

Marjorie identifies herself as a feminist therapist. As a result, Shirley, a lesbian, decided Marjorie would probably be an appropriate therapist for her issues with her mother. During the first five sessions, Marjorie was very facilitative, and Shirley was pleased with her progress. At the sixth session Shirley talked about her partner, Ann. This was the first time Marjorie had any idea that Shirley was a lesbian and soon found herself thinking about Shirley's issues with her mother in different ways. She now viewed Shirley as questioning her sexuality and began to redirect the therapy into discussions about Shirley's choice to be lesbian.

RESPONDENT 1

When Shirley mentioned her lifestyle, Marjorie's buttons got pushed. This was a time when Marjorie should have advised Shirley of her biases regarding homosexuality and referred her to an appropriate therapist (I). As a self-proclaimed "feminist therapist," Marjorie had, perhaps unintentionally, misrepresented herself. Shirley rightfully assumed that a feminist therapist would be accepting of her lifestyle and not "blame" her sexuality on a negative relationship with her mother. Marjorie had the responsiblity for advising Shirley of her theoretical background and in what ways it differed from a feminist orientation (IV). In addition,

Marjorie clearly did not evaluate her own reaction to Shirley's now disclosed orientation as marked by her shift in focus. (Lee Fogarty)

RESPONDENT 2

The information that the client is a lesbian without any other indications would not seem to be enough for a therapist to decide that the client is questioning her sexuality, although it is probably sufficient for the therapist to rethink her formulations about the client's relationship to her mother, at least somewhat. The issue implied here is possible stereotyping on the part of the therapist, something feminist therapists watch themselves for carefully (I). (Hannah Lerman)

RESPONDENT 3

In this case it is clear that Marjorie has biases against lesbians. The fact is that she is now evaluating the client's relationship with her mother based on new information about Shirley's sexual orientation (I, IV). Considering that the first sessions were facilitative, and now the therapy is being redirected based on lesbianism, the therapist is reflecting negative stereotypes and prejudices. To believe that Shirley is now questioning her sexuality is a value-based assumption that may not be linked to reality. Marjorie is projecting her judgments and stereotypes onto Shirley, diminishing the effectiveness of the therapy. The therapist is also abusing her power (II). Because there is an inherent power differential in all therapeutic relationships, when Marjorie refocuses the therapy to discussion of the client's choice to be a lesbian, she is taking control and misusing her power. The therapist is attempting to make the client rethink her lifestyle and is not respecting the client's position. The power she has here is as a heterosexual and as a therapist. She is using an element of coercion, albeit a subtle one. Uninformed heterosexual therapists often bring these biases into therapy, but it is unacceptable for a feminist therapist to do so. She has broken the ethical Code by taking power and control as well as not understanding the impact of her own sexual orientation upon the therapy. (Elaine Leeder)

DILEMMA D

Theodora announces in the first session that she is a "borderline personality disorder." She has had a number of therapists, has previously been hospitalized, and been on psychiatric medication. She is chronically suicidal and physically self-mutilative, often on an impulsive basis. She is aware of severe sexual and physical abuse by a stepfather during her teenage years, but these issues have not been dealt with by her previous therapists.

RESPONDENT 1

There is more and more evidence that behaviors resulting in a diagnosis of borderline personality disorder are a likely result of chronic and severe abuse of some sort. It is a major difference in conceptualization to switch from borderline personality disorder, which describes what someone is, to chronic, severe posttraumatic stress disorder where the focus is on what the woman experienced. It is a more feminist approach to clients and their experiences (I, IV).

Although safety needs are the clear treatment priority in this case, reframing from the individual deficit borderline to posttraumatic reaction along with the accompaning therapist attitude change is essential to a feminist treatment. (Hannah Lerman)

RESPONDENT 2

Although the diagnosis of borderline personality disorder has been predominantly assigned to women, the etiology of the disorder still inspires debate among theorists. The feminist therapist needs to possess knowledge and understanding of the more traditional views of this disorder in order to then integrate knowledge gained from a feminist perspective (IV).

Specifically because this diagnosis is given to women more than to men, a feminist therapist needs to question the reasons behind such discrepancy (I). Is it the different perspectives on causation or the diagnosis itself that requires examination given the stigma (and norming) attached to such a diagnosis? Within the current mental health field one attaches a set of ideas when informed that a client has a diagnosis of borderline personality disorder. These sets of ideas are often negativistic and often do not contribute to positive change within the client. The name holds certain norms. Is it the naming or the norming that is harmful, and what responsibility do feminist therapists have for affecting change in traditional norming (V)? (Beth Lewis)

RESPONDENT 3

In addition to generating legitimate discussions of diagnostic accuracy and conceptual revision, this case demonstrates justifiable anger at those previous treaters who were complicit with an extension of Theodora's abuse. Violence against women is endemic! In Theodora's case, abuse was rendered not only by the stepfather but by the therapists, hospital(s), and diagnostic system itself. How dare her previous therapists not deal with her physical and sexual abuse! Not only is there this omission in Theodora's case, but the commission of self-shame taught through DSM labeling. The traditional mental health establishment with its diagnostic system and individualistic deficit views of causation has reabused this woman. Theodora has not been offered a relationship through which to change her coping strategies, heal the trauma, and decode the woman-hate within her violations. Ethical guidelines I, IV, and V are all involved. (Mary Ballou)

IMPLICATIONS

The cases in this section demonstrate subtly the introductory discussion of naming and norming. Each of the cases reflects difficulties in and the relationship between what a thing is called and how it is evaluated. Elsie's case shows the need to deal with nosologies beyond a feminist reach. The naming and evaluative criteria of the mainstream wield power and must be contended with. Rhonda's assertion of codependency and the evaluation of the husband's weekend drinking as primary in the client's problem constitute a naming and norming of a different sort. But the power here is no less unnegotiated. The cases of Marjorie and Theodora have a bit more emphasis on clinical judgments, understandings, and treatments. As a result, they offer a view of how clinical work is inseparable from ethics.

Ethical analyses, then, must precede and be concurrent with practice mechanics, therapists' values, and therapy in both diagnosis and treatment. Feminist ethics, unlike the "thou shall and thou shall not" of mainstream ethics, are not just a set of rules through which the profession seeks to control its members' behaviors. Rather, feminist ethics aim to integrate feminist principles into the mechanics, theory, practice, values, and decision-making processes in mental health. In so doing, principled decisions become therapy, and therapy becomes principled decisions. But in fact, at the present state of development, the naming and norming so essential to diagnosis and treatment do not have accurate and just models. So feminists are faced with ethical dilemmas often and importantly and are therefore in need of ethical decision-making models. They need models based in developing theory and articulated feminist principles, which offer thoughtful guiding structure for the act of making ethical decisions.

The similarity of respondents' discussions to the cases is quite interesting and leads in two different directions. The first is that the Feminist

Therapy Code of Ethics is well known and integrated into the evaluative processes of the reactors; or that the Code makes intuitive sense and hence has captured essential decision making. The second direction is that the code has become a new naming and normative standard. This direction is at once both gratifying and troublesome. Naming and norming, as already discussed, shape thinking, inform evaluation, set rules, govern actions, and cover over foundational values. In either event, feminists need continually to act justly and accurately for the welfare of clients as ongoing and perhaps changing ethical decisions are reached.

The Feminist Therapy Code of Ethics is meant to provide guidelines for thinking through situations and valuing feminist principles. The guidelines are educational, prescriptive of client rights, and feminist principled. They ought not to be a codified set of rules but, rather, remain guidelines that bring feminist principles into the therapeutic enterprise. Feminist principles of pluralism, egalitarian relationship, harmful external environment, and questioning stance must be applied to ethical decision making within the feminist code as they must within traditional therapy. Equally valid differences, the power to name and the right to bargain, authority of women's experiences, many external causes of which gender ascription is one, and questioning, are principles that feminists must value and apply to traditional mental health, to clients, to therapy, to naming and norming, to themselves, and their evolving creations.

RESPONDENTS

Lee Fogarty, PhD in counselor education, is in private practice in Pittsburgh, PA, and is active in numerous local and national women's organizations.

Elaine Leeder, PhD, Associate Professor and Chair of the Sociology Department at Ithaca College, Ithaca, NY, is the author of *Feminist Therapy with Abuse in Families: Bringing in the Community* (Springer, 1994).

Hannah Lerman, PhD in clinical psychology, is in private practice in Los Angeles, CA, and is active in state and national feminist psychology associations.

Beth Lewis, MS, is a community mental health worker and a doctoral student in counseling psychology at Northeastern University.

REFERENCES

Ballou, M. (1990). Approaching a feminist-principled paradigm in the construction of personality theory. In L. Brown & M. Root (Eds.), *Diversity and complexity in feminist therapy* (pp. 23–40). Binghamton, NY: Harrington, Park Press.

Ballou, M., & Gabalac, N. (1985). A feminist position on mental health. Springfield, IL: Charles C. Thomas.

Bem, S. L. (1983). Gender schema theory and its implications for child development. Signs, 8, 598–616.

Brown, L. S., & Ballou, M. (1992). Personality and psychopathology: Feminist reappraisals. New York: Guilford Press.

Brown, L., & Root, M. (1990). Diversity and complexity in feminist therapy. New York: Haworth Press.

Chodorow, N. J. (1978). The reproduction of mothering: Psychoanalysis and the sociology of gender. Berkeley, CA: University of California Press.

Enns, C. Z. (1993). Twenty years of feminist counseling and therapy: From naming the biases to implementing multifaceted practice. Counseling Psychologist, 21, 3–87.

Lerman, H. (1976). What happens in feminist therapy. In S. Cox (Ed.), Female psychology: The emerging self (pp. 378–384). Chicago: Science Research Associates.

Sturdivant, S. (1980). Therapy with women. New York: Springer.

Sue, D. W. (1981). Counseling the culturally different. New York: Wiley.

FIVE

Monetary Issues

Ruth Parvin
Gail Anderson

Currently few subscribe to the psychoanalytic notion that
money equals feces and is, therefore, unclean.
—KLEBANOW (1991, p. 51)

M onetary issues in therapy have become inextri-
cably bound to treatment decisions and the
quality of care provided to the therapy client. In
the United States, about 50% of the pretax profits of large corporations
are spent on health costs (McWilliams, 1994). Attempts to contain
medical costs are being made in a number of countries, both where
medical care is privatized and where it is nationalized or socialized.
These attempts increasingly shape the definition of professional relationships between the care provider and the client, third-party payers,
other health care providers, and society itself (Webb, 1989). During the
1990s, drastic changes in the provision of mental health care services
are being proposed and tried in the United States and Canada. It will
be necessary to look at the ethical ramifications of these changes on
therapeutic relationships, setting of fees, and provision of pro-bono,
sliding-fee, and bartered services. The ethics of care may be increasingly
determined by the cost of care.

THE CONTEXT OF INSURANCE REFORM

The client's ability to pay for therapy, rather than the client's needs, may
drive decisions about whether a person will get therapy, what diagnosis
will be assigned, and what method of therapy will be used. Individuals
have come to rely on therapy subsidized by insurance, charitable agencies, or the government. As a result, the payer has increasingly gained

the right to dictate the terms of therapy. The resulting cost containment is called *managed care*.

With its use of *triage* and *rationing of services* to keep costs down, managed care is rapidly replacing fee-for-service payments (Ghertner, 1993). Two models being proposed by some insurance policy makers are referred to as "shared risk" and "capitation by diagnosis." (Muszynski & Marshall, 1993; Payton, 1993). In these models, therapists and agencies would contract with the insurer to provide mental health services to a specific population (e.g., the employees of XYZ Corporation) for a year.

In the *shared-risk model*, therapists would have to belong to a multidisiplinary group that would compete with other groups of thera- pists for contracts to provide all mental health care for a "population of lives" for a set fee per person (life) per month. Thus, "shared risk" refers to (1) the risk taken by the therapists of underestimating the services needed (if they bid too low for the contract, they have to carry the losses for the entire length of the contract) and (2) the risk taken by the payer of overestimating the services needed. (they would therefore pay for sessions that are not used). In this model, the group practice members would decide among themselves how to allocate their resources rather than being told by the third-party payer how many sessions they could provide to any one client. In most "risk" contracts, there is also a "withhold," a proportion of the contract payment that is paid at the end of the year as a bonus to the therapists who have used their time most "efficiently" (i.e., seen the most clients for the shortest time while maintaining client satisfaction).

In the second model of *capitation by diagnosis*, reimbursement would be based on the diagnosis assigned to the client, similar to the diagno- sis-related groups (DRG) concept in medicine. Each diagnosis would have a specified number of sessions for which the therapist would be reimbursed and possibly a specification of what types of therapy could be provided, including required medication where appropriate. (These parameters would be determined by outcome studies demonstrating the most efficient treatments.) Once the allotted sessions have been used or if the specified treatment did not work for the client, the therapist might find her- or himself in the bind of terminating a client whose needs exceed the parameters established for the diagnosis or continuing to see the client without insurance reimbursement. Therapists who regularly exceed the recommended amount of time for treatment would be excluded from lists of approved providers.

The ethics of care is also tied to broader economic trends. Low- to no-cost mental health care is increasingly difficult to find in the United States because of an economic recession and decreased federal support for community mental health. Anecdotal information suggests that when such treatment is found, it is often provided by paraprofessionals and student trainees; and it suggests that the amount of supervision provided to these caretakers has decreased as the number of supervisory faculty and personnel has been reduced, due to cost-cutting measures and recent tax revolts. In addition, under the lower payments provided by managed health care, therapists must increase the number of direct care hours provided weekly to maintain the income of their agencies, further cutting into time that was once used to supervise students and paraprofessionals.

The remaining government funding for mental health programs comes from diverse sources, all with specialized paperwork and requirements. Often the regulations limit the type of provider who can qualify for reimbursement. Thus, when the government makes money available primarily for children, adult slots decrease dramatically. When there is a focus on chronically mentally ill patients, there may be little funding for children's services. When funds are particularly scarce, there is a move to increased use of medication.

These economic and insurance trends run counter to values held by many therapists. Traditionally, the therapist's responsibility has been to advocate for the individual client. Under capitated programs, the therapist will have to make decisions weighing the need of one client against another for the limited resources available (Saultz, 1994). The therapist's responsibility will be for the whole population.

This is a major paradigm shift that creates special difficulties for feminist therapists whose work has evolved from analyses of the effects of sexism, financial handicaps, and power differentials on the mental health status of people, especially women and people of color who often have lesser status and power in society.

Historically, feminist therapy has eschewed the medical model of mental illness in favor of an environmental approach. The use of medication and diagnoses has been critiqued from the viewpoint of social control and the effects on the patient/client; for instance, women, poor people, and minorities tend to be overdiagnosed and overmedicated in comparison with white males with adequate income (Chesler, 1972; Lott, 1987). Strong advocacy for the individual has been a major tenet of feminist therapy, and appreciation of diversity has been a cornerstone (Parvin & Biaggio, 1991). While, in the best of all scenarios, employer-paid, managed health care combined with some type of universal, government-sponsored health care promise to extend treatment to a far larger proportion of people, some feminist therapists are concerned that the current focus of managed care is (1) reductionary and not respectful of a variety of ways to treat and understand the client and (2) causing renewed pressures to conform to a more traditional medical model of care. They worry that if they do not conform, they will not be able to help their clients access what limited funding the client may be entitled to or to protect the therapist's or their agency's stream of income.

FEE SETTING

There is a conflict around fee setting that is both an ethical and an intrapsychic one since it is connected to protecting the therapist's income. As well-educated professionals, therapists expect and are expected to earn a decent living. As healers, therapists expect and are expected to temper economic interests with altruism (Klebanow, 1991). Further complicating this issue, historic professional ethics around fee setting and advertising have been changing as a result of the threat of antitrust proceedings. These changes are, however, in flux: one insurance reformer has stated that the current U.S. administration has decided not to pursue antitrust concerns in the health arena because national health care will require linkages that could not withstand antitrust challenges (Payton, 1993).

Surveys of various groups of therapists reflect the ambivalence and difficulty of fee-setting issues: the questions about fee setting are among those that receive the least agreement about whether specific practices are unethical (Tabachnick, Keith-Spiegel, & Pope, 1991; Oordt, 1990). Furthermore, Borys and Pope (1989) found in a national survey in the United States that there are significant differences in this area of decision making based on the therapist orientation. For instance, psychodynamic therapists rated social/financial involvement with clients as less ethical than did respondents of other orientations. Psychiatrists rated social/financial involvement as more problematic than did psychologists or social workers. Solo therapists were more cautious than group practitioners about monetary boundaries. Rural therapists were more forgiving than urban ones in their evaluations of financial ethical conduct. Women had more stringent definitions in this area than did men.

In an informal study of 60 psychotherapists, Lasky (1985) found that two-thirds expressed considerable discomfort around fee setting. She attributes this discomfort to their original motivation for entering the field—the desire to help others. Therapists may feel guilt or identification with the oppressor for getting paid because someone is having a hard time coping with life. On the other hand, therapists want to make an adequate income to compensate them for their work. Beyond adequacy of income, social status, power, and reputation can be affected by the level of income and size of fee commanded by the therapist. Thus a practitioner may come to feel excitement, power, or embarrassment when setting a high fee and loss, annoyance, resentment, or guilt at setting a low fee. Furthermore, the higher the fee that a person or agency charges, the fewer direct therapy hours must be provided to cover expenses. Providing too many hours of direct service can lead to a lower quality of work, mistakes in judgment, professional dissatisfaction, and/or burnout.

In another study Lasky (1984) found that 75% of women therapists charged lower fees than their male colleagues with similar education and experience. This finding parallels a number of studies showing that women pay themselves less for the same work than males if each is allowed to set her or his rate of pay (Kahn & Gaedder, 1985), possibly because money has different meanings for or is a less salient reward to women than men or because they are not privy to the standard against which male colleagues measure the value of their work (Lott, 1987).

In her interviews Lasky found that many women were in a three-way conflict over fees. They wanted to support themselves and their families; they wanted both to work extra hours for additional money and also have those hours available for family and friends; and they tended to focus as much on their clients' monetary situations as their own. The men in her survey were more likely to handle their conflict by figuring out how much money they and their families needed and adjusting their fees to cover this amount.

Closely related to the issue of fee setting is that of the relationship between the therapist and third-party payers. The term "third-party payer" is used to describe parties who pay for therapy but are not officially involved in the therapy sessions. Insurance companies, employers, labor unions, and court systems are examples of third-party payers. Provision for mental health benefits by these groups is somewhat new and has raised a multitude of questions about the amount of control the third-party payer has over the way that services are provided, records are kept, confidentiality is extended, and diagnoses are made. Particularly difficult questions have evolved around which therapists are able to secure payment from third parties. Clients who are paying for insurance should be allowed to use those benefits. Yet the insurance companies may specify a particular panel of therapists, a specific profession, or other limitations that may severely constrain the client's choice of treatment.

Another aspect of ethical fee setting involves the exchange of therapy for goods or services, a practice defined as bartering. This practice, historically a part of commerce, has become less common in industrialized society. Pockets of barter exchange continue in rural areas, among people with small disposable incomes, and among groups of people who philosophically embrace barter as a lifestyle alternative. Bartering fell out of popularity in much of the professional community because of the complexity of relationship issues it raised and the potential for exploitation to occur. Feminist therapists may debate the issue more than others because of their commitment to work respectfully with differing social values and a wide forum of lifestyle philosophies and their self-imposed responsibility to provide services for people with limited incomes.

A step beyond trading therapy for goods is the provision of free therapy. The concept of pro bono services probably goes back to the old concept of noblesse oblige—the idea that those who have been blessed with riches, for instance the education and training to be a therapist, owe something to those who have not. For many therapists, the question is not *whether* to do it but rather *how much* and *in what settings*. The question gets more difficult when a therapist is not only giving her time and expertise but is also foregoing income during that time.

TRADITIONAL APPROACHES TO MONETARY ETHICS

Ballou (1992) has described the foundation of traditional mainstream therapy theory as founded on an epistemology where "exclusive rationalism and/or empiricism are the only acceptable modes of obtaining knowledge" (pp. 4–5). She further describes traditional Western metaphysical values as "reduction and atomism, causality and linearity" (p. 5). Perhaps one of the foremost institutions valuing rationalism, causality, and linear thinking is the legal system. In recent years, legal decisions about malfeasance and negligence have driven many ethics developments and decisions. This influence in the area of monetary issues is well demonstrated in a survey of 196 psychologists, conducted by Handelsman, Kemper, Kesson-Craig, McLain, and Johnsrud (1986). The single most common issue addressed by informed consent forms was fees.

As mainstream practice of therapy has become more legalistically oriented, at least one method of making ethics decisions is based on avoidance of law suits. Woody (1989), a teacher and trainer on the business aspects of mental health, provides an example of ethics decisions driven by malfeasance avoidance. He advocates a firmly set policy for handling financial issues because mental health is seen by the public as part of a huge health care industry where all forms of immunity for the caretaker have eroded, and a malpractice crisis exists. He specifies that the client should be clearly informed of financial expectations at or before first contact, kept fully informed of the status of her or his account, and be expected to pay regularly. He states that as payments lag, the likelihood of a malpractice claim increases. Woody's Rule is "If [a] communication or service (1) relies on the expertise of the professional, (2) is intended to benefit the client, and (3) creates potential ethical, regulatory, or legal liability for the practitioner, a professional fee is justified" (p. 152). He also addresses pro bono services from the standpoint of legal liability and states that pro bono services should not be given directly to clients but, rather, should be spent in agency supervision or political work in the support of government subsidized services.

Traditionally, therapists have been exhorted to take on some pro bono work. Some have addressed this responsibility by seeing a client for free or at reduced fee, others by doing supervision or volunteering their expertise at a local university or agency. Woody points out that, even with pro bono work, a therapist is held financially liable for any mistakes, and Woody therefore abnegates "feeling ethically or morally obligated to fulfill social service by free or reduced fee arrangements for clinical services" (p. 154). He writes that accepting a client who cannot pay is detrimental to the client and bad business. Other writers of a traditional therapy stance have addressed the issue of taking non- or low-paying clients, suggesting that it shames the client, puts them in a position to feel guilty if they feel anger toward the therapist, or sets them up for countertransference from their therapist as a result of the therapist's economic dependency on the client's paying for services (Drelich, 1991; Shainess, 1991). This position assumes that these same issues are lacking in clients who silently pay fees to get help for problems they feel they should be able to solve themselves without the help of some outsider. Decision making regarding monetary concerns that is based almost entirely on the flow of cash provides a number of rationalizations that protect the status quo.

FEMINIST APPROACHES
TO MONETARY ETHICS

Certainly avoidance of malpractice suits is an advisable practice; however the use of legal decisions to determine ethical practices is giving the issues back to a system that has long been patriarchal. By contrast, the cornerstone of feminist thinking and therapy is phenomenological experience, for example, "the personal is political," and political action, for example, affecting systemic change, advocacy, pro bono service. Ballou (1992) states:

> Feminist analysis is political, in that it is essentially an identification and assessment of power relations located centrally in gender ... [and] contains an important focus on the social, economic, cultural, and institutional contexts that form and define individuals' lives, values, cognitions, emotions, motivations, and work and kinship patterns. (p. 6)

She further describes how feminist philosophers and researchers are calling the sole reliance on the underlying bases of traditional episte- mology (linearity, causality, empiricism, reductionism) into question. These issues are reflected also in feminist therapy.

To examine, analyze, and address power differentials are at the core of feminist therapy ethics, and the distribution of money is one of the major determinants of power. Feminist therapists believe that all people have a right to adequate mental and physical health care, the opportu- nity to reach those goals they are capable of reaching, and choices about how they will live their lives. The macro expression of this is through political change; the micro level is through ensuring that counseling is made available to all people by providing adequate pro bono and sliding-fee hours. Yet as Brown (1990) points out, feminist therapists get caught in a bind when trying to apply a political analysis to the conduct of business because the business of therapy is earning a living by dealing with human pain and despair that is often accentuated by lack of client resources. Thus the business of political change is funded with dollars earned from client pain and despair.

MAINSTREAM CODES OF ETHICS

A review of the codes of ethics from the major therapy-related profes- sional associations reveals varying attention to the monetary dilemmas between the therapist and the client. Ethical standards of the American Psychological Association (APA), the American Psychiatric Associa- tion, the American Association for Counseling and Development (AACD), the American Association for Marriage and Family Therapy (AAMFT), and National Association of Social Workers (NASW) were compared on monetary issues, using both specific references and the larger spirit of each code.

The most recently revised codes are more fully developed in terms of being sensitive to and contextualizing oppression and power differ- entials including economic diversity and responsibility. The Feminist Therapy Institute (FTI) Feminist Therapy Code of Ethics predates all of these revisions, suggesting that feminist principles are being brought into the mainstream of the mental health field.

Some codes address the issue of power differentials under the heading of nondiscrimination and advocate varying degrees of proac- tivity. APA, in its Preamble, states, "Psychologists respect and protect human and civil rights, and do not knowingly participate in or condone unfair discriminatory practices" (American Psychological Association, 1992). Principle [D] outlines respect for "cultural, individual and role differences, including those due to age, gender, race, ethnicity, national origin, religion, sexual orientation, disability, language, and socioeconomic status." The APA Code discerns, "Psychologists are sensitive to real and ascribed differences in power between themselves and others, and they do not exploit or mislead other people during or after professional relationships."

The American Psychiatric Association (1992) Code states that psychiatrists should not be party to any policy that "excludes, segregates, or demeans the dignity of any patient due to socioeconomic status" (1.2). The AAMFT Code of Ethics (1991) states that members do not discriminate against oppressed groups (1.1) and that marriage and family therapists are aware of their influential position with respect to clients. They must avoid exploiting the trust and dependency of such persons (1.2).

NASW (1990) lists a number of forms of discrimination that are not allowed, although socioeconomic class is not explicitly listed. However under the section on the social worker's ethical responsibility to society, NASW provides the strongest context that members are expected to work toward goals where services are provided to all people on the basis of need.

No mainstream code is as specific as NASW (1990) in its commitment to activism. Italics have been added by the authors to highlight that these commitments involve active participation on the part of the therapist:

1. The social worker should *act* to prevent and eliminate discrimination against any person or group on basis of race, color, sex, sexual orientation, age, religion, national origin, marital status, political belief, mental or physical handicap, or any other preference or personal characteristic, condition, or status. 2. The social worker should *act* to ensure that all persons have access to the resources, services, and opportunities which they require. 3. The social worker should *act* to expand choice and opportunity for all persons, with special regard for disadvantaged or oppressed groups and persons. 4. The social worker should *promote* conditions that encourage respect for the diversity of cultures which constitute American society. 5. The social worker should *provide* appropriate professional services in public emergencies. 6. The social worker should *advocate* changes in policy and legislation to improve social conditions and to promote social justice. 7. The social worker should *encourage informed participation by the public* in shaping social policies and institutions. (VI, 1–7)

In general, the professional codes are concerned about clear disclosure regarding fees and avoidance of exploitation of the client. For instance, the APA (1992) Code states that psychologists should not exploit the recipient or the payers through the fees set for services. They are forbidden to make false and deceptive statements about fees, must disclose fees and limitations on services based on monetary difficulties, and must provide other contractual information to the recipient of services at the earliest feasible point. Clients must be informed of plans to turn unpaid bills over to a collection agent and be provided with ample opportunity to make prompt payment. AAMFT (1991) forbids excessive fees and requires disclosure of compensation and billing arrangements at the beginning of services.

The American Psychiatric Association (1992), AACD (1988), and NASW (1990) are silent on the explicit discussion of fees with the client. NASW states that fees should be "fair, reasonable, considerate, and commensurate with the service performed and with due regard for the clients' ability to pay," and AACD directs its members to consider the financial status and locality of their clients in setting fees. The American Psychiatric Association states only that contractual arrangements with clients should be explicitly established.

Another area of concern for some professions is that of fee splitting, the practice where a supervisor, referral source, or office provider takes a designated percentage of each client's fee in exchange for the services they render. Previously, the APA Code eschewed fee splitting. However as part of a settlement related to antitrust regulations, the organization promulgated a new standard that requires that fee splitting be based on actual services provided, not merely for referral. The American Psychiatric Association (1992) states that fee splitting, defined as fees based on a percentage of the intake of another professional, is not acceptable: fees for administration, supervision, education, or consultation should be based on a set amount. Fees for referral are explicitly forbidden by AAMFT, NASW, and AACD.

There is increasing interest in defining the relationships among the client, the therapist, and the additional parties (i.e., an insurance company or employer) that pay some or all of the fee. Many third-party payers limit payments to certain professionals who are already licensed, to specific diagnoses, and to limited types of services. In the past, a billing might have been made under the name of a supervisor for services rendered by a student so that services to a client could be covered by the client's insurance. These practices are changing radically.

Psychologists are forbidden from misrepresenting fees or exploiting *any* payers. They must accurately state "the nature of the .. service provided, the fees or charges, and where applicable, the identity of the provider, the findings, and the diagnosis" (American Psychological Association, 1992, 1.25b). AAMFT (1991) notes that facts about services rendered must be truthfully represented.

The NASW (1990) Code of Ethics does not specifically address the issues around third party payers. The American Psychiatric Association (1992) also refrains from mentioning third-party payments, but when psychiatrists assume a collaborative or supervisory role, they must spend the time to ensure that proper care is given. "It is contrary to the interests of the patient and to patient care if [the psychiatrist] allows himself/herself to be used as a figurehead" (5.3).

The APA (1992) Code is the only one to explicitly address bartering, and it indicates that generally the exchange of psychological services for goods, services, or other nonmonetary remuneration is not advisable because of the inherent risk of conflict, exploitation, and contamination of the professional relationship. Under the revised Code, if bartering does occur, the practitioner should be able to show that there are no clinical contraindications and that the relationship is nonexploitative. This new guideline reflects a more explicit, and probably more lenient standard, than existed in previous APA Codes.

The APA (1992) Code encourages the contribution of professional time and expertise for "little or no personal advantage" (Principle [F]). NASW (1990) does not specifically address pro bono work but requires its practitioners to work for access to services for all people; AACD (1988) requires members to consider the financial status of clients in setting fees. The other mainstream codes do not refer to pro bono services.

THE FEMINIST THERAPY CODE OF ETHICS

The Feminist Therapy Code of Ethics (Feminist Therapy Institute, 1987) is intended to be added to rather than replace the ethical principles of the various professions in which feminist therapists practice. At first glance, it says little about monetary transactions; however, careful reading suggests a clear orientation from which to approach ethical concerns around monetary relationships with clients.

A fundamental way the FTI Code differs from the above codes is the focus on egalitarian valuing, which requires the feminist therapist to examine carefully the power differentials in the client/therapist relationship and to use that power differential to the benefit of the client. Only the FTI Code recognizes the pervasive effects of patriarchy and oppression on people's lives (Feminist Therapy Institute, 1987, Preamble).

The Preamble states that a feminist analysis must be integrated into "all spheres of work as therapists, educators, consultants, administrators, and/or researchers" (1987). Such power analysis requires feminist therapists to understand the interactive effects of the client's internal and external worlds and to take a proactive stance to challenge patriarchy, classism, and the other forms of oppression. This degree of sensitivity to and responsibility for power differential analysis and egalitarian system change deeply informs the FTI Code, setting it apart from mainstream ethics codes.

The FTI Code uses specific language when referring to access and flexibility of services for a wide range of clients. The monetary implications for the feminist therapist are broad and require that she examine all monetary transactions for classism or other oppressions. She acknowledges the power imbalance directly to her clients, and she models effective use of personal power. A feminist therapist not only conducts an analysis at the outset but continues to negotiate and renegotiate formal and/or informal contracts in an ongoing mutual process including monetary transactions.

Further, a feminist therapist questions other therapeutic transactions in her community that appear monetarily abusive to clients or therapists. She assists clients in intervening when it facilitates their growth. She serves as an advocate for her client and for herself regarding monetary issues.

How do fee guidelines reflect power differentials? Fee structures need to increase the feminist therapist's accessibility to and for a wide range of clients. They should model effective use of personal power in an ongoing way. They should reflect the therapist's ability to engage in financial self-care, balancing her self-interest with that of the client. Carefully negotiated fee setting, responsive to both the context of the client and the needs of the therapist, can set an egalitarian tone to the relationship.

There are no specific references to third-party payers or fee splitting in the FTI Code. Many feminist therapists have difficulty with the medical model of diagnosis and with insurance requirements for *Diagnostic and Statistical Manual of Mental Disorders* (DSM) labels on clients, opting out of receiving third-party payments. Others, in a mild form of guerrilla warfare, always choose V code (conditions not attributable to a mental disorder) or adjustment diagnoses to avoid negative labels. (Some of these issues are addressed in a 1992 reader response column of *Interchange*, the FTI newsletter.) Still others think that both these choices carry a flavor of unethical practices. With the rapid growth of managed care, there will be a need to address these issues more explicitly.

Although there are no specific references to pro bono services in the FTI Code, it is generally accepted that the therapist will offer some pro bono services in her attempts to provide accessibility of services to a wide range of clients. The FTI Code also makes no direct references to barter; however, an argument can be made for barter in terms of increasing accessibility through flexible delivery of services. Opposing arguments identify barter as a monetary transaction rife with opportunities for abuse of power.

Although the FTI Code enjoys broad endorsement among feminist therapists, there is not always agreement, even among experienced feminist therapists about how to implement its principles. In the dilemmas below, the respondents illustrate some of the differences.

DILEMMA A

Terri works in a private agency on hourly contract. Therapists are paid a percentage of the fees collected. The agency will allow therapists to slide their fee no lower than $40 an hour based on need. The agency is in a small community an hour's drive from county-funded mental health agencies. The client, Ali, is a single parent who left high school at age 15. He is under court supervision, and continued therapy will be looked upon as a positive factor. Ali makes minimum wage so that the lowest therapy fee is the equivalent of a full day's wages. Some therapists in the agency suggest that Terri explain to the client that the agency will not pursue clients who do not pay their bills and that she tell Ali to pay what he can afford and not worry about the balance.

RESPONDENT 1

In the absence of a public agency within easy client access, Terri's private agency does not have a fee schedule flexible enough to meet the needs of the community (IA). The agency deals with the dilemma by the informal practice of "forgiving" unpaid bills, placing the low-income client in an oppressive power relationship (IIA), burdened with an unpaid debt if she or he wishes to use agency services. The agency practice of charging the client more than she or he can afford and more than the agency expects to collect is disrespectful and dishonest. This kind of seemingly generous intention intensifies the existing power differential. It is ultimately humiliating to the client; and it models an irresponsible coping mechanism, none of which is good therapy. The client's situation is exacerbated by court supervision that expects the client to be in therapy. This agency's unstated double message also puts Terri in an ethically uncomfortable middle position between her client and her agency (IVB).

Advocacy for change within the agency and/or change in public delivery of services would meet Terri's ethical obligations to her client, herself, and her agency. Terri could insist that the agency discuss the ethical and practical issues involved, using this dilemma as the catalyst for necessary change (IIC, VA). She needs to ask herself and her colleagues if the agency has an ethical obligation to fill the void created by the absence of a publicly funded agency (IA, VB).

Among the multiple avenues for promoting change, Terri could look into and suggest the following options: (1) advocate for a more flexible fee schedule within the agency and suggest that the agency set aside a clearly defined number of slots for low-income, low-fee clients, while raising fees for highest-income clients; (2) submit a proposal for an agency contract with the county or state for underwriting low-income clients; (3) encourage her agency to advocate for a more accessible delivery of public services such as bus service to the nearest public agency or the development of a part-time, satellite public agency in her community.

In taking responsibility for effecting change at the agency or public level, Terri will need to be mindful of her own energy level and to take care of herself in view of the professional and financial consequences to herself and her colleagues (IVB, D). She can mitigate the risk-taking aspect of being a change agent by enlisting support among immediate colleagues, feminist colleagues in other agencies or communities, and/or from feminist professional literature such as the FTI Code. (Rachel Josefowitz Siegel)

RESPONDENT 2

An agency cannot, and should not, try to be everything to everyone. It takes concerted thought, effort, and clarity to identify and state, "I'm sorry; I can't do what you ask; it is outside of my role." Once an agency becomes clear about roles and boundaries, the staff can give up the need to meet ongoing, changing, and endless expectations from their professions, public, and colleagues, and focus on what they can and must do well.

The issues in Terri's dilemma can be simplified and addressed by applying a standard framework for assessing the appropriateness of an agency's service delivery. A standard framework provides clear roles and boundaries and facilitates feedback and consistent decision making. One such model, based on work by Biele and Jacobson (1988), is useful because it differentiates between a personal and professional relationship. The professional relationship is time limited, structured, and other (client) focused. It has an inherent imbalance of power. The relationship with the professional is a contract for services. Once these limitations are understood, the contracting agency can identify its mission by defining its role and responsibilities. The staff roles and responsibilities are then defined. The agency's mission, the expectations of the community, the funding sources, and employment contracts all define staff roles. Finally, once the roles are defined, all parties involved clarify the boundaries of their roles.

These boundaries can be specified by asking to whom, what, where, when, and how services are or cannot be provided.

In this dilemma, there are several areas that need to be clarified on the agency level. First, is the mission of the agency to provide mental health services to all, or only to insured, persons? An agency evaluation should identify what services are available to whom. If the mission is to be available to all, the sliding-fee scale and the availability of county funding must be reexamined. This scrutiny could require a concerted effort to obtain some county funding to subsidize service fees, given the distance between the client and a subsidized program (IA, VB). The sliding-fee scale must be examined to reach a balance between the client's and the agency's financial needs. If the sliding scale is set too low, the agency can no longer operate, affecting the availability of services to all persons in the community (IVB).

The staff's obligations to the agency are a key problem in this dilemma. When staff contract to work for an agency, they agree to uphold the mission, policies, and procedures. If there are policy problems, they should be addressed in an overall policy review. Staff instructing clients to ignore policy is a set-up for other, and more damaging, boundary violations (IC).

The professional is always responsible for maintaining boundaries. Staff who encourage clients to ignore their therapy debts model inappropriate behavior. If staff members have personal standards of service that include providing services regardless of income, they can work independently and provide services pro bono at their discretion. However, once staff accept a contract, they should not subvert that agreement by encouraging the client to ignore agency policies (IIIA).

The therapist must act within the confines of agency mission, policy, and personal standards. Salaries are based on the percentage of fees collected. Does the therapist support the unwritten procedure that the agency does not actively pursue unpaid fees? Currently when service fees are not collected, pro bono services are already provided in an unstated manner. Was this Terri's understanding or the employment contract? Can the therapist renegotiate the contract to legitimize planned pro bono work? Finally, what is the limit to the therapist's pro bono ability? If she is unable to support herself, she, like the agency, will be unable to provide services to the greater community (IVD).

Once the agency's mission and staff responsibilities are clarified, then they must be applied to the needs of individual clients. In this dilemma, what are Ali's needs? The only need stated in this vignette is that Ali continue in therapy because it will look good to the court. Being a single parent, working in a low-paying position, and being involved with the court system are reasons in and of themselves to seek outside support. Ali needs to find accessible services he can afford.

The agency, through its staff, can assist Ali to identify and prioritize his needs and resources (IA, IID, VA). If Ali decides that he needs therapy for court supervision, he might utilize the services of the county-funded agencies, support services, transportation, and child care. If Ali gives a high priority to continuing services with his current therapist and agency, he would then need to negotiate a payment schedule that he could afford (IIC). Ali's income is low, and the agency's fees are high. Knowing the fee schedule, he can contract services in a manner that balances both his needs and resources. Ali could choose to have fewer sessions monthly and use lower-cost community services that address nontherapeutic issues (i.e., parenting or employment). This expansion of support could enhance his personal development and standing with the court. (Danna R. Farabee)

DILEMMA B

Beth has established her private practice using a sliding scale for fees. She negotiates her fee with each new client who is unable to pay a full fee and then renegotiates each six-month period. Shortly after determining fees for the next six-month period with Joan, a long-time client, Beth learned from a second therapy client (who is a friend of Joan) that Joan recently won $100,000 on a trip to Reno.

After five additional sessions with Joan and no mention of her improved financial status, Beth is getting resentful of working with Joan at a reduced fee. Because she is having difficulty relating to Joan, Beth determines she must confront Joan about the fee she is paying and decides to tell her that she heard from some other source that Joan had come into a large sum of money.

RESPONDENT 1

External observers face difficulty in trying to make a decision about whether a therapist's action is ethical. They can raise questions, but some of these can be answered within the given context or only by the therapist given her particular values, therapy theory, and definitions.

Beth is to be commended for recognizing and naming her countertransference with Joan elicited by the fee issue (IC). She needs to think about how much the countertransference is due to the fee issue versus the extent to which the fees have triggered preexisting feelings of resentment, related perhaps to the length of treatment and/or therapy issues? What has Joan's progress in therapy been recently, and does Beth believe that Joan is or should be finished with therapy? What ongoing contracts have been implicitly or explicitly made (IIC)?

Once Beth knows about the windfall, she cannot ignore Joan's silence regarding her change in economic status as a therapeutic issue. Prior to initiating such a discussion in therapy with Joan, however, Beth should clarify in her own mind and with consultation (IVB) her intentions and plan for all likely outcomes of the discussion. For instance, does she intend to require that Joan move to a full-scale fee? Will it be at all retroactive? If Joan refuses to increase the fee she pays, does Beth intend to terminate therapy? What are the transference issues to be expected? How does Beth intend to deal with Joan's reaction?

Beyond the countertransference issues there are fee-setting issues to be addressed. Feminist therapy guidelines require the practitioner to be accessible to a wide range of clients, including low-income, through flexible delivery of services (i.e., using a sliding-scale fee structure) (IA). How many clients are waiting for a sliding-scale place on Beth's case load? It is probable that Joan, a client who is no longer in need, is taking a sliding-scale place that another client, truly in need, could use.

The responsibility for accessibility must also be balanced against the therapist's income needs (IVB, D). Beth needs to ask if her approach to fee setting is satisfying her income needs or if her resentment toward Joan is enhanced because she generally feels underpaid for the work she does.

Beth also needs to examine her fee contract: does she have an agreement with clients that they inform her of changes in their fortunes in addition to the six-month renegotiations? (IIC). If she has not explicitly outlined this requirement in advance with Joan, she may need to take a loss on the sessions from now until the six-month renegotiation time, and in future, she will have to change her fee-setting policy to include such an agreement.

Another issue is raised by the way that Beth learned of Joan's windfall. It is reality that there is gossip in the therapy community—therapist–therapist gossip about other therapists, about clients (sometimes referred to as "consultation"), client–client gossip about therapists, and client–therapist gossip about other clients and other therapists. Client–therapist gossip about other clients should be avoided (IIIB), but the therapist's intention not to be a party to such gossip must be balanced against the client's need and right to bring into therapy any issue or information that she believes to be relevant to her own work (IIIA). In addition, there is the question of *how* such gossip should be avoided. In this situation, should Beth have interrupted the informant client midsentence to stop her from passing on the information about Joan's windfall? What does this do to confidentiality?

A general policy not to incorporate information gleaned from gossip into the therapy hour is recommended. In this case, the fact that the information about Joan's windfall comes from another client is problematic. The countertransference issue, however, takes precedence over avoiding the use of information gleaned from gossip. Given that she will act on the information she has, Beth's apparent intention not to name her source is appropriate. She must decide how will she respond when Joan asks her who told her about the Reno win.

This dilemma involving client–therapist gossip about another client brings to light another boundary issue for therapists to consider (IIIA, B). Beth heard about the windfall because two of her clients are friends. A therapist must decide what boundaries to exercise regarding taking a new client who is part of a current client's social, familial, or employment network, if indeed the therapist or even the prospective new client knows prior to beginning therapy that such a relationship exists. (Lynn M. Sloane)

RESPONDENT 2

Beth's first step is to explore what she has contributed to the situation. Some therapists (Sears, 1990) ask clients not to talk with them about other clients. Other therapists believe this request constrains a client's necessary freedom to deal with whatever may be of concern to her. It is up to Beth to work through her anger and resentment in her own therapy or in consultation until she can deal with the issue as she would with any other information she thinks a client is withholding (IVB).

Preventive ethics in this dilemma would start with the meaning and implication of "full fee" within sliding scale. It is potentially humiliating to a prospective client if the therapist states a "full fee" and adds that she "slides" for people who cannot afford what others pay (IA, IIC, D). A therapist who subscribes to the principle of a sliding scale can conceptualize the *range* of fees *as* her fee, so that she will indicate a fee that slides from *x* (the low figure, mentioned first) to *y*, depending on a client's *resources*, not income.

Beth might also reconsider her contract. Rather than building in a six-month renegotiation period, a therapist can indicate to her clients that openness on all matters, including monetary matters, is most helpful to therapy and that the client is to accept responsibility for notifying the therapist if her resources change. The therapist can then correspondingly indicate *her* (considered) responsibilities around money (IIB), issues she will have worked out for herself over time by thinking through her own money issues, by making mistakes and learning from them, and through professional books, seminars, or/and consultation. Krueger (1986), though not feminist, offers both wide-ranging and in-depth chapters on this issue, which many women find difficult to negotiate.

In therapy, the therapist must also keep in mind that "truth" is always subjective and relative, not absolute. In this dilemma, exploration of the meaning of the information giving is integral to Joan's therapy. Thus, in determining the ethical issues, Beth must ask: How accurate is the information? What is the client's investment in telling Beth? Is this friend breaking Joan's confidence? Does Joan know the therapist has been given this information? If not, why not? Is the implication of gambling ("Reno") a factor in the disclosure, in Beth's reaction, and if so how? Is it perhaps a ploy to test Beth's ability to protect confidentiality? What might happen if Joan learns, not from Beth, that the friend has told Beth? If Joan does not know what her friend has said, Beth can decide whether it might be in the best interests of both Joan and the friend for the second client to be open with Joan. Is the friend paying a higher fee to Beth than Joan is, and if so, how has that contributed? The answers to these questions all affect the decisions that Beth must make. (Jeanne Adleman)

DILEMMA C

Dr. White is supervising Dr. Martinez as she completes her residency prior to being licensed. Dr. Martinez has a client who works for a company whose insurance will not reimburse a nonlicensed psychologist. Although Dr. White meets with her supervisee weekly and discusses all of her dilemmas during the hour-long supervision session, she has not met with the client. As the supervisor, Dr. White signs the necessary insurance forms as though she has delivered the therapy to assure that the client gets insurance coverage.

RESPONDENT 1

Dr. Martinez needs to establish the agreement for compensation and billing as early as feasible in the professional relationship and to discuss any limitation of services that can be anticipated because of financing (American Psychological Association, 1992, 1.25 a, e). In today's health care climate, providers need to clarify whether the client's insurance will pay for the services during the initial client contact. Many clients are not fully cognizant of their benefit plans, requiring the provider to verify the benefit or to instruct the client on appropriate questions to ask the insurer. In so doing, Dr. Martinez would have become aware of the insurance reimbursement problem her client faced in seeking treatment with an unlicensed therapist. The client could then have made an informed decision about whether or not to pursue therapy with Dr. Martinez (IID).

Therapists must not exploit the recipients or payers of services with respect to fees. They must accurately state the nature of the service, fees, and must identify the provider in reports to payers for services (American Psychological Association, 1992, 1.26). In signing off on the insurance without noting that Dr. Martinez is the actual provider, Dr. White leads the insurance company to pay for services for which it would not otherwise have paid. Securing payment for services in this way is fraudulent.

Dr. White may be able to help the client to obtain the insurance benefit by proactively contacting the insurance company and indicating that she is closely supervising the therapy provided by Dr. Martinez (VB). She might want to indicate she has seen psychological testing results or has listened to audio tapes of the sessions. The goal would be to convince the insurance company that the quality of care provided by Dr. Martinez is not compromised by the fact that Dr. Martinez is not yet licensed. An argument for cost effectiveness might be made. For instance, if there has been a strong therapeutic alliance, it may be difficult for the client to switch therapists midstream, possibly to the point of the client not seeking needed services and thus ending up hospitalized. (Kathleen A. Mack)

RESPONDENT 2

This is a fairly straightforward dilemma involving a supervisor who "signs off" on the work of a supervisee. This occurrence used to happen a great deal in therapy settings and may still occur in certain locales.

The APA (1992, 1.26) as well as individual state psychological associations specifically state that "signing off" on another person's work is unethical. However, a review of other professional codes shows that such unequivocal statements are not common. If this dilemma involved nonpsychologist therapists/supervisors, the ethical considerations might differ. In those dilemmas where "signing off" is not specifically prohibited by professional codes of ethics, the counselor/therapist would be advised to check with state law and the third-party payer in question as many third-party payers (e.g., Blue Cross and Blue Shield of Minnesota) prohibit the practice of "signing off" to receive insurance coverage. Indeed, to do so in the face of such a prohibition could constitute fraud and be criminally prosecuted, as it has been in Minnesota.

For feminist therapists who are not psychologists, the dilemma poses important ethical questions. The issues involved raise fundamental questions of accessibility to diverse therapeutic approaches, especially for rural and underserved populations (IA). The practice of "signing off" by a supervisor for unlicensed therapists who offer a different therapeutic or cultural perspective expands the accessibility of services to people who have third-party coverage but need to have that service provided by a practitioner with a specific degree or license. Complicating the issue for feminist therapists is that in this particular dilemma, the clinical responsibility seems to be very completely met by both Drs. White and Martinez. Therefore, from a clinical standpoint, the professionals involved have met their responsibilities; and from a feminist standpoint, their practice has increased clients' accessibility to the services of Dr. Martinez.

A question that remains unanswered and that is relevant to good feminist therapy practice is whether Dr. Martinez has fully informed her client that Dr. White is providing supervision and is "signing off" on the insurance forms (IIB). Although it could be argued that this particular information does not facilitate the therapeutic process, feminist principles advocate full disclosure unless it is specifically not in the client's best interests.

With continuously decreasing financial resources and decreasing support for mental health services being covered by medical insurance plans, the likelihood of a third-party payer allowing an unlicensed practitioner to receive reimbursement under any circumstances grows increasingly small. Therefore, the issues of accessibility to which feminist therapists are particularly sensitive are going to be acute in the next decade. Questioning therapeutic practices and seeking multiple avenues of impacting social change, including lobbying, advocacy, and public education will continue to be essential (VA, B). (Katherine H. Speare)

The following two dilemmas are related to barter and are presented together to help clarify the issues through comparison and contrast.

DILEMMA D

Mitsuye began seeing her therapist Dr. Roland several months before she lost her job as an accountant as the result of her company's closing its local office. Mitsuye has a great deal of respect for Dr. Roland as a therapist and felt she was making progress. She was paying $60 an hour for therapy but continued to fall behind in her payments. Dr. Roland told her that her part-time bookkeeper had resigned and that she thought it made sense for Mitsuye to fill in at the salary she had been paying. Her bookkeeper had been earning $15 an hour. This salary would be applied to her therapy debt. Mitsuye thought she had to accept her offer since she owed Dr. Roland money but has become increasingly disenchanted with the arrangement. She has decided to quit *therapy with Dr. Roland and to consult with a second therapist about the situation.*

DILEMMA E

Linda Fineday, a counselor, was seeing Danny, a client whose economic circumstances were marginal: he worked sporadically at entry-level jobs. The therapist had reduced Danny's fee to $20 an hour, but even at that rate, he was accruing an increasing balance.

Danny was a client who had difficulty negotiating the vicissitudes of daily life because of his intellectual limitations and used his therapy primarily to sort through his responses to life situations. Over time in therapy, he had gradually developed a set of internalized guidelines that enabled him to approach life in a more functional way. His transference response to the therapist was mild: he valued her as a reliable, supportive, and helpful person in his life. At one point, feeling uncomfortable about his bill, he offered to pay for part of his therapy by giving Linda Fineday cheese that he had gotten as part of his benefits from the cheese factory where he worked.

RESPONDENT 1

Bartering is a particularly rural phenomenon: a personalized economic practice commonly used in parts of the country where human interactions of all kinds are perhaps more personal than in more populated areas. But more important than this is the issue of class. To insist on being paid with money is to ignore the reality of how difficult it may be for some people to come by money. It is classist to assume (without other evidence) that difficulty in paying the fee, even a reduced fee, is necessarily some form of therapeutic resistance (IB, C). One of the primary ethical imperatives regarding any financial transaction with a client is to avoid exploitation, and bartering can easily be exploitative in any number of ways.

Therapy is expensive. A client may well earn a fraction of what the therapist earns. A client who would be likely to consider a bartering arrangement is, almost by definition, likely to be at a financial disadvantage relative to the therapist.

One solution might be to see the client for free or for a very token amount of money as long as the therapist does not feel burdened or resentful and as long as the client is comfortable with this arrangement. However, some clients may feel infantilized if seen for free and may wish to recompense the therapist out of a sense of healthy pride and fairness. In addition, a therapist who can occasionally barter appropriately and feels fairly paid in this way may be able comfortably to see a greater number of low-income people (IA). Thus, complicated though it may be, finding a way to barter nonexploitatively is an ethically responsible position.

In an everyday bartering situation, the matter of exploitation is generally taken care of by the (presumably) equal power between the two participants. If either feels that she is being taken advantage of, she simply does not agree to the arrangement. In therapy, the transferential or symbolic aspect of the relationship may add to the already existing power difference. In addition, the therapist should remember that therapy is her "turf," and that she generally will be seen by the client as having the power to make the rules, including defining what is appropriate or fair.

When sorting through whether a particular barter arrangement is fair, the therapist should be guided by the following considerations (Hill, 1993).

1. *What is the nature of the transference, or the symbolic aspects of the relationship with the client? Given this, what does the bartering arrangement mean to the client?* In the dilemmas above, Mitsuye's "great deal of respect" for her therapist should signal greater caution in making bartering arrangements than might be necessary for Danny, whose transference is milder. In addition, Dr. Roland shows poor judgment in suggesting a barter that would give Mitsuye access to information about other clients. At the very least, such information is likely to complicate the transferential aspects of therapy.

2. *What is the nature of the dual relationship involved?* In Mitsuye's case, Dr. Roland's decision meant that she was employing a client as her bookkeeper.

3. *What is the economic context? Is it clear that the client would be unduly burdened by having to pay?* Although both clients in these dilemmas had trouble paying for therapy, only Danny's therapist had already tried to resolve this situation by lowering the fee.

4. *What is the relative cost of the barter arrangement to the therapist and to the client?* Mitsuye's side of the agreement cost her four hours of professional labor for every hour of therapy. Danny's cost was more reasonable, since the cheese he bartered for therapy was not excessively expensive to him in either time or money.

5. *Are there other power differences between therapist and client?* In these dilemmas, there is no information about race, age, sexual orientation, or physical disability. Mitsuye, as a woman, has less gender-related power, although, as a professional accountant, her social class relative to her therapist may be less of an issue. Danny's gender may actually soften the impact of the power differences with his female therapist. However, he clearly is at a disadvantage in terms of social class

and intellectual ability. Whether the idea of bartering and the specifics of the agreement are suggested by the therapist or by the client are also important factors in terms of power. Mitsuye clearly felt unable to reject or change the proposal made by her therapist, while Danny was more in control of the agreement that he suggested to his therapist.

6. *If a bartering agreement is made, how will the problem of evaluation be handled?* Bartering for impersonal items, such as the cheese suggested by Danny, is safer than bartering for personal services. When in doubt, the therapist and client should discuss, as part of the agreement, how any conflict in the area of evaluation will be handled. One possible solution is to arrange a three-way barter in which the therapist receives something from a third individual who in turn receives something from the client. With goods, a third person might be used to assign the monetary value of the goods.

As in all ethical decisions, the therapist will make the best choice if she uses both her intuitive and logical knowing, especially when it comes to personal biases (such as countertransference or feelings about money) that may be involved. Any bartering agreement should be discussed carefully with the client, considering especially what the client thinks is fair, potential problems, and any way in which the client's feelings about the therapist are a factor. Finally, consultation with a colleague is the best way to ensure that any bartering arrangement is nonexploitative. (Marcia Hill)

RESPONDENT 2

Accepting goods or services as substitution for part or full monetary payment is fraught with implications for the progress of psychotherapy. For this reason, many practitioners refuse to enter into such arrangements. Others work with persons of very low income pro bono, asking the client to pay whatever she or he can afford from week to week. One interesting variation is accepting nominal cash payment plus mutually agreed-on community service work by the client. Such a plan eliminates the de facto employer–therapist duality, has a potential for increasing the client's self-esteem, and helps some clients move out of isolation.

Still other therapists hold a clear value of being available to at least some clients via exchange. To the extent that it can be done honorably and respectfully, with a "contract" to explore its impact on therapy on an ongoing basis, it can be productive (IC, IIC). The therapist needs time before confirming an agreement to explore what it will mean *to her* to use her time in this way (IVD) and what it will mean to the self-esteem of the client if dollar values are very unequal (IIA, C). It is difficult but not impossible to find a language that is realistic and not demeaning for discussion of these issues. Neither monetary nor other arrangements are problem-free. Therapists are accountable for how they prioritize ethical and value conflicts.

In the dilemmas at hand, Dr. Roland has suggested an exchange of therapy for professional services. She is clearly in violation of virtually any code of ethics when she makes such a proposal. This plan would require Mitsuye to know the names of Dr. Roland's other clients, the amount of each person's fee, and the status of each one's account, a clear breach of the confidentiality of those clients. It is up to Mitsuye to figure out the means to pay her overdue bill. Mitsuye has made a good decision about ending therapy with Dr. Roland. When she finds a new therapist, her first task may well be to work on her perception that she "had to accept" Dr. Roland's "offer since she owed her money." The exploitive "suggestion" may have carried an implied threat that Mitsuye did not recognize. Additionally, if Mitsuye is of Japanese origin, the therapist's "offer" may betray a racist stereotyping (IB) of Japanese women as submissive and accommodating.

The second dilemma, where the client suggests an exchange of goods for therapy, is also problematic. A therapist who accepts goods she does not really want, or that are too personal, is not being helpful to the client (IIA, IIIA). Linda Fineday has a responsibility to deal respectfully with Danny. If she is unwilling to work for barter, she might tell him she is unable to accept his offer of partial payment in cheese because it violates conditions of her profession. She might alternatively establish with him a period during which he will focus on working toward employment at which time he will be better paid, simultaneously expressing trust in him to pay off his accrued bill on a modest but regular basis later. Or she may work with him toward a reasonable termination date, on the realistic grounds that he seems unable to afford therapy at this time but that he may return in the future when he can. Finally, if she is unable to work out the financial issues in a mutually satisfying manner, she should help Danny find even less expensive local services to meet his needs. (Jeanne Adleman)

DILEMMA F

When Jean Smith was first starting her practice and building a clientele, she offered a certain number of hours monthly of pro bono therapy to clients of the local women's shelter and a women's addiction treatment program. Although with her paid clientele she tended to do long term, insight-oriented therapy, with the pro bono clients she used problem-solving, short-term therapy of four sessions or less.

As Jean's practice expanded and her professional reputation grew, she could fill her entire practice with full-fee and insurance-covered clients. She had less time to volunteer with the grassroots programs. In addition, she was regularly asked to sit on boards for various feminist organizations. Gradually all of her pro bono work was on this organizational level and none was direct service.

RESPONDENT 1

The first issue raised by this dilemma is that of offering different services dependent on the clients' ability to pay full fees. One of the appeals of private practice is that the therapist can choose the kind of work she does. A therapist may choose to work largely with lesbians, for example. Doing long-term therapy with full-pay clients and short-term therapy with pro bono clients is different and problematic because the therapist's interests are given priority over those of the client. The client's well being should be the guiding principle (FTI Preamble). Jean's decision is also discriminatory, based on socioeconomic class (IC), and she probably is not negotiating with the client in a mutual process (IIA, C).

An argument can be made that Jean Smith's policy may be acceptable if she is offering a triage system where people needing longer-term therapy are referred to comparable services. If her pro bono clients are referred to her only when a brief, more directive intervention is needed and they are able to get longer-term supportive assistance from case workers or volunteers at the referring agencies, she may be able to offer services to more people over a shorter period of time.

In all cases, the therapist has an ethical requirement to inform the client as early as possible of the limitation of services resulting from limitations in financing (American Psychological Association, 1992). In the best of all possible worlds, Jean Smith's low income clients then have the option to go elsewhere for longer-term therapy at an affordable price.

The second issue raised by this dilemma is the philosophical question all feminist therapists face: how to balance feminist commitment and paid work? Therapists have many layers of ethical obligations: (1) as feminists, (2) as feminist therapists to clients, and (3) as feminist therapists to self-care. Fulfilling all of these can be exhausting and sometimes seem impossible or mutually exclusive. Often as they focus more on careers, feminist therapists devote less time and energy to feminist political involvement. One solution is to find some way to merge the two. Some feminist therapists, for example, may take the position that providing pro bono work to other women and doing a politicized therapy satisfies their feminist obligations. At the other end, Jean Smith seems to hold that fulfilling her obligations to a feminist ethic (sitting on boards of feminist organizations) also satisfies her ethical responsibilities to her profession by impacting change (VB). Nevertheless, other guidelines (IA, C, IIC) remain unsatisfied or violated. Jean Smith is left with an obligation to make her services as a therapist accessible to a wide range of clients, including low-income ones, in addition to her political involvement at a board level. (Lynn M. Sloane)

RESPONDENT 2

Offering pro bono therapy solely to build a practice and discontinuing when it is no longer necessary to meet the therapist's needs violates feminist values (FTI Preamble). Such a practice is self-serving and does not represent a genuine attempt to meet the health needs of clients who are in crisis (IA). Presumably, if the therapist in question had provided pro bono work from a proactive stance to reduce the oppression of women, she would continue to do so even when she could fill the hours with paying clients. The amount of time she has available for pro bono work may decrease as her practice becomes more mature, but the commitment to provide the assistance should remain strong.

Jean Smith's practice of sitting on boards of various feminist organizations with goals to create a genuinely egalitarian society is acceptable as pro bono work. When she filled her practice with only full-fee and insurance-covered clients and discontinued seeing pro-bono clients, she was no longer accessible to a wide range of clients (IA). A committed feminist therapist has a flexible fee schedule.

The most serious ethical violation, in terms of an immediate harmful impact on clients, is Jean Smith's practice of providing only problem-solving, short-term therapy of four sessions or less to the pro bono clients. This practice is exploitative of these clients, could result in serious harm, may constitute abandonment in the legal sense, and is indicative of the same self-serving attitude mentioned above and of a class bias on the therapist's part. This bias impairs her judgment and clinical competency. She has a duty to confront and change her biases (IIC).

To the extent that she has limited hours and offers only short term work for pro bono clients as a way of working with more people, she should help the shelter personnel screen for clients for whom these services are most appropriate. In setting up the therapeutic contract, she should be explicit about the limitations, the possibility of referrals, and the reasons for these limitations (IIC). She should work to ensure that other resources are available in the community (IA, VA). (Barbara McCandlish)

IMPLICATIONS

The feminist ethical decision-making model engendered by Hill, Glaser, and Harden (Section 2, this volume) acknowledges two different ways of knowing as basic components of the feminist therapist's ethics discernment tasks: the feeling–intuitive and the rational–evaluative. It is interesting to notice the differences between respondents who approach the questions in terms of a process of decision making versus those who are primarily code oriented. Some responses indicate a difference of opinion, which may reflect individual differences in the background of respondents as well as contextual, intuitive, and emotional elements they perceive in the case material. Such differences may be disturbing to readers who want a solid answer to an ethical dilemma. However, these differences illustrate the difficulty and ambiguity of monetary transactions and underscore the importance of a dynamic and ongoing consultative process.

These dilemmas and responses beg a number of other troubling questions. As a result of (1) limited therapy resources in rural areas, (2) changing priorities of U.S. government funding, and (3) hit-or-miss insurance for mental health problems, many people in need of counseling cannot afford even the lower levels of sliding-fee rates. A $30-an-hour therapy charge can equal a full day's take home pay for those working for minimum wage. These same people are less likely to have good insurance, child care, and sick/doctor leave. Women, people of color, and people with health problems form a disproportionately large part of this pool. As poor people, many feel disenfranchised and disempowered in the process of finding adequate mental health care, let alone be able to exercise choice about the person who provides it.

This issue gets entangled in other fairness issues on an entirely different level. For instance, in many places, only psychiatrists and psychologists get insurance reimbursement. These same practitioners tend to bill at the highest hourly rates. In addition, insurance companies pay according to specialty, so that allowable charges are higher for psychiatrists as compared to other mental health workers, leading to various professional advocacy groups' demands of equity and inclusion in government and insurance plans. Thus a psychologist may look with hunger at the hourly rate of a psychiatrist but forget to look at the other side of the social equation, in comparing her or his salary to the hourly pay of the client.

The therapist who tries to respond to the client's economics is put in a position of engaging in questionable billing practices, that is, billing full fee and later discounting the client's share of copayment. Therapists who have the most favorable sliding fees can quickly have a practice of only the lowest-income clients who cannot afford therapy elsewhere and who are referred by colleagues and other clients. In addition, therapists who charge more reasonable fees are often criticized by their colleagues for not practicing self-care.

Perhaps it is time for the very face of therapy to change. Changing it is—but not necessarily in ways that enhance practicing feminist therapy principles. Every feminist therapist needs to be alert and active in the highly political process of determining mental health provision. As proposals are critiqued, a power analysis needs to be applied. Are therapy delivery plans sensitive to women's needs? Does any proposed plan reflect that women are more likely to use mental health services, that women are particularly susceptible to emotional, physical and sexual abuse, and poverty, all risk factors for increased need for services? Are members of nondominant groups discriminated against: lesbians and gays, racial and ethnic cultures, children?

Essentially this section is about feminist therapists trying to balance class and quality-of-care issues with their need for income. It is important that women as feminist therapists not get so caught up in responsibilities to others that the issue of self-care, including income, is lost. What is fair to the client needs to be weighed with what is fair to the therapist. It is perhaps more than coincidental that as more women enter the field of providing therapy, managed care and government intervention work to lower income in the profession. Comparing incomes in traditionally male careers to those in mental health reinforces that Western society does not value care taking highly.

RESPONDENTS

Jeanne Adleman, MA, is an educator-turned-feminist therapist born in 1919 who taught and supervised teacher training at several universities and now maintains an active practice in San Francisco.

Danna R. Farabee is Director of the Sexual Assault Program of Beltrami, Cass, and Hubbard Counties of MN.

Marcia Hill, EdD, is a psychologist in private practice in Montpelier, VT, and a feminist therapist for 20 years who also teaches, writes, and consults in the area of feminist therapy, theory, and practice.

Kathleen A. Mack, PsyD, has 15 years of experience as a therapist in private practice in Dayton and Cincinnati, OH, with specialties in feminist therapy, neuropsychology, and lesbian/gay concerns.

Barbara McCandlish, PhD, is a feminist therapist practicing in Santa Fe, NM, is a founding member of the Berkeley Women's Health Collective, and has published several articles on lesbian mother families and lesbian couples.

Rachel Josefowitz Siegel, MSW, BCSW, is a feminist therapist in private practice in Ithaca, NY, whose lifelong search for ethical behavior involves an ongoing process of questioning and clarifying her own Jewish and feminist values.

Lynn M. Sloane, PhD, is a lesbian feminist therapist in private practice in Calgary, Alberta.

Katherine H. Speare, PhD, with 15 years of experience working as a psychologist and therapist, is currently in private practice in Duluth, MN, and rural Wisconsin.

REFERENCES

American Association for Counseling and Development. (1988). *Ethical standards.* Alexandria, VA: Author.

American Association for Marriage and Family Therapy. (1991). *AAMFT code of ethics.* Washington, DC: Author.

American Psychiatric Association. (1992). *Addendum to the 1992 edition of the principles of medical ethics.* Washington DC: Author.

American Psychological Association. (1992). Ethical principles of psychologists and code of conduct. *American Psychologist, 47,* 1597–1611.

Ballou, M. (1992). Introduction. In L. S. Brown & M. Ballou (Eds.), *Personality and psychopathology: Feminist reappraisals* (pp. 5–6). New York: Guilford Press.

Biele, N., & Jacobson, N. (1988). *Framework for service delivery in nonprofit community agencies.* Presentation to the Sexual Assault Program, Beltrami, MN.

Borys, D. S., & Pope, K. S. (1989). Dual relationships between therapist and client: A national study of psychologists, psychiatrists, and social workers. *Professional Psychology: Research and Practice, 20,* 283–293.

Brown, L. S. (1990). Ethical issues and the business of therapy. In H. Lerman & N. Porter (Eds.), *Feminist ethics in psychotherapy,* (pp. 60–69). New York: Springer.

Chesler, P. (1972). *Women and madness.* New York: Avon Books.

Drellich, M. G. (1991). Money and counter transference. In S. Klebanow & E. L. Lowenkepf (Eds.), *Money and mind* (pp. 155–163). New York: Plenum Press.

Feminist Therapy Institute. (1987). *Feminist therapy code of ethics.* Denver: Author.

Feminist Therapy Institute. (1992). Questioning times. *Interchange, 10,* 11.

Ghertner, S. J. (1993, December). *How to form, capitalize and thrive in a multi-disciplinary group practice.* Paper presented at Psychotherapy under Managed Care Conference, San Francisco.

Handlesman, M. M., Kemper, M. B., Kesson-Craig, P., McLain, J., & Johnsrud, C. (1986). Use, content, and readability of written informed consent forms for treatment. *Professional Psychology: Research and Practice, 17,* 514–518.

Hill, M. (1993). *Bartering.* Unpublished manuscript.

Kahn, A. S., & Gaedder, W. P. (1985). Theories of equity to theories of justice:

The liberating consequences of studying women. In V. E. O'Leary, R. K. Unger, & B. S. Wallston (Eds.), *Women, gender, social psychology* (pp. 237–244). Hillsdale, NJ: Erlbaum.

Klebanow, S. (1991). Power, gender and money. In S. Klebanow & E. L. Lowenkepf (Eds.), *Money and mind* (pp. 51–61). New York: Plenum Press.

Kreuger, D. W. (1986). *The last taboo: Money as symbol and reality in psychotherapy and psychoanalysis.* New York: Brunner/Mazel.

Lasky, E. (1984). Psychoanalysts and psychotherapists: Conflicts about setting fees. *Psychoanalytic Psychology, 4,* 289–300.

Lasky, E. (1985). Psychotherapists' ambivalence about fees. In L. B. Rosewater & L. E. A. Walker (Eds.), *Handbook of feminist therapy: Women's issues in psychotherapy* (pp. 250–256). New York: Springer.

Lott, B. (1987). *Women's lives: Themes and variations in gender learning.* New York: Brooks/Cole.

McWilliams, M. (1994, January). *The future of health care in the United States.* Paper presented for Portlandia, Portland, OR.

Muszynski, I. L., & Marshall, J. W. (1993, December). General considerations associated with provider contracting. In *Conference syllabus, psychotherapy under managed care: Outcomes-oriented treatments of choice.* San Francisco: Institute for Behavioral Healthcare.

National Association of Social Workers. (1990). *Code of ethics: National Association of Social Workers.* Silver Spring, MD: Author.

Oordt, M. S. (1990). Ethics of practice among Christian psychologists: A pilot study. *Journal of Psychology and Theology, 5,* 255–260.

Parvin, R., & Biaggio, M. K. (1991). Paradoxes in the practice of feminist therapy. *Women and Therapy, 10,* 1–12.

Payton, P. (1993, November). *NuPLAN 1994.* Paper presented at the Oregon Association for Marriage and Family Therapy Annual Membership Meeting, Eugene, OR.

Saultz, J. (1994, February). *Face to face with primary health care.* Paper presented at The Future Is Now: The Managed Mental Health Care Conversation Continues conference, Portland, OR.

Sears, V. (1990). Ethics in small minority communities. In H. Lerman & N. Porter (Eds.), *Feminist ethics in psychotherapy* (pp. 204–213). New York: Springer.

Shainess, N. (1991). Countertransference problems with money. In S. Klebanow & E. L. Lowenkepf (Eds.), *Money and mind* (pp. 163–175). New York: Plenum Press.

Tabachnick, B. G., Keith-Spiegel, P., & Pope, K. S. (1991). Ethics of teaching: Beliefs and behaviors of psychologists as educators. *American Psychologist, 46,* 506–515.

Webb, W. L. (1989). Ethical psychiatric practice in a new economic climate. *Psychiatric Annals, 19,* 443–447.

Woody, R. H. (1989). *Business success in mental health practice.* San Francisco: Jossey-Bass.

SIX

Overlapping/Dual Relationships

Maryka Biaggio
Beverly Greene

Overlapping and dual relationships present therapists with a range of complex but unavoidable ethical and practical dilemmas. Although all mental health professionals must be aware of the potential for overlapping relationships, feminist therapists may be especially likely to encounter a wide variety of such relationships. Because feminist therapists are often members of the same communities that they serve professionally, and because these communities are often small or inclusive, feminist therapists may have interactions with clients in various contexts. For these reasons, it is especially important for feminist therapists to exercise good decision making when monitoring personal and professional relationships and to have carefully thought through the ethical, personal, and professional issues associated with overlapping and dual relationships. Examples of communities in which complete avoidance of clients is not always possible include the lesbian community (Smith, 1990), rural communities (Gates & Speare, 1990), and ethnic minority communities (Sears, 1990).

Most professional mental health organizations have ethical codes that deem dual relationships problematic because of their propensity to create conflicts of interest in the therapy relationship. This view is supported by Keith-Spiegel and Koocher (1985), Pope and Vasquez (1991), and others who observe that disagreements arising out of dual relationships between therapist and client form the largest group of consumer complaints, actions of licensing and professional disciplinary boards, and financial losses in malpractice cases involving psychologists and other mental health professionals.

According to Pope (1991, p. 21), "a dual relationship in psycho-therapy occurs when the therapist engages in another, significantly different relationship with the patient. The two relationships may be concurrent or sequential." The 1981 and 1989 editions of the Ethical Principles of Psychologists exhorted psychologists to "make every effort to avoid dual relationships that could impair their professional judgment or increase the risk of exploitation" (American Psychological Association, 1990, p. 393).

In 1985 feminist therapist Berman coined the term "overlapping relationships" to refer to the often unavoidable overlap of relationships or roles for therapists and their clients (Brown, 1991). In effect, Berman contended that it is not always possible for therapists to anticipate or have control over all the ways in which their lives may overlap with those of their clients. Interestingly, the most recent issue of the Ethical Principles of Psychologists employs the term "multiple relationships" to address concerns over what had been previously characterized as dual relationships. This version of the Ethical Principles also recognizes that "In many communities and situations, it may not be feasible or reason-able for psychologists to avoid social or other nonprofessional contacts with persons such as patients, clients, students, supervisees, or research participants" (American Psychological Association, 1992, p. 1601). Thus, the feminist perspective that overlapping relationships are inevitable and must be recognized and managed as such is now included in the approach taken by the American Psychological Association in its Ethical Guidelines.

In an article specifically discussing dual relationships in psycho-therapy, Pope points out a number of major difficulties with dual relationships:

> First, the dual relationship erodes and distorts the professional nature of the therapeutic relationship. . . . Second, dual relationships create con-flicts of interest and, thus, compromise the disinterest (not lack of interest) necessary for sound professional judgment. . . . Third, both during the course of therapy and at any time thereafter, the therapist may be invited or compelled (through subpoena or court order) to offer testimony regard-ing the patient's diagnosis, treatment, prognosis, and so forth. . . . Fourth, because of the therapist–patient relationship, the patient cannot enter into a business or other secondary relationship with the therapist on equal footing. . . . Fifth, if it became acceptable practice for therapists to engage in dual financial, social, and professional relationships with their patients, whether prior or subsequent to termination, then the nature of psycho-therapy would be drastically changed. . . . Sixth, dual relationships would affect the cognitive processes that research has shown to play a role in the beneficial effects of therapy after termination. (1991, pp. 23–25)

The conflict of interest to which Pope alludes is the central problem in dual relationships. A conflict of interest in therapy has been defined as the therapist's pursuit or engagement in another significant relationship with the client during the course of therapy or a previous significant relationship with a person that the therapist currently treats as a client (Greene, 1994; Keith-Spiegel & Koocher, 1985; Pope & Vasquez, 1991). This definition also applies to the therapist's deliberate termination of a client's therapy for the specific purpose of pursuing some other relationship with the client (Brown, 1988; Gabbard & Pope, 1989). Many mental health organizations include as a conflict of interest the therapist's promises or assurances, whether subtle or overt, that some other relationship between the therapist and client could or will take place after therapy is terminated (Corey, Corey, & Callanan, 1993).

Many professional organizations contend that the therapist's responsibility to the client does not end when therapy is terminated and discourage the practice of establishing social or other relationships with clients after termination. The therapist is not only expected to establish a reliable set of boundaries that the client can depend on but is expected to maintain those boundaries as well (Brown, 1985; Gartrell, 1994; Pope & Vasquez, 1991).

Dual relationships bring an additional set of interests other than the clients' into the therapy. There is a potential for the therapist's needs to compete or conflict with the needs of the client and confuse the boundaries of the professional relationship with the client. It is that professional relationship that the therapist seeks to protect. The erosion of appropriate boundaries in therapy frequently leads to alterations and confusion in the therapy relationship and may even result in the therapist's use of his or her unequal position to exploit the client (Brown, 1985; Gartrell, 1994; Greene, 1994; Pope & Vasquez, 1991).

THE THERAPEUTIC ALLIANCE AND OVERLAPPING RELATIONSHIPS

Comprehending the nature of conflicted interests in this context requires an understanding of the nature and complex constituents of the therapeutic alliance. It additionally includes an acknowledgment of the power differential between therapist and client that leaves the client vulnerable to the therapist's actions in many ways (Keith-Spiegel & Koocher, 1985; Pope & Vasquez, 1991). In the therapeutic alliance, the therapist is ethically responsible for the therapy relationship and for taking care of her own personal and professional needs (Adleman & Barrett, 1990).

The client's needs are expected to be the paramount focus of therapeutic inquiries and the therapy relationship. In relationships that are truly mutual, each participant engages in a mutual process of responding to and taking care of the other's needs. In therapy it is the therapist's responsibility to address the client's needs. The client is not responsible for addressing the therapist's needs in a similar fashion. This lack of mutuality is an important variable in the relationship and in the difference between therapy and other relationships. It contributes to another important and distinct dimension of psychotherapy, the symbolic relationship. In psychoanalytic models this process is understood as the client's transference to the therapist, and refers to feelings, fantasies, or memories the client experiences for the therapist that have their origins in previous significant relationships with important figures in the client's life.

According to Brown (1983), this component of psychotherapy is one in which the therapist represents or symbolizes something or someone that the client needs her to symbolize. In reality, neither the therapist nor the therapy relationship is exactly that which it symbolically represents to the client. Realistic aspects of the therapist as a person are used by the client, in conjunction with elements of the client's own needs and history, in the construction of a symbolic figure in the therapist. The client may experience and respond to the symbolic nature of the relationship as if it were totally realistic. The fact that the client is not always responding to the realistic aspects of the therapist or the therapy relationship does not diminish its importance to the therapy. Understanding and unraveling the various components of the client's response may in fact be very helpful and are often central features of some therapies. These symbolic representations in the therapy relationship offer clients the opportunity to use therapy to reexperience and examine old feelings and memories in the safety of the therapy relationship.

Clients may respond to realistic aspects of the therapist as a person, and therapists have responsibility to attend to real aspects of their own behavior and its realistic, not fantasized, impact on clients in therapy. Both realistic and symbolic aspects of the therapist are concurrent components of the client's response. Clients respond to and use both the realistic and symbolic or representative aspects of the therapist as important resources in therapy.

When the therapist is engaged in other relationships with the client, these outside relationships can take two problematic directions. Brown (1983) points out that both therapist and client may continue to enact their therapy roles outside of therapy. In this scenario, there is a potential for the therapist to minimize her own needs, which may be unacknowledged, and to use the client to substitute or avoid meeting those needs more directly (Adleman & Barrett, 1990). As Adleman and Barrett (1990) point out, neither party participates in such a relationship in an authentic way. In another scenario, the therapist may make her own needs the focus of the outside relationship and, in doing so, not only abdicate her primary role as therapist but may also interfere with the client's ability to participate in the symbolic aspect of the relationship (Adleman & Barrett, 1990). Furthermore, the dual relationship may give the client access to personal information about the therapist and the therapist's emotional life that makes it difficult for the client to create a symbolic representation of the therapist and use the symbolic aspect of the therapy relationship.

Another important factor to consider is the power differential between therapists and clients. Although feminist therapists seek to develop relationships with clients that are not hierarchical, their roles and responsibilities in the therapy imbue them with power over the client. The therapist is privy to information about the client that the client does not have about the therapist. This "information" is not simply a range of facts about the client but may include an understanding of the client that is based on information the client has both consciously and unconsciously communicated, and that the therapist has been trained to appreciate in particular ways. A similar power differential exists in other professional relationships, for example, the professor–student relationship. For instance, professors have power over students in that they evaluate students' performance; any requests they may make of students to assist them with research and other academic tasks may be considered obligatory to students because of this power differential.

The feminist therapy literature has extensively explored the problems associated with the failure to acknowledge power differentials in therapy and the resulting potential for recapitulating society's normative power inequities within therapy itself. Ethical guidelines for most professionals, including those for feminist therapists, compel therapists both to monitor and use the inherent power differential between client and therapist in ways that benefit the client. These guidelines further admonish therapists to explicitly structure the therapy relationship in ways that facilitate the therapist's ability to put the needs of the client first and to minimize the potential for situations that would compromise the therapist's ability to fulfill this imperative. The therapist must understand the nature and extent of her own needs and be able to make important distinctions between actions in therapy that are designed to meet her own needs and not the client's needs. Therapists must understand these parameters in order to develop a working therapeutic alliance with the client that is not exploitive.

TYPES OF OVERLAPPING/DUAL RELATIONSHIPS

Overlapping/dual relationships may be separated into two broad categories, sexual and nonsexual relationships, and the 1993 Report of the Ethics Committee (American Psychological Association, 1993) provides incidences of dual relationships for these two categories. This report indicates that for 1990, 1991, and 1992, 68% of dual relationship complaints were sexual in nature, and 32% were nonsexual.

Ethical codes of professional mental health associations and the Feminist Therapy Code of Ethics explicitly define sexual relationships with clients as exploitive and offer them as examples of the most flagrant abuses of the therapist's power (Brown, 1988; Pope, 1991; Pope & Vasquez, 1991). However, such prohibitions have not always been explicit, since the professions have only addressed this topic in the past few decades. In their book examining sexual feelings in psychotherapy, Pope, Sonne, and Holroyd (1993, p. 24) note, "The profession historically has demonstrated great resistance to acknowledging the problem of therapist–patient sexual intimacies." These authors point out that it is only since the 1970s that the psychotherapy profession has begun to acknowledge openly violations of the prohibition against therapist–patient sex and to study the incidence and effects of those violations. For instance, it was not until 1973 that the first survey providing evidence of therapist–patient sexual intimacies was published (Kardener, Fuller, & Mensh, 1973). The first explicit reference to a prohibition of therapist-client sexual relations in the American Psychological Association's Ethical Principles of Psychologists occurred in the 1977 edition.

According to Brodsky (1989), sex between therapist and client was not clearly defined as unethical by the mental health professions until the mid-1970s. In fact, during the late 1960s and early 1970s two professionals published accounts of therapist–client sexual interactions: James McCarthy (1966) obtained consent from clients and their families for having sex with clients; and Martin Shepard (1971) wrote a book entitled *The Love Treatment*, suggesting that there were benefits to therapist–client sex. Brodsky notes that although both these psychiatrists were widely read, they were negatively sanctioned by their profession. Brodsky also traces the history of client malpractice claims for therapist–client sex. The first large awards occurred in the early 1970s, with the most media attention given to the case of the New York psychiatrist Renatus Hartogs. This case was popularized in the book *Betrayal*, which was written by the therapy client (Freeman & Roy, 1976). The first research examining sexual intimacy in psychology training found that 10% of the respondents reported sexual contact as students with their educators; gender differences were significant, with 16.5% of the women, compared with 3% of the men, reporting such contact (Pope, Levenson, & Schover, 1979).

Pope and Vasquez (1991) and Pope (1991) review research pertinent to dual/overlapping relationships and raise relevant questions about the continued occurrence of sexual dual relationships between therapists and clients despite both condemnation of the practice by professional mental health organizations and evidence that clients are harmed by them. In their analysis, they note that the perpetrators of such behavior are overwhelmingly male and the victims overwhelmingly female. According to the 1993 Report of the Ethics Committee (American Psychological Association, 1993), of all sexual and non-sexual dual relationship complaints, 72% involved male perpetrators and female victims, with all other possible gender-pair permutations accounting for 28% of the complaints. Pope and Vasquez (1991) suggest that mental health institutions have historically trivialized or denied the destructive nature of behavior when perpetrators are male and victims are female. Such behavior and trends reflect the recapitulation in the therapy process itself of gender-based social power inequities found in the patriarchal cultures of the United States and Canada.

This trend, however, should not imply that female therapists do not engage in such behavior. Gartrell, Herman, Olarte, Feldstein, and Localio (1986) cite female therapist–female client abuses as the second most common of this type of client abuse. Benowitz (1994) and Gartrell and Sanderson (1994) note that a common belief among victims of female therapist–female client abuse was that women are not abusive. It was suggested that this belief made it more difficult for clients to identify abusive situations as such. Clients in the Benowitz study (1994) reported feeling that if the therapist had been male they would have been suspicious or correctly identified the exploitive nature of the relationship earlier on in its course. Other myths were that female therapists who engage in such behavior do so only once, and they do so only after prolonged involvement as a therapist with the client.

According to reports from clients who have been abused by female therapists, over half of those in the Benowitz study reported having heard that their therapist had been in overtly sexual relationships with at least one other client at some time. It was also determined that female therapists in the Benowitz (1994) sample not only initiated sexual contact at a rate of 93%, compared to their male counterparts who did so at a rate of 72%, but that they initiated this contact earlier on in the course of therapy than did their male counterparts (six-and-a-half months vs. nine months). Female therapists who are uncomfortable with their own same-gender attractions, particularly when paired with clients who have questions about their own sexual orientation were found to be at higher risk for sexual experimentation with female clients (Benowitz, 1994; Brown, 1985). The hidden context of therapy may have been perceived by therapists as a safer place to engage in such experimentation than in same-gender relationships conducted in the open with their peers. Benowitz (1994), Brown (1988), Gartrell et al. (1986), Gartrell and Sanderson (1994), and Pope and Vasquez (1991) document the harmful nature of such relationships as well as risk factors specific to female client–female therapist pairs.

The realistic, symbolic, and intense nature of the therapy process may elicit many feelings in the therapist and client, some of them sexual. It is understood, however, that such feelings often emerge out of the symbolic and highly private nature of the process. While such feelings are important to explore and understand, it is considered inappropriate and exploitive for the therapist to act on them or to permit the client to act on them with the therapist (Lerman & Rigby, 1990). Many naive therapists may presume that if the client introduces such feelings into therapy or initiates a sexual relationship, that the therapist is absolved of any responsibility for exploiting the client. After all, they may ask, if the client is a consenting adult and wishes it, why is it harmful? Such thinking emphasizes the importance of the therapist's having adequately considered the symbolic relationship between the two, the possibility that the client's feelings are based on the symbolic and not realistic aspects of the therapist, and the unequal power differential in the therapy process itself that leaves the client more vulnerable.

The next question that arises is that of the appropriateness of sexual relationships after the therapy relationship has ceased. Brown (1988) speaks to this issue and elaborates on the problematic aspects of post termination sexual and romantic relationships between therapists and their former clients. In her analysis, the negative effects of such relationships do not affect the therapist and client alone but extend to other clients as well. The therapeutic alliance depends to a large degree on the client's ability to explore fantasies and feelings of all kinds, even if they are directed at the therapist, without needing to be concerned that the therapist is either listening vicariously or using the information to manipulate the client. Neither should the client protect the therapist from the client's feelings (Gabbard & Pope, 1989; Pope, 1991).

Perhaps of even greater import is the need for clients to feel assured that the therapist would never encourage or require them to act on feelings expressed for the therapist, no matter what the therapist's needs may be. Brown (1988) notes that when therapists engage in such behavior they abdicate their primary role, which is to focus on the client's needs. Because such relationships are deemed professionally inappropriate, they often take place in secrecy, putting the client in the position of having to protect the therapist from discovery, as well as depriving the client of a relationship that need not be conducted in secrecy. When these relationships are conducted openly, other clients are often aware of them, and it would be naive to think that their therapy remains unaffected. Further, clients who wish to have similar relationships with the therapist, but who are not "chosen" by the therapist, may experience this behavior as personally and profoundly rejecting. These same comments could be made about professor and supervisor relationships as well.

Although the propensity for negative effects in sexual relationships is usually clear, many therapists do not see how bartering, business, teacher–therapist, social, or other nonsexual dual relationships would be harmful to the client. One of the ways that nonsexual overlapping relationships have the potential for harm is in their tendency to erode the boundaries of therapy to the degree that they can make the relationship vulnerable to even more serious erosions. The most egregious violations of boundaries in therapy usually occur in the context of more "innocuous" violations. Sexual dual relationships often have their origins in seemingly harmless exchanges of favors or gifts, meetings or encounters between the therapist and client outside of the therapy, physical touching or contact during therapy, or the therapist's disclosures of her personal problems to the client. These behaviors can often facilitate, rather than mitigate against, a further erosion of boundaries in the relationship (Benowitz, 1994; Gartrell & Sanderson, 1994; Greene, 1994).

Even if the relationship may not be explicitly sexual at a given time, it may contain seductive elements that the therapist expresses or uses to manipulate the client rather than seek to understand her. Nonsexual dual/overlapping relationships do not invariably become sexual. However, many sexual dual relationships have had their origins in far less flagrant erosions of boundaries. The therapist must carefully scrutinize behavior or impulses to behave in ways that seek to minimize the maintenance of such boundaries. In addition to their propensity to create a climate in which the development of sexual dual relationships is facilitated, nonsexual dual relationships are often problematic in and of themselves. In examining such relationships, one ultimately discovers a confusion and erosion of clarity regarding expectations in the therapy. That sense of clarity and predictability is one of the crucial elements of the relationship, and its absence or erosion renders therapy less safe and often less helpful.

MANAGING OVERLAPPING/DUAL RELATIONSHIPS IN VARIOUS CONTEXTS

The Feminist Therapy Code of Ethics (Feminist Therapy Institute, 1987) recognize the unavoidable nature of overlapping relationships provide clear guidelines regarding their management (IIIA, B, C). For the feminist therapist, overlapping relationships can occur in various settings or communities, and the particular challenges of such relationships vary as a function of these settings or circumstances.

Smith (1990) has discussed the dilemma of overlapping relationships in the lesbian community. In her analysis, lesbian therapists must be cognizant of the fact that they are role models for members of the lesbian community. They must also be comfortable with the assumption that their lives are open to public discussion within that community. Because they will inevitably see clients at social events, they should plan for such encounters, whenever possible, by having discussions with their clients prior to such encounters. These discussions should include both the client's feelings about the potential meeting and the client's preferences about how to handle these situations (Subcommittees, Boundary Dilemmas Conference, 1987). Smith (1990, pp. 95–96) concludes, "We are the ones responsible for maintaining appropriate boundaries between ourselves and our clients and between our role as therapist and our other roles."

Overlapping relationships in rural communities also present special challenges, as discussed by Gates and Speare (1990). In their rural community they have been forced to develop clear guidelines about how to offer clinical services, taking their relationship with the prospective client and the availability of other comparable services into account. The fact that many people in rural communities are somewhat suspicious of counseling and psychotherapy requires that therapists be willing to provide information and informal consultation to members of the community. To do so they may have to become actual members of the community. Gates and Speare contend that rural practitioners must regularly seek appropriate consultation to remain alert to the potential for dual relationships.

Because feminist therapists are highly likely to be politically active, it is also highly likely that they will encounter overlaps between their professional and activist roles. Berman (1990) provides an elaboration of some of the challenges presented by overlapping relationships in the political community. For example, an overlapping political relationship often implies an actual or potential overlapping social relationship, and the therapist may have to consider whether or not it is appropriate to attend social gatherings that may include clients. The therapist must evaluate whether the contact outside the therapy setting will interfere with the therapeutic relationship. Berman (1990, p. 108) asks, "What effect on the therapeutic relationship would there be, for example, if they [client and therapist] were on different sides of an intense faction fight within an organization?" Berman (1990) contends that the therapist must be vigilant about the ways in which she may exert influence over her client and suggests that the client and therapist discuss how to define limits and establish parameters for their dual relationship.

Feminist therapists who are members of communities of color may experience divided loyalties or differing expectations when addressing dual relationships. For instance, what if the norms for interpersonal relating in the community of color are different from the guidelines offered by one's profession or its professional ethics? When such discrepancies arise how does the feminist therapist of color sort through the expectations so as to be loyal to and remain a part of her community and at the same time conduct herself in a professionally responsible manner?

Sears (1990) attends to the complexity and the difficulties of being an "only" one. As the only Native American, lesbian feminist therapist living in a three-state area, she is often singled out to provide information about Native American gays and lesbians or asked to serve on "political panels or task forces where an 'Indian' and a lesbian are needed" (Sears, 1990, pp. 102–103). Sears points out that as a member of a tribal community, one has expectations that are a function of her culture, as well as overt and covert expectations imposed from the dominant culture. Like most people of color, she also experiences "pressure to be a 'good' Native person" (p. 103). Sears stresses the inherent challenges of addressing dual or overlapping relationships when those relationships bridge different cultures or different expectations.

It is clear that feminist therapists often grapple with the issue of dual and overlapping relationships in the practice of psychotherapy. They may also, however, engage in other professional roles that raise similar challenges, for example, as academician, consultant, or administrator. Academicians must extend confidentiality to students outside of their educational institution, and feminist instructors may find themselves working with feminist students on activist projects within as well as outside of the educational setting. Students in clinical training programs may be supervised by feminist instructors in a relationship that is certainly characterized by a power differential. A consultant may find herself offering recommendations to a feminist organization in which one of the board members is a colleague with whom she is coauthoring an article. Feminist administrators may be required to supervise and evaluate employees who view them as colleagues or friends in other settings. These other feminist professionals must also carefully consider the potential for actual or perceived exploitation in their professional relationships and the means to minimize it.

As the Preamble of the Feminist Therapy Code of Ethics (Feminist Therapy Institute, 1987) indicates, the well-being of clients is the guiding principle underlying the Code. That well-being should be the foremost consideration in decision making when therapists are confronted with dual/overlapping relationships or the potential for them. The dilemmas that follow demonstrate some of the challenges presented by dual and overlapping relationships in therapy and training. The respondents discuss the ethical dilemmas and ways to sort out the questions presented by these cases.

DILEMMA A

June, a therapist, has been seeing Elsie as a client for approximately eight months. June has a live-in partner named Dan, with whom she has been living for two years. They at one point had discussed marriage. However, they both decided marriage was not a viable option for either of them for some time. At a local environmental organization meeting, Dan and Elsie met and began seeing each other. Neither told June about their relationship. Eventually Dan and Elsie became sexually involved and decided they needed to tell June about their relationship. Dan did so at dinner with June in their apartment. June will be seeing Elsie for her regular therapy appointment the next day.

RESPONDENT 1

The case of June, Dan, and Elsie presents a situation in which several ethical issues emerge. One is clearly the mandate that the therapist evaluate ongoing interactions with clients for evidence of therapeutic biases (IC). Certainly the significant change in the relationship between Dan and June (resulting from Dan's recent involvement with Elsie) will impact June's ability to be an unbiased listener for Elsie and to be able to maintain therapeutic neutrality. June also needs to be aware of her bias.

Thus June should not continue to work with Elsie. This action needs to be communicated in a way that facilitates the therapeutic process (IIB) rather than serving as an evaluation of Elsie's behavior. June needs to let Elsie know that her feelings related to the situation are going to interfere with her ability to work with Elsie and that ethically it is not appropriate to continue to work with a client when the therapist's feelings are likely to interfere with the client's needs. It is also important that June not abandon Elsie as a client and see to it that she is provided with a list of other therapists who could work with her.

A third issue is the need for June to take care of herself. A therapist must recognize her personal and professional needs, utilizing a variety of methods to maintain and improve her work with clients, her competency, and her emotional well-being. The abandonment by Dan is likely to have a significant emotional impact on June, and she will need to take whatever action she needs to help herself through the healing process. (Kathleen A. Mack)

RESPONDENT 2

At this point the therapist has not engaged in any unethical behavior. However, the agenda at the next appointment with Elsie should have as its focus the disclosure of the change in the nature of their relationship and the necessity for termination. To continue as Elsie's therapist and to be a part of the triangle with Elsie and Dan is to sustain a dual relationship with her client in which there is a clear conflict of interest (III). June's ability to be objective has been compromised. A therapist is supposed to recognize her own vulnerabilities and make every effort to take care of her personal needs outside of the therapeutic relationship. Despite June's probable distress, she cannot abandon the client. Her final obligation to her client would be to provide her with referrals to another therapist. (Janet Brice-Baker)

DILEMMA B

Dr. Quimby is a well-respected and charismatic faculty member at a major university. When Dr. Quimby is research advisor for a doctoral student, he prefers to get to know the student informally. Although Dr. Quimby has never become sexually involved with a student, the majority of his female students have become enamored with him. In fact, most of his female students take a year or more longer than his male students to complete their dissertations. Dr. Grant, a colleague of Dr. Quimby's, has expressed her concerns about his behavior to Dr. Quimby and to other members of the faculty. Dr. Grant is one of two female faculty members in the department; her concerns about Dr. Quimby have been minimized by the rest of the faculty, and she has been called "jealous" of Dr. Quimby. A female doctoral student of Dr. Grant's has similar concerns about Dr. Quimby after taking two courses with him. She asks Dr. Grant for advice on how to proceed with a complaint. Because of her experiences with other faculty members, Dr. Grant discourages the student from taking any action against Dr. Quimby.

RESPONDENT 1

Central to this discussion is the issue of power. There are two ways in which the impact of power differentials are evident in this case—Dr. Quimby's desire to get to know his students, and Dr. Grant's retreat from an opportunity to use her power to help a student.

Dr. Quimby risks abuse of power in his practice of getting to know students informally. Such meetings may set the stage for mixed messages and abuse of power by virtue of unclear and potentially vacillating boundaries. Feminist therapists and faculty should acknowledge the inherent power differential between therapist and client and teacher and student and model the effective use of personal power (IIA).

Dr. Grant's behavior offers a second example of the impact of a power differential. She is retreating from an opportunity to use her greater power as a faculty member to assist a student to assert herself within the academic institution and to model effective use of personal power. If Dr. Grant's student continues her professional career, these battles regarding power abuse will, in all likelihood, be part of her professional life. Shrinking from support of the student's request because of a failure of a previous attempt to raise Dr. Quimby's consciousness represents a form of neglect as an advisor to a student.

Associated with the responsibility to attend to power differentials is the responsibility of feminist therapists to actively question the practices in their communities that appear abusive and, when possible, to intervene or assist clients to intervene (VA). The same principle applies to academe. The wheels of change are often incredibly slow within institutions, but time and again the gradual building of a body of evidence regarding the need for action proves helpful. Dr. Grant's support of her student's wish to take action by instructing her as to the proper procedures could contribute to greater awareness on the part of the department. Multiple complaints may contribute to a developing awareness and some action regarding the need for Dr. Quimby to examine the impact of his relationships with students.

A third ethical issue in this case stems from the fact that many of Dr. Quimby's female students become enamored with him. This state of affairs suggests one of the consequences of his informal boundaries. Although the reasons that female students take longer to finish their work are not specified (it could be in part that many women students do not have spouses who support them as they go to graduate school), there is the inference that these somehow result from the relationship that Dr. Quimby develops with his female students. The fact that they become enamored with him suggests the possibility of covert and possibly overt sexual behavior. Whose needs are met and whose ego is stroked at the expense of another's success? As clearly indicated in the Code (IIIC), feminist therapists should be aware of the impact of such behaviors and should not engage in them. This by far is one of the more dangerous issues to bring up with colleagues, but it may be among those hidden examples of behavior that is experienced as unwelcome and harassing. Raising this issue may be instructive for Dr. Quimby, as men often claim that they were not aware that their behavior was having an adverse impact on the women around them. (Kathleen A. Mack)

RESPONDENT 2

Although the Feminist Therapy Code of Ethics says little that specifically addresses educators, it is clear that the duty of a feminist psychologist in any setting is to act in the best interest of those she serves, in
this case, her students (Preamble). It is also her obligation to "assume a
proactive stance toward the eradication of oppression" and to "work
toward empowering women" (Preamble).

This particular situation is a difficult one because Dr. Grant is
herself a victim of the sexist tactics with which her student is struggling
in the department. In order to fulfill her ethical obligation to her
student, she must not only take steps to overcome her own isolation and
feelings of powerlessness, but she must also be careful in handling the
dual relationship she now has with her student, that is, as covictim.
While it is important that she offer her student some resources and
support in addressing the behavior of Dr. Quimby, it is also important
that she simultaneously protect and preserve her educational relationship with her student. She could begin by consulting with profeminist
faculty in other departments or outside the university and with experts
in sexual harassment and by sharing these resources with her student.
In view of her own experiences of marginalization within the department, she should try to get outside support for herself and also encourage
the student to work closely with someone else outside the department
on this issue. Doing so will accomplish two things: first, it may keep Dr.
Grant and her student from being further victimized by being stigma-
tized in the department because of her collaboration on a politically
sensitive project, and it will allow Dr. Grant to continue to function in
her primary role as doctoral advisor to her student.

If the situation evolves such that Dr. Grant and her student need
to cooperate more extensively on this issue, Dr. Grant will need to talk
with her about how their academic relationship will be impacted and
what steps can be taken to keep that relationship distinct from their
activism. If at some point the Dr. Quimby issue begins to overshadow
their academic relationship, Dr. Grant will need to evaluate whether
her usefulness to her student has been compromised and assess with the
student the advisability of her transferring to another academic advisor
(IIIA). The feminist practitioner recognizes the "conflicting priorities
inherent in overlapping relationships" and "monitors such relationships
to prevent potential abuse or harm to the client" (IIIA). (Mary Hayden)

DILEMMA C

*Celia, a Hispanic therapist who works in a hospital, has been seeing Margue-
rite, a Hispanic adolescent, in both individual and family therapy. After a*

six-month stay in the hospital, Marguerite is discharged and referred to Gail, an Anglo therapist, for outpatient therapy. Marguerite's mother is extraordinarily grateful to Celia for "saving" the adolescent and the family. Gail learns through Marguerite that Celia is now employing Marguerite's mother on a weekly basis for house-cleaning services.

RESPONDENT 1

There are three ethical issues raised by this example: (1) employment of a former client by Celia; (2) respect for client Marguerite's confidentiality; and (3) the relationship between ethical and cultural considerations. Any intervention on Gail's part should be driven by the advisability of actively questioning another therapist's therapeutic practices and intervening when appropriate (VA).

Celia is jeopardizing a therapeutic relationship with her former client by employing her as a house cleaner (IIIA). Because of the power differential between client and therapist, the onus of responsibility is always on the therapist to ensure that the present or former client can relate as freely as possible to the therapist, unfettered by overlapping relationships in which the client may feel threatened in terms of self-expression, confidentiality, and so forth. Employing a former client does not allow for that freedom.

The second issue is one of respecting Marguerite's confidentiality. Why did Marguerite tell Gail about Celia employing her mother? It may or may not bother her. But if Gail is to go to Celia and discuss this issue, she must ensure that Marguerite endorses such action. It is important to consider the relative importance of two key issues involved here: the desirability of addressing the ethical issue and the importance of protecting Marguerite's confidentiality. Gail should not simply address the ethical issue at the expense of Marguerite's confidentiality or her (Marguerite's) own power (IIA). In addition, Gail could (depending on Marguerite's feelings about the relationship between Celia and her mother) educate Marguerite about her rights as a former client of Celia and about how to resolve differences and/or file a grievance (IID).

Having said all of the above, it should be recognized that these comments come from a white, ethnocentric viewpoint that considers the actions of Celia as problematic. Some discussion needs to take place between Gail and Marguerite about Gail's values regarding therapists employing present or former clients (I). A similar discussion needs to take place between Gail and Celia. It is possible that the arrangement between Celia and Marguerite's mother is acceptable within their cultural context (IB). Nonetheless, it is imperative that Gail explore this issue and its consequences for the therapeutic relationship. (Nikki Gerrard)

RESPONDENT 2

This case illustrates some of the complex cultural dynamics that can have an impact on the therapeutic relationship. From a pragmatic perspective, Celia has engaged her former client's mother, in a service for pay, which not only has the appearance of a violation of professional boundaries (maintaining in another context a client–provider relationship that has formally been terminated), but which also may be unduly advantageous to the former therapist.

From a cultural perspective, the overlapping relationship between Celia and her client may be attributable to a number of factors. Depending on the size of the Hispanic community in this case, it may not be unusual for Hispanic therapists and clients to have external and continuing contact after termination of the professional relationship. In addition, the norms of Hispanic/Latino and other cultural groups are not always bound by the same views of the patient–provider relationship as those historically defined by the European–American dominated mental health system (IB). Especially given the traditional scarcity of Hispanic mental health professionals, a competent provider who is perceived as helping a Hispanic family might be expected to be held in some regard not only by the client, but by other ethnic community members. Such regard for the *context* in which the relationship was established—a positive helping one—might influence the provider's perspective on the advisability of maintaining a connection after the formal mental health relationship was terminated.

Any intervention by Gail, the outpatient therapist, could take a number of forms. Depending on the strength of her relationship with Marguerite, she might further explore the extent and scope of the mother's continued connection with Celia, including Marguerite's feelings about their relationship (VA, IIA). Does Marguerite also have contact with Celia, either informally (in the "community") or formally? Is any such involvement independent of her mother or dependent upon her mother's employment connection with Celia? Is there any significant negative impact upon Marguerite's mental health caused by her mother's connection to Celia? After assessing the influence, if any, of her mother's relationship with Celia, Gail might adjust their therapeutic contract accordingly. In addition, such an assessment would help determine whether or not Gail should actively pursue any further direct action with Celia regarding their overlapping relationship (VA). (Valli Kanuha)

DILEMMA D

Betty has been in therapy with Elaine, a heterosexual feminist therapist, for over a year. Betty has wanted to come out as a lesbian and has several issues

*around the process that Elaine was concerned she would not be competent to
facilitate effectively. As a result, Elaine referred Betty to Marilyn, a lesbian
therapist. Elaine later learned from Betty that Marilyn and Betty had become
romantically involved. When Elaine confronted Marilyn about possible ethical
violations, Marilyn maintained she had not formed a therapeutic relationship
with Betty but instead had provided consultation services only. In addition,
Marilyn had returned the consultation fee to Betty and insisted there had been
no ethical violations.*

RESPONDENT 1

It seems likely that Marilyn has committed an ethical violation (IIIC)
and that Elaine was acting appropriately in confronting her (VA). In
terms of preventative ethics, what were Elaine's alternatives? She might
have indicated to Betty her perceived inability to handle issues of
"coming out" adequately (IVA) and have encouraged Betty to move
toward terminating their relationship and finding a lesbian feminist
therapist (IA).

Alternately, Elaine might have sought consultation herself with a
feminist lesbian therapist and thereby educated herself further on issues
(presumably) outside her competence (IVB). Minimally, Elaine could
have established a clear contract with both Betty and Marilyn as to the
nature of work those two would do together and its relationship to any
ongoing therapy with Elaine.

It is extraordinarily difficult for a homophobia-conscious heterosexual feminist therapist to find an ethical path through the often
thorny process of a client wanting to "come out as a lesbian." The report
does not say to what extent Elaine and Betty had together explored the
meanings for Betty of "coming out." It might have been very important,
if termination were under consideration, for Elaine to give referrals to
more than one lesbian therapist for Betty to interview and then make
her own decision (IA). If only one lesbian therapist is available or if the
original therapeutic alliance is to be retained, then it would seem
especially important that boundaries be clarified in advance, along with
details about how much information would be shared, by whom, and
when (IIIA). (Jeanne Adleman)

RESPONDENT 2

The Feminist Therapy Code of Ethics specifies principles that are clearly
violated by Marilyn. Less clear are any ethical transgressions on the part
of Elaine, although her ethical predicament is clearly evident.

Sexual involvement with a client clearly has potential to harm, and
the code prohibits sexual intimacy with clients (IIIC). Whether acting

primarily as a consultant or a therapist, Marilyn does indeed accept Betty as a client, and her romantic involvement is therefore unethical. Returning fees to the client after the fact does not retroactively cancel the existence of this professional relationship, as Marilyn would like to believe. Further, the action of returning fees suggests that Marilyn is aware of the inappropriateness of her relationship with Betty and attempts to reframe it instead of seeking peer consultation to sort out her ethical dilemma (IVB).

Both therapists contributed to the potential for client injury by not more clearly defining the nature of the referral and the appropriate reporting/collaboration procedures. These specifics lay the groundwork that facilitates ethical decision making. Reporting/collaboration might have resulted in earlier identification of the romantic relationship and limited the potential for harm to Betty.

Elaine recognizes the need to restrict her therapy to her areas of competency and arranges a referral to Marilyn (IVA). This referral was motivated by Elaine's acknowledgement of and respect for the cultural differences that exist as a function of sexual orientation (IB). Once Elaine became aware of the inappropriate therapeutic practices of Marilyn, she was ethically bound to intervene (VA), which she accomplished by confronting Marilyn. Since Marilyn denied any wrongdoing, Elaine must decide whether to pursue the issue further by educating the client of her rights and grievance procedures (IID) and/or by reporting the ethical infraction to a professional association.

In summary, it appears that Marilyn clearly violates several ethical principles. Elaine generally abides by the Feminist Therapy Code of Ethics but could have improved her management of the referral process to further safeguard the rights of her client. (Dorothy Holden)

DILEMMA E

Rachel is a lesbian therapist who has been working with Angie, a lesbian client, for four years. Both Rachel and Angie have five-year-old sons. Coincidentally, over the summer, Angie has moved into the same school catchment area as Rachel. Unknown to Rachel or Angie, their sons have been enrolled in the same class at school. Rachel and Angie end up running into each other at the second parent meeting of the year and also learn they are now attending the same church.

RESPONDENT 1

This report indicates a solidly-established therapeutic relationship with no apparent ethical irregularities so far; however, this situation now holds many potential dilemmas for the therapist. Resolution will depend in part on how well the two women have previously negotiated and "contracted" with each other about possible encounters (IIC) in what is usually referred to as "the lesbian community" (which is typically not a singular community).

The apparent coincidence of Angie having moved into the same school catchment area as Rachel would need to be a topic of exploration in therapy (IIIA). Had Angie never discussed that she might be moving, and where she might move? Had therapist and client ever negotiated the risks and possible benefits of encountering each other unexpectedly *or* predictably (IIC)?

How does the present situation reflect the initial circumstances of their entering a therapy agreement? Four years ago, each would (presumably) have been a lesbian with (again presumably) a one-year-old son. Was this a factor for Angie in deciding she wanted Rachel for a therapist, or for Rachel in deciding to accept Angie as a client? It is often the case that people seeking therapy look for a therapist as much like themselves as possible; sometimes it works well, and sometimes it impedes the client's need for differentiation and eventual separation from the therapist.

After four years, was Angie's move a conscious or unconscious indication of her readiness to bring an end to her therapy with Rachel? It is not, after all, unlikely that at some point in those four years Angie might have learned something about where Rachel lived. If the issues that initially led Angie to seek therapy have by now been relatively well resolved, this apparent coincidence might be a good time for the two women to work toward closure of the therapy relationship.

A therapist takes risks in being present at events where current or past clients are likely to appear (IIIB). She may feel confined by or constrained within her professional role, but surely it is not entirely negative if clients see her as a real human being who holds more than her current or past symbolic meaning for them.

A client also takes risks, especially if encounters are unexpected or if her rights to privacy have not previously been discussed. She is subject to embarrassment, may feel "found out" (justifiably or not), and may not know whether to acknowledge any connection. The benefit to the client is that her therapist has an opportunity to see her in the larger world among others with whom she variously interacts, thus enriching the therapist's total picture of the client. (Jeanne Adleman)

RESPONDENT 2

In this situation therapist Rachel must resolve potential conflicts between her duty to promote the well-being of her client Angie (Preamble) and her duty to provide herself with good self-care (IVD) in the context of multiple overlaps with the client. In this case there are so many role conflicts and so much potential for extratherapeutic exposure to one another that Rachel must consider with Angie whether continuing their therapy will be beneficial or whether termination and referral to another therapist would be preferable.

In making this decision, they should consider the amount of unavoidable exposure to each other's private lives and the extent to which such exposure will be manageable for each of them. Rachel will need to identify any feelings of resentment she may have about Angie's presence in what was formerly her own "territory." If there are activities or groups at school or church that she wishes not to share with Angie, she should let Angie know about these, thus helping her to avoid acting out any hostile feelings toward Angie. As Angie identifies her interests in each setting, further discussions will be needed about which events will be exclusively for one or the other and which can be comfortably shared by both. By being careful about respecting her own need for private space, Rachel is being accountable (IVA) for her own self-care and respecting Angie's needs as well.

Rachel should talk with Angie about how they will respond when they run into each other at school or church, letting Angie know that she will do her utmost to maintain her confidentiality (IIIB). She will need to find out whether Angie wants to introduce her to her family and/or friends and, if so, whether she will be identified as Angie's therapist. Here Rachel must clarify her own feelings about the extent to which she is comfortable meeting members of Angie's social network. Because their sons may also develop some kind of relationship, Rachel must be alert to feelings of envy or competition that could arise in either of them, since they will be relating as mothers as well as client and therapist. If, in assessing all these dimensions, Rachel and Angie decide to continue their therapeutic relationship, they will need to engage in an ongoing process of working through the information Angie will no doubt be exposed to about Rachel's personal life. Because of the many conflicts that Rachel is likely to experience as she attempts to remain clear about her own self-care needs, the needs of her son, and her concern to foster Angie's welfare in treatment, it would be wise for her to engage in ongoing consultation as treatment proceeds (IVB). (Mary Hayden)

DILEMMA F

Audrey has been in therapy with Carolyn for five months. Audrey has a history of extreme physical abuse, with her early years spent in several foster homes, and she has been addressing these issues in therapy. She is presently trying to reconcile with her mother, who had been extremely abusive to Audrey during her childhood. Audrey, who is a social worker by profession, serves on the board of the local battered women's shelter. Carolyn, not knowing Audrey was on the board, arranged with the shelter to organize and run a fund-raising garage sale at her home. Audrey later informs Carolyn that she will be at her home to help with the sale.

RESPONDENT 1

There is no ethical issue in this example, save for the fact that Carolyn should ensure Audrey that she will respect confidentiality and not say or do anything that would reveal their therapeutic relationship (IIIB). In this section's overview, the authors refer to the issue of overlapping relationships in the context of social activism. As Berman (1990) is quoted as suggesting, Audrey and Carolyn should engage in a discussion about defining limits and establishing parameters for their dual relationship in the context of their mutual activism. (Nikki Gerrard)

RESPONDENT 2

This is, unfortunately, not an uncommon situation for feminist therapists or other health providers who work in a small or closely-knit geographic, political, or social network. It is typically the therapist's responsibility to anticipate the potential for any situations that may involve overlapping relationships with clients (IIIA). In anticipating such potential conflicts, the therapist may want to discuss even the possibility of overlapping social or political contexts with her client at the earliest appropriate time in therapy (IIC). For example, were there any indications of possible overlap for Carolyn and Audrey? They are both mental health providers, and both are obviously experienced and interested in domestic violence issues. It is possible that there might have been an earlier opportunity to discuss the impact of some of their shared political and social values on the therapeutic relationship.

However, lacking that opportunity, there are a number of alternatives each could consider. Based on the case description, it appears that Audrey was aware of Carolyn's involvement before Carolyn was of Audrey's. For Audrey to "inform" Carolyn that she would be at her home appears to be her attempt to push the boundaries of the therapeutic alliance, perhaps towards more intimacy. First and most importantly, Carolyn should decide whether or not to pursue the process of Audrey's "informing" her of the situation, or the content of the dilemma, or both. In this case, it appears that Audrey's possible transference issues dictate a careful balance to reassure her of the solid and appropriate boundaries necessary for integrity of the therapeutic relationship, while also emphasizing the insecurity, fears, and other possible feelings of rejection that Audrey might experience as a result of merely discussing such an awkward situation.

In any case, Carolyn should consider the therapeutic context of her relationship with Audrey to determine the range of possible options she might consider and/or discuss with Audrey. Depending on the nature, timing, and history of Audrey and Carolyn's therapy relationship, Carolyn might opt to take the position of recommending a particular option. Or, she may prioritize a number of options and present them to Audrey for the two to discuss and mutually agree upon. It appears that a final decision would be primarily and foremost dependent on the meaning of the social interaction for Audrey (IIA). Finally, factors such as the extent or kind of interaction both would have at the event, the feasibility of Carolyn's "graciously" postponing or canceling the event, and perhaps whether or not Carolyn's practice was in her home (which might affect the nature of the boundaries regarding Carolyn's personal vs. professional space) are all additional aspects to be considered in resolving this situation. (Valli Kanuha)

DILEMMA G

Mrs. Alexander is a 50-year-old African-American woman. She is divorced with three minor children. The divorce was a very acrimonious one and left Mrs. Alexander in severe financial straits. She was referred to a community mental health center by her internist. He was treating her for insomnia, loss of appetite with a weight loss of 30 pounds, decreased concentration, frequent crying spells, anhedonia, withdrawal, headaches, and various stomach complaints. A thorough gastrointestinal series revealed negative results, and her internist concluded that her symptoms were probably related to depression.

When Mrs. Alexander began treatment with Dr. Hope Chester, a clinical psychologist, they both agreed that therapy should focus on (1) allowing her to grieve the loss of her husband and the breakup of her marriage, (2) helping her adjust to the demands of being a single parent, (3) helping her to return to the work force, and finally, (4) eliminating the vegetative symptoms mentioned above. Part of the treatment plan involved sending Mrs. Alexander to a psychiatrist for a medication evaluation.

After approximately two months in treatment, Mrs. Alexander reported that she was sleeping a little better and her appetite had returned. As the debilitating physical symptoms dissipated, she was able to put more energy into raising her children and looking for a job. In the meantime, a friend of hers, who was a Mary Kay Cosmetics consultant, suggested that Mrs. Alexander get involved in the business as a way to earn extra money. Lacking self-con-

fidence, Mrs. Alexander was hesitant to do the makeup demonstrations required of a consultant. During one therapy session she brought the demonstration kit with her and spoke about some of her concerns. In an attempt to encourage Mrs. Alexander, Dr. Chester paid for her to do a skin consultation and purchased several of the cosmetics. Dr. Chester believed that by doing so she was encouraging Mrs. Alexander's vocational development.

RESPONDENT 1

The therapist in this scenario is clearly behaving in an unethical manner. The therapist's willingness to become a customer of her client is in direct violation of the standards of both the Feminist Therapy Institute (III) and the American Psychological Association (1992, APA 1.17). Both principles prohibit therapists from knowingly forming another relationship with the client, be it business or professional. In this case the purchase of cosmetics from the client creates a business relationship that may automatically alter the nature of the therapeutic relationship. What if the therapist were dissatisfied with the client's performance? How would she seek redress and how could any further action not adversely affect the therapy relationship? Even though the client may indeed benefit from the encouragement of her vocational goals, the therapist need not be her first customer to encourage her. It may have been more helpful to the client to encourage her in other ways. The therapist may have done well to scrutinize more closely her own need to be the client's first customer. (Janet Brice-Baker)

RESPONDENT 2

Dr. Chester's attempt to bolster her client's confidence was certainly well intentioned. It does, however, raise questions regarding conformity to these codes (American Psychological Association, 1992; Feminist Therapy Institute, 1987). Dr. Chester should have negotiated and renegotiated formal and/or informal contacts more carefully with her client (III). The underlying issue appears to be an impulsive gesture that was not thoroughly considered in terms of its therapeutic consequences and was not explicitly discussed by client and therapist. Dr. Chester would have done better to consider the source of the offer in terms of how she views the client, what the client elicits, and what the client would conclude from the exchange. Whenever clinicians act impulsively, the possibility exists that there is a tension in the relationship that requires discussion rather than action. Is the behavior standard practice with all or many clients, and if not, why is it occurring at the present time with this client? In addition therapists need to consider alternatives that might have better long-term clinical outcomes. By acting impulsively on such inclinations, therapists often rule out more effective alternatives.

Mrs. Alexander, for example, might appreciate the offer and find it helpful, a vote of confidence clearly meant to empower the client and to avoid rigidity in therapeutic roles. However, she may have felt patronized or indulged, anxious and on trial, or as if she were perceived as someone who needed extra caretaking who could not be encouraged to go out and practice the demonstration with friends or even a potential client. The gesture could be perceived in ways that undermine her confidence. This is yet another reason to gather information about what this action might mean to the client before acting on impulse.

This gesture could compromise the therapeutic relationship because it places the client and therapist in dual roles as customer and client. It also involved physical contact which might prove to be uncomfortable for either or both parties involved. Dr. Chester might have been left feeling uncomfortable or dissatisfied with the demonstration or the products. She may have felt subsequently trapped in terms of what she could say authentically to her client. Hence, the usefulness of what amounts to a role reversal should have been considered. The client might also not find this a realistic practice, given that she might interpret any positive feedback from her therapist as less than credible.

If this were behavior therapy where "coaching" or in vitro techniques were standard, it would be more clearly defensible. Since the vignette does not suggest that this is the case, a more appropriate intervention probably would have been to encourage the client to practice with friends and to work with her reluctance to take that step. Ultimately, that might have been less ambiguous, more empowering, and expressed more confidence in the client's ability to go out into the world and pursue this new vocation. (Sheila Bob)

DILEMMA H

Dr. Louise Zane is a first-year assistant professor in a counseling program at a state university. At the end of the first semester of the academic year, one of the other professors becomes seriously ill and must take a leave for the second semester. Dr. Marilyn Dixie, the department chair, asks Dr. Zane to teach the group counseling class and supervise doctoral students who lead the group counseling practicum. Dr. Dixie realizes group counseling is not Dr. Zane's specialty but explains that everyone must pull together in this time of crisis, and other faculty members are temporarily adding to their work loads. Dr. Zane reluctantly agrees to take on the added responsibilities. During her preparations, Dr. Zane discovers that all students are not only required to take the group counseling class but must also participate in group counseling sessions throughout the semester. Students are assigned to groups that are facilitated by doctoral students whom the group counseling instructor supervises. Students receive a letter grade (A–F) for the class, but the group counseling sessions are graded Pass/Fail. Dr. Zane is extremely concerned about the dual relationships involved in the situation and the potential for abuse of those relationships. She discusses her ethical concerns with Dr. Dixie. Dr. Dixie not only discounts the concerns about dual relationships but emphasizes how much better the situation is than a decade earlier when the group counseling class and sessions were combined, letter grades were given, and one professor taught everything. Dr. Dixie says any changes would have to go through the department and university curriculum committees and be put into the university catalog, a process that would take two to three years.

RESPONDENT 1

Dr. Zane is in a difficult and complex situation. She has been asked, for expediency, to fill a university teaching position whose course content is not in her area of specialty. The central problem in this scenario is each person involved in this class will have overlapping relationships (III) and power differentials (II). Students in the class will be both clients and students; the PhD students will be therapists, instructors, evaluators, and students; Dr. Zane will be an instructor, supervisor, and evaluator, and as a first-year assistant professor will be under pressure to comply with Dr. Dixie's direction. The question of whether personal material revealed in the group therapy sessions might impact an evaluation of a student is an issue. Having students participate in group therapy is beneficial, as they can experience what it is like to participate in a therapy group. The experience is important in their training to be therapists and allows Dr. Zane to monitor issues that may impact students' abilities to be therapists.

However, feminist ethics make it clear that a therapist's responsibility is to protect the rights and interests of the client (IIIA, B). Dr. Zane should also take responsibility to acknowledge the inherent power differentials (IIA) and to inform the students of their rights (IID). She would be required to discuss the implications of the dual relationships (IIIA, B) and to monitor the situation to see that there are no abuses.

Dr. Zane's reluctance to teach the class demonstrates her awareness of the principle of therapist accountability (IV). An ethical instructor is committed to working only within the realm of her competencies (IVA). Dr. Zane's training as a counselor qualifies her to some extent to teach this course, but does she have sufficient skill and understanding in relation to the issues of group therapy? Are her own counseling skills and knowledge adequate to supervise the PhD students doing group counseling?

Dr. Zane has several courses of action. She could decline the assignment, but by doing so, she may risk her own position. She could accept the assignment, trusting her own competence to read and become sufficiently informed to do an adequate job (IVB). She could seek supervision and direction from a colleague trained in group counseling. She could discuss the situation with both the PhD students and the group counseling class to see how they all can contribute to ensuring the class is managed responsibly so that the implications and consequences are known and potential problems anticipated. There is also a need for modeling and monitoring feminist ethics in the areas of theory development, research, and professional training.

Dr. Zane has an opportunity to participate in changes that would improve awareness of ethical issues (V). She could take action to articulate the issues (VA) and begin meetings with people to develop an ethical system of teaching this class (VB). Although her actions may not change the situation for the current class, it is worthwhile to start the process so that future students will be assured of ethical treatment. (Margaret McLeod)

RESPONDENT 2

The well-being of Dr. Zane's students is the guiding principle underlying this application of the ethics to the educational setting. The most problematic aspect of Dr. Zane's situation centers on the overlapping relationships (III) created by the department's historic approach to the group counseling class and practicum. The requirement that students take the group counseling class and participate in a group counseling experience facilitated by fellow students and supervised by the instructor creates a multilevel set of dual relationships. Dr. Zane is placed in the awkward and unethical situation of evaluating students about whom she likely has gained personal information through her supervision of the doctoral student therapists. By serving as clients in the practicum for doctoral student therapists, students in the group counseling class are being asked to compromise their right to privacy within the student group. The doctoral student therapists may find themselves conducting therapy with social acquaintances or friends.

At the departmental level, students' lower position of power in the organization is being exploited, without their informed consent, in order to provide practicum experiences for doctoral student therapists. The overlapping relationships within this group counseling training model clearly set the stage for abuses of power. By raising concerns about these multiple dual-role issues with Dr. Dixie, Dr. Zane demonstrates sensitivity to student confidentiality (IIIB) and willingness to take action (IIIA).

In addition to issues of student well-being, Dr. Zane's situation highlights challenges to her own well-being as an educator. Being asked by her chairperson to teach a course out of her area of specialization without adequate preparation, retraining time, or clear provisions for mentoring and/or supervision raises the issue of exploitation. There is an inherent power differential (IIA) between Dr. Dixie, the chairperson, and Dr. Zane, the young assistant professor, such that Dr. Zane may not feel she has the power to refuse Dr. Dixie's request. To further complicate the situation and jeopardize Dr. Zane's practice as an ethical educator, her agreement to teach the course violates the accountability guidelines to acknowledge the limits of her competencies (IVC) and work only with those issues within the realm of her competencies (IVA).

To Dr. Zane's credit, however, is her attempt to seek consultation (IVB) from her chairperson to resolve the multiple dual relationships created by her department's approach to group counseling training. Since it appears that Dr. Dixie may be contributing to the maintenance of a system of abusive educational practices, it would be wise for Dr. Zane to seek additional consultation from other senior, preferably feminist, members of her own or another faculty who might be able to offer additional direction for facilitating change within the department. It might be possible for her to identify practicum clients through a departmental clinic, the university counseling center, or community agencies. Such a change in practicum participants would eliminate many of the overlapping relationships present in her current departmental situation.

Dr. Zane's actions are also very much in concert with the social change principle to actively question practices in her community that appear to be abusive (VA). She models the "effective use of personal power" (IIA) by beginning the process of questioning the departmental status quo in this area of training. (Michele C. Boyer)

DILEMMA I

Joan has been a client of Helen's for three weeks. She came to see Helen because she has been depressed and because her marriage has been "falling apart." She says her husband has been very critical of her housekeeping and says she isn't taking proper care of the children. He refuses to have sex with her, which hurts Joan deeply. Joan thinks if her husband would stop blaming her, things would be a lot better between them. Joan seems to be avoiding having her husband come in so they can work on the marriage. Joan denies any history of previous emotional or substance abuse other than her use of cigarettes and coffee. One of Joan's friends called Helen and blurted out that Joan is a "hopeless" alcoholic who is ruining her own life and that of her family.

Helen makes it a policy not to talk to friends and family of her clients but, in this instance, she was unable to stop Joan's friend before she got her message out.

RESPONDENT 1

The primary ethical dilemma involved in this case centers on the unsolicited information that Helen has received from Joan's friend. The information about Joan's alleged abuse of alcohol is crucial in correctly evaluating and dealing with Joan's depression and marital problems. Two dimensions of this dilemma must be considered. First, because the therapeutic relationship is in its early stages, primary goals are defining the basic issues to be worked on and establishing trust and rapport in the relationship. Since Joan has denied abusing alcohol, Helen must find an assertive way to reveal the "new" and conflicting information in a manner that supports, rather than undermines, Joan's sense of well-being, as well as the developing relationship (IIA, B). If alcohol abuse is substantiated, it provides one explanation for the presenting depression and marital stress. If Helen does not feel competent to deal with the alcohol abuse issues, she should assist Joan in finding a substance abuse therapist and other appropriate services, such as support groups, in the community (IVA, IA).

The second dimension of the ethical dilemma concerns the confidentiality issue. Even though Helen has a policy not to talk to friends or family of her clients (IIIB), she did not have the opportunity to end the phone call before receiving potentially important information about Joan. Helen is ethically bound to protect the confidentiality of her relationship with Joan but has no ethical obligation to protect the friend and thus should inform Joan about the phone call and the information she received. This provision of information models honest and assertive communication, respect for Joan as an individual and creates an opportunity for Joan to feel an alliance with Helen (IIA). Because of the complex nature of this ethical dilemma, Helen may want to discuss this matter in professional supervision (IVB). (D. Brooks Cowan and Cheryl L. Haller)

RESPONDENT 2

The most significant ethical dilemma confronting the therapist is what to do *with* and *about* the phone call from the client's friend. The issues concern the matter of overlapping relationships (III).

Helen, the therapist, seems sensitive to the problem of overlapping relationships and has established boundaries for herself: for example, she has a policy of not talking to family and friends of clients. In spite of her best intentions, she is now confronted with a problem, not an uncommon dilemma, especially for therapists who find themselves working (and often simultaneously living) in smaller communities.

The first issue that Helen must address is confidentiality (IIIB). Even if Joan has told this friend that she was seeing Helen, it is the therapist's responsibility to ensure that both the fact and process of her client's therapy are kept confidential, unless the client gives her informed consent for release of information. Helen must make clear to Joan's friend that she is not at liberty to discuss this matter.

The second issue concerns what to do with the information that has already been received (IIIA). It is the therapist's responsibility to model both clear, direct, and open communication as well as appropriate boundaries and limits. But the issue is complicated. If Joan's friend called Helen about an unrelated matter and inadvertently or spontaneously let this information slip, Helen may feel comfortable ignoring the information as gossip until such time as Joan is ready to address it (IIA), allowing Joan to determine the course of her therapy. The situation is somewhat different if the friend called Helen specifically to discuss Joan. If Helen does not acknowledge the information she has been given and does nothing, she may well feel triangulated, or feel as if she, too, has been coopted into an unhealthy relational system. In either case, Helen may "wonder" about Joan's truth-telling, which could affect the therapeutic relationship. On the other hand, if Helen believes she has received crucial information and confronts Joan, Joan may feel hurt, betrayed, and abused by both her therapist and her friend.

It is important to remember that Joan has been seeing Helen for only three weeks, probably an insufficient amount of time for trust to have developed between Joan and Helen. It is not only understandable but also important that clients feel there is trust before revealing significant information about themselves. To confront a client prematurely would indicate disrespect and entail disempowerment of the client; the therapist would effectively be taking control of the therapeutic process (IIA).

So what might Helen do to demonstrate both respect and truth-telling? Much, of course, would depend on the context, on the particulars of this situation, and these people. Helen might suggest to the friend that perhaps the best way to show her concern is to speak to Joan directly and tell her that she called Helen. Helen might also calmly describe her own discomfort and position on secret-keeping and on third-party information. If the call were specifically about Joan, Helen might tell Joan, in a nonconfrontational and fully respectful manner, that she received a call from someone who thought she should know about Joan's drinking. Helen could then explain to Joan that she is telling her because of Helen's *own* need to not keep secrets. She could state her intent to respect Joan's wishes concerning whether, when, or how Joan chooses to discuss the issue. Helen then must honor Joan's decision concerning the direction of the discussion. Communication such as described is not always possible or advisable. However, Helen's behavior in this instance would model personal accountability, open communication, and effective respectful use of power. (Rosa Spricer)

IMPLICATIONS

Responses to the ethical dilemmas presented in this section share a range of concerns. The respondents note that unclear or vacillating boundaries in professional relationships carry the risk of sending mixed messages to clients. In a climate where the signals are unclear, there is a potential for harm to the client. There is general agreement that overlapping/dual relationships can facilitate the erosion of those boundaries. Despite agreement that therapists should not knowingly form such relationships, respondents acknowledge that they may occur regardless of the best intentions of any therapist. They advocate conducting an open discussion with clients when there is a propensity for overlap in the therapy relationship, preferably early on in treatment. There is similar agreement on the importance of therapists' understanding the nature of the power differential between themselves and clients so that they can develop conscious strategies to avoid misusing their power. Therapists are encouraged to be effective models of personal power and to use their power for the benefit of clients as well as students and colleagues.

The therapist whose client and romantic partner engaged in an intimate relationship (Dilemma A) faced an unexpected and painful personal dilemma. In the midst of her own pain and confusion the therapist was nonetheless required to discharge her responsibilities to her client appropriately. While the therapist must end this professional relationship, her responsibility does not end there. She must terminate the relationship in a way that facilitates the therapy process and not evaluate the client's behavior or punish the client for playing either an intentional or unwitting role in the therapist's personal pain. Some of the respondents address the need for self-care in therapists, acknowledging that therapists become more vulnerable to boundary violations when they fail to attend to their own needs.

Overall, respondents agree that the range of issues confronting therapists who attempt to conduct psychotherapy in overlapping communities is wide-reaching and cannot be addressed with a simple set of rules. In a recent volume on feminist ethics, Brown (1994) offers a conceptual formulation to assist in deciding when important boundaries are jeopardized. In this formulation, boundary violations share three important characteristics. They objectify the client (e.g., the therapist views the client as an object of entertainment or education), they are an indication of the therapist acting on an impulse that has its origin in the therapist's need, and they invariably make the needs of the therapist primary (Brown, 1994). In Dilemma G, Dr. Chester acted on her impulse to bolster her client's confidence and may have intended well. However, she did not explore the client's feelings about her actions, nor did she anticipate how the client would experience these actions. The assumption that the client would interpret her gesture in precisely the way she consciously intended it, despite many other possible interpretations reflects the kind of seemingly innocuous boundary violation that Brown (1994) describes. In this case, the therapist in effect volunteers to be a client of her client, when she has never ascertained what the client will make of this reversal or how it will affect the therapy relationship. When the therapist fails to explore the client's needs and the client's experience of the therapist's actions, she runs the risk of using the client to respond to her own needs.

A number of authors have provided guidance for managing overlapping relationships or monitoring possible boundary violations. Lerman and Rigby (1990, p. 51), in an analysis of therapist power, contend that "the lack of awareness of power we hold is intrinsically related to therapists' lack of recognition of the appropriate therapist–client boundaries, and hence to power abuses and violations of such boundaries." These authors point out that some feminist therapists initially felt that power issues did not exist for them because both therapist and client were women. Unfortunately, this was a naive perspective, and often was associated with boundary violations. Lerman and Rigby thus warn against the denial of the inherent therapist–client power imbalance and exhort feminist therapists to examine their own power needs and be aware of how they act on them. In addition to continued self-examination, they point out the importance of consulting with ethically informed colleagues in preventing boundary violations.

Brown (1991) has also specified some steps toward ethical boundary management. First, therapists must acknowledge and validate the existence of overlapping relationships. They should also deal in a deliberate manner with those overlapping relationships that can be anticipated. In addition, feminist therapists should develop a more complex concept of the therapeutic frame than is currently the norm. That is, Brown urges recognition of the complex nature of the therapy relationship and development of a core set of norms to guide decision making given the specific needs, diagnosis, and setting of the particular client. Brown also thinks it important that a feminist analysis of power in therapy be applied to the ethical maintenance of boundaries and that the ethics of therapy be considered an integral part of the practice of therapy.

Adleman and Barrett note, "Overlapping relationships do contain potential hazards for boundary violations and ethical missteps" (1990, p. 89), and they offer a number of guidelines:

> 1. The therapist needs friends and associates in the community who are not and have not been clients. . . . 2. The therapist should have other seasoned therapists with whom she consciously discusses issues of concern in overlapping relationships. . . . 3. The therapist and client should discuss the potential for overlap early in therapy. . . . 4. The therapist should have means of meeting her social and emotional needs other than those exclusively provided in the shared community. 5. The therapist assumes responsibility and is accountable for her choices in this ethically complex area. (p. 90)

As the above authors have pointed out, it is extremely important that therapists recognize and responsibly manage dual and overlapping relationships. Feminist therapists, perhaps more than therapists who practice in larger communities, face the inevitability of overlapping relationships in their work. They have attempted to develop criteria that are both sensitive and flexible to guide therapists' thinking in both anticipating and formulating responses to problems that may arise in overlapping relationships. The respondents in this section and the feminist therapy literature strongly encourage the use of supervision and consultation to minimize therapists' likelihood of responding to these dilemmas in ways that may be harmful to their clients. As society becomes more diverse and more is learned about the therapy process itself, the principles will be viewed as guidelines in a constant state of revision.

RESPONDENTS

Jeanne Adleman, MA, is a feminist therapist and partner of Multicultural Associates in San Francisco.

Sheila Bob, PhD, is on the faculty of the School of Professional Psychology at Pacific University in Forest Grove, OR, where she teaches Ethics and Professional Issues.

Michele C. Boyer, PhD, a woman of color, is Professor and Director of Training in Counseling Psychology in the Department of Counseling at Indiana State University, Terre Haute, IN.

Janet Brice-Baker, PhD, African/West Indian–American, is a clinical psychologist and Clinical Coordinator of Adult Outpatient Services at the University of Medicine and Dentistry's Community Mental Health Center in Newark, NJ.

D. Brooks Cowan, PhD, Lecturer in the Department of Sociology at the University of Vermont, has been in private practice as a clinical sociologist for 10 years.

Nikki Gerrard, PhD, immigrated to Canada from the United States 20 years ago and is Caucasian and a community psychologist at the Saskatoon Mental Health Clinic, specializing in rural mental health and interactions of racism and sexism in mental health systems.

Cheryl Haller, MS, a licensed clinical mental health counselor in private practice, specializes in incest survival, adult children of alcoholics, and bereavement.

Mary Hayden, PhD, is a clinical psychologist in private practice in Pasadena, CA, with a special interest in work with survivors of childhood abuse and with lesbian issues, particularly relationship enhancement.

Dorothy Holden, MSc, is a psychologist in Calgary, Alberta, specializing in career and personal development by conducting workshops for women considering career planning, management, and transition issues and by teaching in the Career Development Certificate Program and the University of Calgary.

Valli Kanuha, MSW, of Japanese and Hawaiian-Chinese descent, is affiliated with the Center on AIDS, Drugs, and Community Health of the Brookdale Health Science Center, Hunter College of the City University of New York.

Kathleen Mack, PsyD, has 15 years of experience as a therapist and has a private practice in Dayton and Cincinnati, OH, specializing in feminist therapy, neuropsychology, and lesbian/gay issues.

Margaret McLeod, MEd, is a psychologist in private practice in Calgary, Alberta, working with individuals, couples, and families with a spiritually based approach using hypnosis and body-focused therapy.

Rosa Spricer, PhD, a feminist therapist in private practice in Edmonton, Alberta, specializes in eating disorders and issues pertaining to abuse and promotion of self-esteem.

REFERENCES

Adleman, J., & Barrett, S. E. (1990). Overlapping relationships: Importance of the feminist ethical perspective. In H. Lerman & N. Porter (Eds.), *Feminist ethics in psychotherapy* (pp. 87–91). New York: Springer.

American Psychological Association. (1990). Ethical principles of psychologists (Amended June 2, 1989). *American Psychologist, 45,* 390–395.

American Psychological Association. (1992). Ethical principles of psychologists. *American Psychologist, 47,* 1597–1611.

American Psychological Association. (1993). Report of the Ethics Committee, 1991 and 1992. *American Psychologist, 48,* 811–820.

Benowitz, M. (1994). Comparing the experiences of women clients sexually exploited by female versus male psychotherapists. *Women and Therapy*, *15*, 69–83.

Berman, J. S. (1990). The problems of overlapping relationships in the political community. In H. Lerman & N. Porter (Eds.), *Feminist ethics in psychotherapy* (pp. 106–110). New York: Springer.

Brodsky, A. N. (1989). Sex between patient and therapist: Psychology's data and response. In G. O. Gabbard (Ed.), *Sexual exploitation in professional relationships* (pp. 15–25). Washington, DC: American Psychiatric Press.

Brown, L. S. (1983). Finding new language: Getting beyond analytic verbal shorthand in feminist therapy. *Women and Therapy*, *3*, 73–80.

Brown, L. S. (1985). Power, responsibility, boundaries: Ethical concerns for the lesbian feminist therapist. *Lesbian Ethics*, *1*(3), 30–45.

Brown, L. S. (1988). Harmful effects of post-termination sexual and romantic relationships between therapists and their former clients. *Psychotherapy*, *25*, 249–257.

Brown, L. S. (1991). Ethical issues in feminist therapy. *Psychology of Women Quarterly*, *15*, 323–336.

Brown, L. S. (1994). Boundaries in feminist therapy: A conceptual formulation. *Women and Therapy*, *15*, 29–38.

Corey, G., Corey, M. S., & Callanan, P. (1993). *Issues and ethics in the helping professions*, (4th ed.). Belmont, CA: Brooks/Cole.

Feminist Therapy Institute. (1987). *Feminist therapy code of ethics*. Denver: Author.

Freeman, L., & Roy, J. (1976). *Betrayal*. New York: Stein and Day.

Gabbard, G. O., & Pope, K. S. (1989). Sexual intimacies after termination: Clinical, ethical and legal aspects. In G. O. Gabbard (Ed.), *Sexual exploitation in professional relationships* (pp. 115–127). Washington, DC: American Psychiatric Press.

Gartrell, N. (1994). Boundaries in lesbian therapist–client relationships. In B. Greene & G. Herek (Eds.), *Lesbian and gay psychology: Theory, research and clinical applications* (pp. 98–117). Thousand Oaks, CA: Sage.

Gartrell, N., Herman, J., Olarte, S., Feldstein, M., & Localio, R. (1986). Psychiatrist–patient sexual contact: Results of a national survey, I: Prevalence. *American Journal of Psychiatry*, *143*, 1126–1131.

Gartrell, H., & Sanderson, B. (1994). Sexual abuse of women by women in psychotherapy: Counseling and advocacy. *Women and Therapy*, *15*(1), 39–54.

Gates, K. P., & Speare, K. H. (1990). Overlapping relationships in rural communities. In H. Lerman & N. Porter (Eds.), *Feminist ethics in psychotherapy* (pp. 97–101). New York: Springer.

Greene, B. (1994). Teaching ethics in psychotherapy. *Women and Therapy*, *15*, 17–27.

Kardener, S. H., Fuller, M., & Mensh, I. N. (1973). A survey of physicians' attitudes and practices regarding erotic and nonerotic contact with patients. *American Journal of Psychiatry*, *133*, 1324–1325.

Keith-Spiegel, P., & Koocher, G. (1985). *Ethics in psychology: Professional standards and cases*. New York: Random House.

Lerman, H., & Rigby, D. (1990). Boundary violations: Misuse of the power of the therapist. In H. Lerman & N. Porter (Eds.), *Feminist ethics in psychotherapy* (pp. 51–59). New York: Springer.

McCarthy, J. (1966). Overt transference. *Journal of Sex Research, 2,* 227–237.

Pope, K. S. (1991). Dual relationships in psychotherapy. *Ethics and Behavior, 1,* 21–34.

Pope, K., Levenson, H., & Schover, L. R. (1979). Sexual intimacy in psychology training. *American Psychologist, 34,* 682–689.

Pope, K., Sonne, J. L., & Holroyd, J. (1993). *Sexual feelings in psychotherapy: Explorations for therapists and therapists-in-training.* Washington, DC: American Psychological Association.

Pope, K., & Vasquez, M. J. T. (1991). *Ethics in psychotherapy and counseling.* San Francisco: Jossey Bass.

Sears, V. L. (1990). On being an "only" one. In H. Lerman & N. Porter (Eds.), *Feminist ethics in psychotherapy* (pp. 102–105). New York: Springer.

Shepard, M. (1971). *The love treatment: Sexual intimacy between patients and psychotherapists.* New York: Wyden.

Smith, A. J. (1990). Working within the lesbian community: The dilemma of overlapping relationships. In H. Lerman & N. Porter (Eds.), *Feminist ethics in psychotherapy* (pp. 92–96). New York: Springer.

Subcommittees, Boundary Dilemmas Conference. (1987). *Ethical standards and practice in the lesbian community.* Los Angeles: Boundary Dilemmas Conference.

SEVEN

Violence against Women

Susan Contratto
Jane Hassinger

HISTORY AND CURRENT STATUS

Violence against women and their daughters in Western, postindustrial culture is common and includes acquaintance rape, marital rape, sexual assault by strangers, sexual abuse, physical violence in the home, obscene phone calls, sexual harassment in public settings and at work, and sexual objectification in pornography and advertising. In the United States it is estimated that a woman is raped every 1.3 minutes and that 75% of victims know their attacker. Nine out of 10 murdered women are murdered by men, and four out of five are murdered at home. One out of two women will experience sexual harassment during her academic life, and one in four girls are sexually abused before they are 18 (Women's Action Coalition, 1993).

Prior to this wave of the women's movement, violence against women was not named or documented. Women began to talk about the violence in their everyday lives in the safety and security of consciousness-raising groups that sprang up all over the country in the late 1960s and early 1970s. Experiences previously felt to be private, shameful, self-induced, and without words and labels were tentatively shared. Others not only empathized but often said, "That happened to me too." Women began to find a language for violence against themselves and their daughters.

Women were also insisting that their communities respond to these problems. Grassroots activists founded women's centers, shelters, and crisis lines. They influenced legal changes to make partner battering and marital rape illegal. Women insisted that police be trained in domestic violence and that hospital emergency rooms collect appropriate evidence when a woman who had been raped required service. Women at the level of their own communities closed down distributors of pornography and got ordinances passed against obscene advertising. And most recently, women have spearheaded the drive to protect children against sexual abuse.

Concurrent with grassroots activities, feminist scholars such as Susan Brownmiller (1975), Susan Schecter (1982), Sandra Butler (1978), Judith Herman (1981), Lenore Walker (1979), Florence Rush (1980), and Laura Lederer (1980), as well as others, broke the generations of silence about types and frequency of violence against women. Within the academy, there has been a flood of scholarly work. In 1993 alone, there were 58 new articles in journals abstracted by the American Psychological Association that had "women" and "violence" in their titles.

There has been a backlash to acknowledging violence against women and the political actions that surround it. The mainstream media, for example, seems quick to latch onto any reasonably well-argued antifeminist position. The treatment of Katie Roiphe's (1993) book on acquaintance rape by *The New York Times* is a good example. The book is little more than Roiphe's essay elaborating her opinion that acquaintance rape is overestimated because young women frequently act in the moment and then regret their sexual behavior. The book was featured in a *New York Times Sunday Magazine* article, was given a daily and Sunday book review by the same publication, and an interview and picture of Roiphe and her mother were on the front page of the second section. This free publicity is an inestimable gift for any book and any author. Given Roiphe's poor scholarship and inadequate argument (e.g., see Pollitt's [1993] review in *The New Yorker* and Phillips's [1993] in *The Women's Review of Books*), it certainly appears that the editorial decision was primarily sensationalistic and political—irresponsibly stirring the political pot.

Part of the current backlash is the questioning of the validity of repressed and retrieved memory, an experience that is relatively common among adult survivors of childhood sexual abuse. The question of the accuracy of memory is an old one in psychology. Freud himself first believed the incest reports of his patients and then became skeptical and developed a theory of unconscious fantasies and wished-for seduction (Masson, 1984). Recently, psychology has joined the debate again. In *The Harvard Mental Health Letter*, Elizabeth Loftus (1993) encourages therapists to be skeptical of repressed memories of abuse. She reports David Holmes's work where he reviewed 60 years of research "and found no controlled experiments showing that an event can be accurately reproduced in memory after a long period of repression" (p. 4). Judith Herman and Mary Harvey take a diametrically opposed view in the April 1993 issue of *The Harvard Mental Health Letter*. In the midst of this scholarly controversy, the American Psychological Association has appointed a committee to compile and review research on repressed memory.

The debate is more than academic or clinical. On the basis of the retrieval of repressed memories, survivors have been suing their perpetrators, in some states winning their lawsuits and in others spearheading changes in laws about the statute of limitations. In reaction to these successful activities, a lobbying group called The False Memory Foundation, originally founded by alleged perpetrators who claimed they were falsely accused, has become increasingly active. This group attempts to influence legislation and media reporting. In Pennsylvania a proposed law would make it a crime to falsely report a case of incest or sexual abuse or to aid someone in making such a report. The bill is sponsored by a legislator who claims to have been falsely accused, and the witnesses at public hearings have been largely in favor of the bill (Williams, 1993). Another example of the group's influence is found in a recent *New Yorker* article (Wright, 1993) This two-part series on a ritual abuse report in Oregon concludes by arguing that the individuals in the case who recovered memories did so under the inappropriate influence of clergy and mental health professionals. The last several pages of the article refer to the False Memory Foundation and its efforts to rein in victims' advocates whom the author of the article portrays as harmful zealots. This kind of backlash activity is on the rise and can only have a chilling effect on survivors, therapists, and advocates.

Often when a feminist talks about violence toward women, she is called upon to include violence toward men or asked about this issue. When she talks or writes about male perpetrators, there is subtle or overt pressure to give equal time to female perpetrators. Many groups experience violence, but more women and female children of all social classes and all ethnic groups experience victimization by men than their male counterparts do by women. This fact can get lost within a postmodern dialogue of diversity and multiple perspectives. The debate can lose its moral anchoring when the damaging effects of one or another particular kind of violence is questioned by contextualizing its social acceptability. For example, the tradition of sexual harassment in the Navy does not make it appropriate. Female genital mutilation, while a part of some ethnic groups' heritage, remains an example of unacceptable violence against women. Questions or concerns are not necessarily wrongheaded, but when they are raised in a climate of backlash, they should always be addressed with caution.

CLINICAL ISSUES

There are two ongoing clinical problems that emerge from the literature on violence against women. The first is victim blaming, which holds the woman situationally or psychologically responsible for her own victimization. The second is diagnostic; many data suggest that certain heavily woman-dominated psychiatric diagnoses are in reality forms of simple or complex posttraumatic stress disorder and that many clinicians continue to use inappropriate categories because they do not recognize the frequency of violence in women's lives, and they do not take a history that asks about incidence of trauma with individual clients (Bart & Moran, 1993; Brown, 1991; Herman, 1992; McGrath, Keita, Strickland, & Russo, 1990). Even as the connections between victimization of women, social and economic status, and psychopathology are more firmly established, it is still uncommon for clinicians to routinely take complete and contextually complex histories with clients. McGrath et al. (1990) recommend a model for a context-relevant assessment that systematically examines the violence and exploitation history of each client as well as class, race, sexual orientation, and cultural/religious background.

The treatment of women who have experienced violence in their lives presents two general ethical dilemmas for currently practicing therapists. First, therapists may frequently find themselves treating beyond their level of competence and second, certain treatments may not be appropriate for victims of violence. While posttraumatic stress disorder (PTSD) is outpacing depression in its frequency of use as a diagnostic category, it has only recently been rediscovered by training institutions (Herman, 1992). Simultaneously, educational efforts have increased recognition of the consequences of violence in women's lives, so that more women are seeking a variety of treatments. Some irresponsible and unethical therapists may see a potential market they can enter without proper training and caution. Hence, another possibility exists for revictimization of already traumatized individuals. Furthermore, the statistical probability is very high that therapists working with women are very likely working with victims of violence, whether or not it has been acknowledged as a treatment issue. They therefore have a responsibility to be trained in this area through additional course work or through continuing education offered by their state or national professional organization.

There has literally been an explosion of treatment articles and books in the area of violence within the last 10 years. Major books and journals on this topic include Judith Herman's book, *Trauma and Recovery* (1992), social psychologist Ronnie Janoff-Bulman's *Shattered Assumptions* (1992), special issues of the journal *Psychotherapy* (Ochberg

& Willis, 1991), a two-volume special issue of *Women and Therapy* (Cole, Rothblum, & Espin, 1992), and review articles in the "Psychology in the Public Forum" section of the *American Psychologist* (1993). Each of these publications is an important resource with excellent and extensive bibliographies. In addition, Herman's book comprehensively describes the explicitly feminist treatment approach that has been developed by her and her colleagues. *Psychotherapy* (Ochberg & Willis, 1991) contains articles that represent a variety of kinds of interventions ranging from groups, to journal keeping, to traditionally psychodynamic, cognitive-behavioral, and other interventions. Although it is an excellent resource, the approaches are not necessarily feminist.

Some of the work developed with hospitalized veterans may violate feminist therapy ethical guidelines. For example, the technique of flooding, bombarding the client with traumatically loaded material in the interests of ultimately desensitizing her, is not a technique of short-term empowerment, and as a process intervention violates the principal of equalizing client–therapist power. Hypnosis is an increasingly popular technique for the recovery of traumatic memories. Used with women who have been victims of violence, it can easily violate the feminist principle of equalizing power in the therapeutic relationship. It may be that in certain instances hypnosis is the only treatment possible. Such a decision should be reached in collaboration with the client and with a consultant, following the steps and the time required in the feminist ethical decision-making model (the section by Hill, Glaser, & Harden, this volume).

There are other kinds of treatments traditionally offered for women who have experienced violence that are questionable within the guidelines of the FTI (Feminist Therapy Institute, 1987) Code. For example, women who have been battered by spouses often find themselves with a therapist who defines the problem as a marital one. Such a therapist may suggest couples therapy. A situation in which a husband is beating up his wife and children may be recast as family violence, and the recommendation may be for family therapy. This reframing avoids several realities. First, a man who is violent is the problem—not the couple or the family. He needs treatment and/or punishment and others deserve protection from him. Second, treatments that put the survivor in the same room as the perpetrator implicitly suggest that it is a two-way problem. Third, it is chilling and intimidating for many survivors to have any contact with perpetrators, and such contact should only be initiated by a fully informed and strong survivor.

Other popular self-help modalities, such as 12-step programs, which rely on a "higher power" and writings, workshops, and groups on codependency, are ethically questionable with women who are survivors of violence. It is essential for their healing that they know both the energy and the limits of their own power because they have been in situations, sometimes chronic ones, that have been disempowering (Walker, 1991). Groups that from the beginning require that individuals acknowledge their powerlessness are not helpful to women who know full well that they have been powerless. Instead, these women need to find their real competencies and strengths. Further, the term codependency suggests an interdependent relationship in which both members have equal access to power and resources. Victimized women have not been in anything approaching equal relationships with the perpetrator. Such a movement, then, can become victim blaming. Codependency–dependency asks, "What did you do to make this happen?" and "What are you doing to sustain its occurrence?" instead of "What kind of person would do this to you?" and "Why does he continue to do it?"

Each of the dilemmas illustrates a number of the ethical responsibilities and dilemmas feminist therapists face when dealing with questions of actual or suspected violence.

DILEMMA A

Carla is a Euro-American therapist in a university counseling center. One of her clients, Sara, is a master's student at the university whose husband is a doctoral student. Both are citizens of India. Sara has expressed difficulty concentrating on her studies. During the second session with Sara, Carla notices dark bruises on Sara's arms. When asked about them, Sara said she fell against a door. Carla has read a little about Sara's culture and knows that the husband is considered the dominant one in the marriage, and wife beating is not uncommon. In an effort to demonstrate respect for the culture, Carla does not pursue the possibility of Sara's being battered.

RESPONDENT 1

Carla experiences a conflict between her duty to promote Sara's well-being (Preamble) and her desire to respect Sara's Indian cultural tradition (IV). In resolving the dilemma, the therapist must use her feminist awareness that almost every cultural tradition is oppressive to women; insofar as any tradition is destructive to women, it is not to be respected but changed so that it will offer full human rights to women. Woman-abuse in any culture must be challenged. Ultimately she will engage with Sara in "challenging oppressive aspects" of the value system in which she was raised (Preamble).

At the outset, however, Carla will need to proceed carefully and respect the extent to which Sara will inevitably feel trapped between her pain and fear about the injuries she has sustained and her loyalty to her husband and their cultural tradition. Carla could begin by engaging in a general discussion with Sara about the value system into which she was born and the one in which she is now living and studying. They can then begin to talk about inevitable conflicts between one's own needs and the dictates of one's culture and the difficult choices that must sometimes be made. After some measure of trust has been established, Carla can ask Sara about the bruises and let her know that she empathizes with the dilemma Sara might feel over what, if anything, to do. As Sara feels more comfortable about being open about her marital situations, she and Carla can discuss the various options she has for protecting herself and dealing with her husband about his violence. (Mary Hayden)

RESPONDENT 2

An ethical dilemma in this example is created by two conflicting responsibilities. They are respect for the client's culture (IB) and ensuring the client's safety (IC). By respecting Sara's culture, Carla is jeopardizing her safety and may be perpetuating her oppression. Sara's silence about her abuse may be an outcome of being away from her support system. It is not uncommon for some men to become abusive when their spouses are away from the extended family. Extended family systems protect women from abuse (in some cases). Moreover, Sara may be feeling isolated. Isolation is a common reality of racialized women in a racist society (Miles, 1989). It is the therapist's responsibility to explore Sara's lived experiences, including racist social treatment (Javed, 1992).

Carla has made little attempt to go beyond stereotypic notions of the Indian culture. There is an abundance of evidence suggesting flaws in the way "the orient" (including India) is constructed and represented in the West (Miles, 1989; Said, 1979). The assumption that Indian culture endorses violence against women and that women are dominated by men creates misunderstandings about a culture that has numerous complexities. Understanding gender relations in the Indian society is not a simple task. Contrasts in Indian women's lives are hard to grasp. On one hand, there are women like Indira Ghandi and, on the other, women who are burnt for dowry. Class differences, religious beliefs, and cultural mythology simultaneously represent women as Goddesses and Dasi (slaves). These contradictory representations of women reveal the intricacy of gender relations that ought to be acknowledged in understanding the client's reality. Carla has ignored this responsibility. (Nayyar S. Javed)

DILEMMA B

Ann is a 15-year-old sophomore in high school. Her grades have dropped considerably over the last two years, and she has lost most of her friends. In junior high school she was very active in school activities and generally was considered a well-adjusted student. Jane is Ann's high school counselor and has approached the subject of sexual assault with Ann who denies vehemently that she is a victim. Because of the changes in Ann's behavior, Jane is convinced Ann must be a sexual assault victim. Although Ann asks Jane not to talk to her parents, Jane decides that she must do so because of the differences in Ann's behavior.

RESPONDENT 1

Although it is technically ethical for therapist Jane to contact Ann's parents about the suspected sexual abuse without Ann's permission (since she is a minor, and parents hold the privilege of confidentiality), it could be both dangerous and an abuse of her power as therapist to do so. Jane, although she is eager to protect Ann's well-being (Preamble), should first respect Ann's expressed request at least until she has given Ann the opportunity to explain why she does not want her parents contacted (IA). Jane should let Ann know that she has a legal right to contact her parents, but that she respects Ann's feelings and wants to understand them. She may find out that Ann fears retaliation from her parents (if indeed they are perpetrating abuse on her), and in this case it would be wise not to contact them first but to report any abuse to the child protective services. In any case, Jane must build trust and convey respect for Ann if she is to obtain any further information from her about being abused, and of course, such a trusting relationship will be even more necessary if she is to assist Ann in healing. (Mary Hayden)

RESPONDENT 2

In this dilemma, Jane is failing to be sensitive to the power differential between client and therapist. Although the counselor is convinced Ann is a sexual assault victim, the example here does not justify that conclusion. However, even if the counselor were correct, taking control from the client (IIA) and failing to develop a cooperative therapeutic alliance (IIC) conflicts with feminist ethical practice. By taking power from the client, the therapist undermines the therapeutic process.

Jane should meaningfully explore with Ann all the possible explanations for her change in behavior, thus helping Ann gain an understanding of her own issues. There are many possible causes of Ann's behavior, including serious problems in the home, drugs, and depression. Without Ann's involvement and understanding, the therapist cannot be effective. The therapist should certainly make every effort to obtain Ann's consent to include her parents, especially if their cooperation is needed for her treatment.

The importance of respecting a child or adolescent's need for privacy is always an issue for therapists. Often therapists resolve the dilemma by having joint sessions with parents and the teenager as part of their treatment approach. Frequently parental involvement and understanding of the therapy is important for therapeutic success. Except for "duty to warn" circumstances when the teenager is suicidal, homicidal, or otherwise self-destructive, every attempt is made to have an intervention carried out with the teenager's cooperation. (Barbara McCandlish)

RESPONDENT 3

If Jane indeed has reason to suspect sexual assault, she must rigorously investigate the meanings of sexuality and sexual violation for members of Ann's cultural groups (IB). In some cultural groups, the victims of sexual assault and violation are viewed as "sullied" women. For others the need for retribution and the potential for the incarceration or death of the avenger may instill fear and silence in a young person. Jane must also be sensitive to biased societal constructions, which she and Ann may have internalized, about women from various class and cultural groups (i.e., the dominant culture vision of African-American or Latina girls from low-income backgrounds as hypersexual, promiscuous, etc.).

Jane needs to be cognizant of and willing to explore other explanations for Ann's behavior. For example, in some communities a 15-year-old girl is in the dangerous stage of her life, a stage when she might become pregnant and "waste her life." In order to safeguard against pregnancy, some parents/guardians become exceedingly strict, forcing girls into isolation and creating frightening narratives to enforce safety (IB). Or Ann may have been a witness to violence in her environment. Perhaps the demographics of her junior high school may have been significantly different from the high school in which she is enrolled; she may have suddenly become a cultural outsider. Similarly, the loss of friends may be the result of her placement in classes in which her friends are not involved, for example classes for exceptional students.

Jane must be willing to ask some questions about her role in this young woman's life. How and under what circumstances was their relationship defined? Jane must be careful to understand Ann's construction of counseling and what it means to go to a school counselor. Ann may be unclear about the boundaries of the relationship between teachers, principals, and school counselors (IID). And, if she is from a culture or class setting that has clear taboos about "therapy" or "airing dirty laundry," these issues must be uncovered and addressed. In the latter case, it may be necessary to engage the assistance of a trusted outsider or an individual whose cultural or class background or sexual identity may make her an easier or more comfortable ally for Ann (IA).

Jane must recognize that while she has the power to inform Ann's parents about her suspicions, in wielding her power in this way she will be taking the risk of retraumatizing/revictimizing Ann. If the agenda behind Jane's actions is Ann's healing and empowerment, then they need to talk about how to incorporate Ann's parents as allies in her healing process. Jane will have to develop language with which to effectively communicate with both Ann and her parents. Jane should reflect candidly on the reasons for her conviction that Ann is a victim of assault. If she or someone close to her is a victim of assault she must insure her own and Ann's safety by seeking support and consultation for herself (IVD).

Jane needs to actively seek out and perhaps establish avenues of proactive support for young women (and men) like Ann. Jane should consider exploring and visiting church groups, community groups, and other mental health services for youth (VB) so she can make informed referrals. (Jacquie Mattis)

DILEMMA C

Marge, a 50-year-old mental health worker, was referred to Norma by the "gatekeeper" of Marge's HMO because of "stress and depression." In therapy, Marge tells Norma about one therapist who has had sexual contact with multiple clients. The therapist was quietly fired by the administration. Other male therapists continue to socialize with female clients. Marge has been asked to provide psychological treatment to one of the sexually abused women, a client of the fired therapist. Marge believes she cannot provide appropriate treatment, which would include encouraging the client to pursue legal action. Nor can Marge refuse to treat the client without jeopardizing her job. Norma is expected to give feedback to the referring person as part of the HMO requirements.

RESPONDENT 1

Marge's cultural background, socioeconomic status, and sexual orientation all must be accounted for in understanding her response to the circumstances with which she is struggling (IB). These factors also influence the way in which the power differentials between Marge and the institution and between Marge and Norma are managed. For example, meaning and power issues vary considerably according to class and status: women of historically marginalized groups in relation to therapists who are white males represent a particular set of issues that differ from those of upper-middle-class women. If Marge herself were struggling with issues related to sexuality/sexual orientation, the ethical and treatment issues are made significantly more complex.

The therapy will necessarily have to include exploration of the relationship between Marge's ethics, spirituality, and construction of her identity. There must be exploration of the possibility that Marge's stress and depression are manifestations of her effort to deny or remedy the disjuncture that she is feeling between her ideal self and the actualities of her work place and its demands. Norma should help Marge understand that the double-consciousness, the incongruity, and the discomfort with which she lives are an outgrowth of the sexual domination of women. The historical patterns of oppression often leave women feeling fragmented and ambivalent about loyalties and responsibilities to others. If the core of Marge's identity is constructed around her professional and political ethics, then she must be helped to explore the ways in which this situation has fractured or shaken her sense of self. Norma must be prepared to consult with or encourage Marge to consult others who can assist in providing alternative supports for her sense of adequate self (IA).

Marge should be helped to think about the meaning of her job to her and the possibility that the constraints of the organization may make it impossible for her to function in a professionally ethical way. Financial constraints must also be given weight in this process. Marge must have the power to control the agenda of this therapy. Norma needs to place the safety of the client over the institutional agreements made with the HMO. If she finds herself unable to do so, she must inform Marge and propose alternate arrangements for Marge's treatment (IIC, D, IIIA, B). (Jacquie Mattis)

RESPONDENT 2

This dilemma is an example of the potentially wide-ranging reverberations that result from a serious boundary violation between a therapist in an agency and a client. Marge may be seen as a secondary victim of the transgression committed by her colleague with his client. Her victimization takes several forms. Marge faces conflicting concerns and finds herself in a double-bind similar to that of the violated client. Her attempts at resolution may put her in a high-risk situation. Efforts to empower her client in assertively confronting her former therapist and/or the agency that has decided against legal action in the case probably will create conflict for Marge in her workplace with her employers. Her integrity as a therapist is at risk as are her comfort and well-being on the job. Furthermore, given the considerable body of evidence that supports the likelihood that therapists who commit sexual transgressions with clients will continue to do so, other clients will most likely be at risk (Brodsky, 1986; Gartrell, Herman, Olarte, Feldstein, & Localio, 1986; Pope & Bouhoutsos, 1986). Marge may legitimately worry for the welfare of future clients of the offending therapist. Workplace pressures and the threat of job loss may function to prevent Marge from acting in accordance with her values and ethical principles.

Another level of trauma may be evident in the organizational response and adaptation to the original violation. Unfortunately, this agency seems to have responded in a fairly typical pattern. The staff person was dismissed, the victimized client was reassigned within the agency, no efforts were made to report the transgression to state licensing boards and/or professional accrediting groups, and no notification of the reasons for dismissal was made to the next place of employment (or so it appears). The agency has inadvertently contributed to the likelihood of further victimization of clients. In its concern with "taking care of its own internal dirty laundry," the agency has created a pathological environment for the remaining staff. Experience shows that such events often lead to demoralization and mistrust among staff, decline in the quality of work, withdrawal of or resignation of some of the best staff members, and in some instances the reactivation of earlier trauma in the lives of certain women staff members. Fearful for its reputation and of legal reprisals, the agency's managers have responded to the situation in a manner that will establish conditions for increasingly hobbling organizational norms with respect to managing conflict, maintaining high standards of practice, rewarding competence, and insuring safety for workers and clients alike. Thus, the agency itself becomes in effect another victim and another victimizer.

Several important areas of confusion about professional role, boundaries, and ethics are further evident in the responses of the players in this complicated situation. For example, Norma makes an automatic assumption that her acceptance of Marge as a client will require that she urge Marge to take legal action against her transgressor (Marge's former colleague). Although it is certainly in keeping with feminist ethical principles to provide education about clients' rights and "procedures for resolving differences and filing grievances" (IID) and to intervene actively in situations that involve the abuse of clients (VA), the empowerment of the client to act on her own behalf and to set her own agendas in and out of therapy is a fundamental premise of ethical feminist practice (IIA). Paradoxically, Norma may be uncritically taking on too much power in relation to Marge and Marge too little in relation to her client. In both cases, the empowerment of the client is of paramount interest. In this process, careful discussion about and evaluation of the pros and cons of legal action need to be pursued. For Marge, it would include sensitive exploration of the double-bind (psychological and ethical) in which she finds herself. Norma must take care to rein in a well-intended but overzealous urge to impose her agenda on her client.

In considering the ethical practice of the organizations involved, the agency for which Norma works, and the HMO for which Marge works, both have performed poorly in protecting their clients and their employees. Institutional requirements lead to institutional blind-spots where, for example, Norma has the obligation to report on the progress of Marge's treatment. Always a vexing concern in increasingly managed-care-driven treatment systems, Marge's confidentiality may not be protected in this example, thereby violating a fundamental feminist practice ethic (IIIB). In addition, the problem of colliding and overlapping boundaries between therapists and clients is unavoidable, especially in small communities and professional groups. To outlaw such occurrences altogether is unrealistic. But both circumstances highlight the need within agencies and across managed-care systems for the careful development of standards and practices grounded in real experiences for the managing of confidentiality and boundary conflicts and transgressions. These standards and practices would necessarily involve the devotion of resources to staff development activities and ongoing peer review and consultation systems for professional staff (IVB). One outcome of an empowering therapy for Marge might be that she is able effectively to inform her agency and the HMO of the double-binds created for her (and others) by this circumstance and work to change these systems.

Finally, this situation strongly argues for the importance of the wide-spread creation of mandatory reporting laws to state and professional regulatory boards. Had the agency been required to report the first therapist's transgression, many of the traumatizing and double-binding consequences that unfolded might have been avoided. Marge and Norma might wisely and ethically (VB) work toward the creation of such legislation. (Joan Zald)

DILEMMA D

Latoya's client Debbie, a battered woman and mother of four, called the police when her husband George beat her. State law provides that an abuser can be arrested on affidavit of the injured party. George has a history of violence that has resulted in previous police reports. When the police came, the couple was separated, and a female officer advised Debbie of her right to arrest her husband. Debbie also reported that the male officer told George he could arrest Debbie as well if George had been hit.

George was taken to jail, and Debbie was arrested. She was advised that if she could not find anyone to care for her children in two hours, they would be turned over to Social Services. George called within two hours, offering to drop his charges if she would drop charges against him. Unable to find anyone to watch the children, Debbie agreed.

After Debbie told her what happened, Latoya contacted the chief of police to inform him that officers had violated her client's right to protection. The chief promised that his officers would be told that only the perpetrator was to be arrested. Latoya promised to check whether or not the chief followed through and would go to the newspaper and domestic violence groups and urge women to seek legal redress against the police if such behavior occurred again.

RESPONDENT 1

The therapist, Latoya, demonstrated an excellent grasp of the systemic abuses to which her client Debbie was subjected. Both her awareness of patriarchal and sexist practices and her determination to change the system are commendable (Preamble, VA). As a feminist therapist she is obligated to take a proactive stance in response to systemic abuses, and she clearly does so.

The difficulty occurs in the way the therapist chooses to act. She resolves the problem by taking direct private action rather than involving and empowering the client (IIA, VA). Such action by the therapist would serve to reinstate the client's sense of helplessness within a patriarchal system where powerful others decide her fate, not herself. Also, it is not clear in this instance whether or not the client has consented to the therapist's action and her right to confidentiality was protected.

From a feminist ethical perspective, the therapist would involve her client in every step of the process from educating her, if necessary, about the nature of the wrong done to her and informing her of steps for legal redress in order to correct this wrong, to offering her support and helping her obtain community support if necessary (IID). In doing so, the client would feel empowered to affect change in her personal life and the system. The only basis for acting as the therapist did would be the argument that her approach and her approach alone would have worked to protect women under similar circumstances in that community. Even so, it is likely that her approach would undermine the desired feminist outcome. (Barbara McCandlish)

RESPONDENT 2

Feminist ethics differ from conventional standards in that it is not sufficient simply "to do no wrong." Advocacy, a proactive rather than strictly reactive approach, is an integral part of the therapy process (Rosewater, 1990). This viewpoint is consistent with Brown's (1985) stance that a feminist therapist has an ethical imperative to use her power and privilege on her client's behalf. In the case of Debbie, the therapist took a proactive stance to address systemic abuse. This intervention was appropriate and clinically helpful, provided that the therapist first sought her client's permission to intervene with the police chief. No intervention should be undertaken without permission, as this behavior parallels the victimization process in which victims are assumed to be unable to manage on their own. To gain permission in a client-respectful manner, the therapist should address the pros and cons of the proposed intervention and let the client decide whether or not she would find such intervention to be helpful and whether or not it would add to her sense of personal danger.

With the client's permission, the therapist's confrontation of the police chief served several constructive purposes. First, the therapist was modeling appropriate assertive behavior; second, she was acknowledging both the client's sense of revictimization when the police failed to protect her and the validity of her realization that she was not safe; and third, she added to her client's sense of empowerment in knowing that she would not be subjected to a repeated incident of having unwarranted charges filed against her. One of the most common forms of revictimization for battered women is the helplessness that is engendered by their unsuccessful attempts to seek assistance (Walker, 1987). The therapist's intervention provided a way of responding that was affirming of the client's frustration with the inadequacies of the criminal justice system. The therapist's use of her power as an expert on domestic violence to coerce the police to follow the intent of the law and to insist that they be held responsible for any future abuse of the domestic violence law was an appropriate way for a therapist to use her power on a client's behalf (IID).

Ultimately, feminist therapists must help make systemic changes, legislative and legal, that aim to distribute equitably social, political, and economic power (VB) (Rosewater, 1990). The symptoms clients present are most often representative of societal rather than individual ills. (Lynn Rosewater)

DILEMMA E

Tracy, a middle-aged professional African-American woman, telephoned Ellen, a well-known, Euro-American feminist therapist in town, for a consultation. At first, Tracy was frightened, inhibited, and shared only a few pertinent pieces of information. She had been referred by her lawyer who would not work with her unless she saw a therapist. Tracy had been sexually abused by a previous therapist and was currently working with the lawyer to stop this person from harassing her. Tracy may or may not take further legal action. She was reluctant to get involved in therapy at all and was doing so only to keep her lawyer working with her. Before leaving the office, she made another appointment and gave Ellen a document the lawyer required that outlined the history of the relationship with her previous therapist. She also said that Ellen had not been her first choice but that other therapists had no time for her.

After Tracy left, Ellen read the document and became intensely upset. The allegations in the document amounted to years of unethical, abusive, and exploitative practice. Ellen found herself wondering if they were true. She was familiar by reputation with the therapist who was the alleged perpetrator. Although this person was unconventional, he had practiced in the community for over 20 years. The document itself suggested the enormous psychological distress that Tracy was experiencing, including suicidality.

RESPONDENT 1

The possibility that Tracy feels coerced into treatment poses the first ethical dilemma. The ethical guidelines specifically address power differentials (IIA). Therapists are advised against taking power that rightfully belongs to the client. However in this scenario, Tracy was ordered into therapy by her lawyer as a condition for legal representation. The first responsibility for the therapist is to clarify to the client that therapy has to be a decision she, and no one else, makes (IIB). In addition, it is the therapist's responsibility to educate Tracy with regard to her "rights as a consumer of therapy, including procedures for resolving differences and filing grievances" (IIC).

It is essential that Ellen clarify with Tracy why Ellen is not her first choice. Are the objections of a type that Ellen can resolve or not (IB)? To what extent are the objections related to identity issues such as sexual orientation, class, or race that Ellen cannot change? It would be unfair to Tracy for Ellen to proceed with therapy without clarifying and resolving Tracy's concerns about working with her. Ellen has an ethical obligation to inform Tracy about her knowledge and competence with respect to any concerns that Tracy may raise (IVA). If Ellen does not feel competent to work with Tracy or if she ascertains that Tracy has strong feelings against working with her, it is Ellen's responsibility to make an appropriate referral.

Another significant issue in this dilemma is the fact that the grievance must be "owned" by the client and not her therapist or attorney (IIA). Again, the control over the choice of action must rest with Tracy. It is essential that Ellen be sensitive to the need to protect Tracy's well-being as she advises her about a possible grievance procedure. It is certainly important to try to investigate Tracy's claims of abuse against her previous therapist and, if valid, to take steps to prevent further abuse of clients (VA). However, the scenario indicates that Tracy is experiencing a great deal of distress including suicidal thoughts. Any steps to protect other clients must be balanced with the protection of Tracy.

A final related issue is confidentiality (IIIB). To what extent can the therapist or the lawyer insure confidentiality if Tracy pursues a grievance against a former therapist? Can confidentiality be maintained in the face of charges that the former therapist is harassing her? If Tracy's suicidal potential increases, confidentiality must clearly be waived. The irony of this case is that Tracy is seeking protection from a therapist who allegedly victimized her and unless Ellen as her new therapist is very careful, she can inadvertantly prolong the victimization process. Ellen must help Tracy take the time to fully explore the implications of any action she might take, particularly as she might end up feeling exploited by publicity or someone else's agenda. (Janis Sanchez-Hucles)

RESPONDENT 2

In Tracy's case, the following ethical dilemmas are apparent:

1. Tracy, whose distrust of therapists is justifiable, is not particularly interested in consulting another therapist. She has been coerced to do so by her lawyer in an effort to pursue legal action against the therapist who is harassing her.

2. Tracy is forced to seek the assistance of Ellen, who was not her first choice, because the therapists she preferred had no time to see her.

3. Ellen is faced with responding ethically to the newly acquired knowledge that an experienced but unconventional therapist, with whom she is familiar, is Tracy's alleged perpetrator.

4. Tracy's enormous psychological distress, including suicidality, revealed by the document certainly intensifies Ellen's professional responsibility to this woman.

Dilemmas 1 and 2 clearly indicate significant power differentials between Tracy, her lawyer, and her therapist(s). Tracy is reluctantly seeking a consultation. Furthermore, even as she complies with the lawyer's recommendation, she does not have access to the counselor she prefers. Therefore, it is important for Ellen to be sensitive to these power differentials and to acknowledge them with Tracy early in their work together (IIA, C, D). Not only would her response convey critical levels of respect and empathy but the probability of gaining trust would be enhanced. Ellen will need to face the reality that controversial issues concerning race in the United States are often transferred into the therapeutic relationship. Since Tracy is African-American, it is particularly crucial for Ellen to acknowledge these conditions early in her contact with Tracy, since building rapport with African-American clients tends to occur rapidly, if at all, within the first two or three sessions (IA, C). In addition, Ellen's willingness to speak openly about this racial difference would model an appropriate use of personal power for Tracy (IIB). Even if she and Tracy were both African-Americans, Ellen would need to be mindful of power differentials between herself and Tracy. Therefore, Ellen should inform Tracy of her rights as a consumer of therapy (IID).

Since sexual intimacies and sexualized behaviors are forbidden between therapists and clients, it is Ellen's ethical responsibility to question the alleged abusive therapeutic practices of Tracy's previous therapist (IIIC, VA). Furthermore, in view of Tracy's enormous psychological distress, it is necessary that Ellen intervene early and as appropriately as possible. (Yvonne M. Jenkins)

DILEMMA F

Sue has seen Rena, a therapist trained in family therapy, for several months in order to work out problems of poor self-esteem, nonassertiveness, occasional rageful outbursts at her children and husband, and problems communicating with her husband. Sue feels intimidated by her husband Sam. Although he has never hit her, he has threatened her, calls her names (dummy and stupid), has said numerous times that he is exasperated with her, and says he will leave if she does not "shape up." Rena has suggested several strategies for improving self-esteem to Sue including taking an aerobics class, an assertiveness-training class, and a class on men's and women's communication styles at the local community college. Rena also has suggested that Sam is trying, albeit inappropriately, to make contact with Sue. She sees him as frustrated, lonely, and inadequately prepared for dealing with conflict. She advises that they work with her in family therapy to help Sam feel more connected and more loved. Rena thinks it will strengthen the marriage and help Sue feel better about herself.

RESPONDENT 1

Sue's case calls for a "proactive stance toward the eradication of oppression" and " working toward empowering women" (Preamble). The therapist has adopted a therapeutic approach that is aimed at enabling

Sue to live in an emotionally abusive marriage rather than actively supporting the client to consider alternatives that allow her greater opportunity to choose other options.

An initial concern is whether or not Rena is practicing outside of her area of competence with Sue. The ethical guidelines are clear in stating that therapists should work within their areas of competency and reevaluate their training with respect to new developments in feminist knowledge (IVA). Rena's approach will undoubtedly border on victim-blame in that her focus is on improving Sue's communication skills and her feelings of competence/confidence through such methods as aerobics classes. This strategy reinforces the idea that Sue's abuse is caused by her behavior and that if her behavior changes, the abuse will end. Literature on abuse indicates that Sue's complaints may most likely be the result of abuse and not the cause (Walker, 1984). Rena may need more training to help her direct her interventions toward what should be the central issue of this therapy, the emotional abuse of Sue and the power differential she feels in relationship to her husband (IVB).

Rena needs to be aware that this power differential and the patriarchal structure of society make it easy for Sue to think that she, rather than her husband's behavior, is the problem. It is common for victims of abuse to feel helpless, powerless, and disempowered. Does Rena recognize this syndrome of powerlessness as a possible feature in the therapeutic alliance? To what extent was there an open discussion of therapeutic goals? Did Rena provide Sue with the safety to make an informed decision about whether she wants to stay in this marriage and stay in this therapy (IID)?

When Rena recommends family therapy, she risks contributing to the normalization of the abuse in Sue's life. Her interpretation of the problems between Sue and Sam puts Sue's abuse in a secondary position to the needs of her husband. The therapeutic strategies are problematic because the central issues of protecting the client's well-being, eradicating the sources of oppression she faces, and empowering her are not being directly addressed. (Janis Sanchez-Hucles)

RESPONDENT 2

The therapist's response to Sue demonstrates dangerously conceived therapy. Because of the verbal abuse and threatening behavior of her husband, Rena places Sue in both psychological and physical peril by suggesting family/couples therapy. Evidently Rena is unaware of the increased potential for violence to erupt during family work where abuse is an issue (Bograd, 1992). If so, Rena is practicing outside the limits of her competence, which entails a departure from ethical practice (IVD).

Rena should explain the safety issues involved for Sue and help her to protect herself (IIA, D). Next, she could begin to educate Sue on the dynamics of power and oppression being acted out in her marriage. Because feminist therapists are also concerned with the empowering aspects of social change efforts for all women, Rena could provide a model for Sue by encouraging her to become involved in other social contexts where emotional and physical abuse of women is addressed. (Gail Civish)

DILEMMA G

Jeanette, obviously frightened and wary, arrived at the college counseling center and requested an appointment as soon as possible. Mary Louise, the walk-in counselor, learns that the night before Jeanette awakened to find John, a friend she had gone out with once or twice and who lived in the same dorm, fondling her and climbing into her bunk. She screamed, John left, and her roommate raced in from the living room to see what was the matter. Jeanette is shaking and distraught as she tells this story. She wants John (who had been drinking beer with her and her roommate before she went to bed) moved out of the dorm, but she does not want to get her roommate or him in trouble. She also does not want her parents to find out. Jeanette, a freshman, is the only daughter of a wealthy Filipino-American engineer and his wife. She says, "This would kill them and they would pull me out of school." She wants the school administration to take action right away. She has not slept, is afraid to be by herself, is convinced she will fail her midterms next week, and is saying that she might as well be dead.

RESPONDENT 1

The first issue of concern in this dilemma is the well-being of Jeanette. Given that she is in college, she is probably 18 years of age and a legal adult. Mary Louise should first evaluate her safety. If Jeanette is a high risk for suicide, normal confidentiality guidelines do not hold. Depending on her response to being informed that she is considered "dangerous to herself," several options should be evaluated. For example, the therapist may decide to initiate involuntary commitment procedures if she determines that Jeanette is highly suicidal and unwilling to enter a hospital. She might also explore setting up a sort of "house arrest" with the collaboration of friends, family, and residence hall staff to protect Jeanette until she is through the dangerous period. Because the client is 18, the clinician is not required to inform her parents, though it may be desirable to do so. Jeanette is Filipino and Mary Louise does not yet know the degree of her family's acculturation. Therefore, Mary Louise would do well to respect the Filipino's need to keep social conflict unexposed, and while remaining sensitive to this need, provide as many options as possible in order to protect the client's safety (IA, B).

After Jeanette is calmed and not in imminent danger to herself, Mary Louise must address her dilemma between not wishing to "get John and her roommate in trouble" and "wanting John removed from the dorm." Mary Louise must explain Jeanette's confidentiality privilege, that she retains the right to disclose what happened to her or not, and that she risks losing some control over the course of events if she does disclose her experience to the university administration (IIC, D). If Jeanette wants Mary Louise's help in revealing the incident (and Mary Louise thinks that this support is clinically indicated), a release of information must be signed by Jeanette. Furthermore, Jeanette needs to understand that even if she does not wish to press charges against John the administration may want to call her as a witness should it decide to pursue the case. Once Jeanette's safety and comfort in therapy are assured, Mary Louise may be able to help her understand how certain cultural values pertaining to keeping personal and family conflict hidden may help perpetuate the ongoing abuse of Filipino women (IB). (Gail Civish)

RESPONDENT 2

Assuming that Jeanette and Mary Louise's backgrounds differ along significant dimensions, Mary Louise's willingness to be of assistance to Jeanette within a culturally relevant framework is essential (IA). Therefore, if necessary Mary Louise should seek culturally competent supervision and not pass her along to a counselor of Asian descent. Of course, Jeanette should be referred to another resource if Mary Louise is at a point in her personal and professional development that precludes her from embracing diversity, lacks the competence to address the issues involved, or does not have culturally competent supervision available to her (IVA). From a cultural standpoint, the concepts of shame, honor, saving face, and the significance of reverence for parents and elders are central to Jeanette's issues. An awareness of gender roles of Asian-American women and awareness of the related oppression they have suffered are also essential to working with her (Chan, 1988). The therapist must take responsibility for educating herself about cultural diversities and the many forms of oppression in her clients' lives (IA, B, IID).

The challenge is to develop a relationship within an atmosphere of mutuality that empowers Jeanette after a very disempowering episode (IIIC). In the process, it is important to protect Jeanette's rights to confidentiality (IIIB) and take appropriate steps to ensure them in as caring and reassuring a manner as possible. Maintaining a caring and trustworthy stance can be particularly significant on a university campus where the counselor may need to collaborate with housing staff or other professionals who may not be governed by clear norms of confidentiality. Procedures for filing a grievance and information about what can be expected administratively and emotionally should be thoroughly explained to Jeanette (VIIA).

As Mary Louise is a walk-in counselor at Jeanette's college counseling center, Mary Louise has multiple avenues for impacting social change in that setting (VB), such as educating students and employees at the college about what constitutes various forms of sexual misconduct, the role of alcohol and drugs in the occurrences of such behavior, how precipitating conditions and actual occurrences may be perceived differently by young men and women, and ways to prevent such episodes in the future. Mary Louise could also participate in lending her expertise to student and administrative bodies that develop and implement policies related to the treatment of these issues on campus in an effort to eradicate further victimization through manifestations of prejudice, discrimination, or forms of unfair treatment. (Yvonne M. Jenkins)

IMPLICATIONS

Victims of violence remain vulnerable to many forms of disempowerment and revictimization. For example, Bessel van der Kolk (1987) reports that sexual abuse survivors describe a shocking array of abusive experiences in adulthood. Twenty to 30% of the women he interviewed were abused by therapists and other health care providers. Sixty-eight percent experienced rape or attempted rape. Fifty-three percent reported unwanted sexual advances from authority figures. Most of the reactors have emphasized the significance of boundary protection, confidentiality, and consent in work with clients. Empowerment of the client emerges as the preeminent concern and must always temper the most well-intended urges to help a client who has been violated. Furthermore, the respondents frequently discuss the importance of incorporating a proactive stance and advocacy/educational functions into the fabric of therapy.

Many respondents speak to the complexities and confusions that are inevitable in working with clients when assumptions about culture, class, race, and sexual orientation are limited and biased. In all cases, an alertness to and understanding of the experience and management of power remain very significant. The therapist must remind herself that her professional role carries multiple meanings regarding power and authority that are anchored in the client's cultural standpoint. The therapist's responses to the client's presentation, equally determined by her position in a gender/class/cultural/racial web, will shape her particular reactions to the client's dilemmas. For example, a client's apparent reluctance to report a sexual violation and/or her seeming passivity in problem solving with the therapist may be wrongly interpreted as evidence of psychological pathology as opposed to a reflection of the client's culturally derived assumptions about her power in relation to persons of authority. Hill, Glaser, and Harden's work on decision making reminds therapists that clinical problem solving must be conducted as a collaboration with the client in which there is a built-in corrective for the development of faulty formulations about the client's status and the likelihood that the therapist could make plans of action without the full participation of the client.

The feminist therapist needs to face her own conscious and unconscious biases. She needs to seek information about any client who is different from her in subtle or obvious ways. Therapists learn from clients, to be sure, but must not rely on them for education about people and ways of life that are unfamiliar. Mainstream therapeutic materials that carefully deal with these issues are sadly scarce. Faculty are often unaware of their biases and make little effort to include helpful readings on diversity (Higginbotham, 1990). Unpacking the knapsack of white privilege (McIntosh, 1986) is an ongoing struggle. Not engaging in the struggle can subtly revictimize clients, increasing their sense of hopelessness, powerlessness, and isolation.

Javed makes an extremely important point when she warns of the "danger of making little attempt to go beyond stereotypic notions of a culture. . . . that eliminate complexities and controversies within the culture." In an effort to respect the client's culture, a therapist may inadvertently create a triple-edged transgression in which she (1) assumes she knows about a given culture's gender arrangements and subsequently fails to develop more complex understandings of the "intricacies of gender relations as they are mediated by class, religion, and cultural mythology" (Hayden); (2) avoids protecting the client from on-going or future violence; and (3) perpetuates limited and prejudiced mythologies about that culture. Mattis, echoing these concerns, adds a note of caution about the possibly precipitous leap to the assumption of sexual violation with a client when her history, social, and cultural situation have not been thoroughly explored. Therapists are accountable for continuing education and consultation, particularly in areas outside their experience and expertise.

In some instances, the therapist is pulled by competing imperatives in which it appears that she must privilege one ethical standard over another. However, feminist therapists assert that any level of violence, regardless of a particular culture's tolerance for violent acts from men toward women and children is personally unacceptable and psychologically damaging for all people. Cultural and class-related traditions require sensitive understanding but not universal respect. It is essential for each therapist to develop a framework for practice that is well anchored in an analysis of violence that incorporates culture but does not bow under the weight of cultural tradition. It is vitally important to remain clear about positions on violence, particularly during periods of cultural disruption and backlash. Cross-cultural studies on domestic violence, for example, show that battering and rape increase in times of economic and political insecurity (Cole et al., 1992). In her essay "The Mind That Burns in Each Body: Women, Rape, and Racial Violence," Jacquelyn Down Hall (1983) theorizes that when highly stratified and rigidly enforced gender ideologies give way to the pressure of liberation movements, violence and racial hatred increase. Currently, in spite of liberalized rape shield laws and increased consciousness about assault in the United States, rape rates have increased (Fairstein, 1993).

Several other themes touched on by the respondents deserve amplification. The probability that therapists will need to work with clinical problems involving violence is high, and in many cases ethical behaviors will include communicating and collaborating with other professionals and organizations. Zald, in her response to Dilemma C, illustrates the ethical dilemmas that evolve from colliding organizational systems that hold staff accountable to policies and procedures (and funding agencies) in such a way as to compromise the protection of the client. Feminist therapists need to develop sophisticated understandings of the systems within which they work and with which they intersect. Organizations, as Zald points out, may traumatize clients when institutional practices overlook the needs of traumatized people. However, organizations themselves can become traumatized when boundary transgressions among staff and between staff and clients occur, thus creating dysfunctional climates for workers and clients. The health of organizations in terms of their protection of vulnerable populations, the education of their staffs on subjects such as violence and sexual harassment, and the ethical construction of policies and procedures should become part of the feminist therapist's concerns.

Therapist abuse of clients is an ongoing concern. Laura Brown, in her discussion of the problem in confronting a colleague, offers an important reminder:

An essential philosophical core of the confrontation of feminist therapy colleagues is the conceptualization of ethical actions as a continuum. . . . All therapists move throughout their work lives from place to place on that continuum; the realization that we carry the potential for abuse is an important one to hold in consciousness when preparing for a confrontation. . . . This awareness is essential for avoiding an internal image of the offending therapist as the existential other. (1990, p. 150)

She points out that all therapists are, for a variety of reasons, vulnerable to engaging in potentially harmful behavior toward clients. There are many disturbing examples of powerful and destructive reenactments of trauma in the therapeutic setting (Brown, 1991; Herman, 1992). For example, ethical self-examination with respect to self-care, continuing education, and peer supervision is essential in the often volatile area of identification with the histories and feelings of clients. One should also carefully consider the wisdom of self-disclosure, contact with a client outside the therapy appointment, intervention with others related to the client, even with permission but most especially without permission. For all clients, but particularly survivors of incest and sexual assault, boundary transgressions including self-disclosure, spontaneously extending sessions, and touching clients are usually to be avoided. Impulses to do otherwise, regardless of the conscious altruistic intent, are often complex responses to very horrific and painful situations that require thoughtful discussions in supervision or with trusted colleagues.

The decision-making model by Hill, Glaser, and Harden offers a strategy for collaboratively discovering the personal significance of powerful responses to clients. They incorporate personal/affective dimensions into the process of making ethical decisions about clinical interventions. The nature of one's feelings toward a client, such as feeling like a friend, a rescuer, a good mother, an overburdened caregiver, or an outraged advocate, must also be seen as ingredients that can support or hinder the goal of doing no harm and offering help. These feelings must be regularly discussed with consulting colleagues before being expressed in the therapy.

Furthermore, ethical feminist practice will offer the possibility for confronting colleagues whose potentially or unequivocally unethical conduct has come to the therapist's attention. Brown (1990) and others discuss the necessity of clarifying and identifying with the same standards to which one would hold others in making a confrontation. Front and center among these should be a concern with abuses of power. Confronting possible abuses of power may set in motion a cascading series of consequences involving further unforeseen compromises to a client's empowerment. For example, consider the situation in which a client reports a boundary violation by a former therapist known to the current therapist, and one's ethics and legal statutes mandate reporting to a state licensing board and/or a professional association. If the client has been unable to confront the former therapist and remains unready to do so, the therapist faces a thorny ethical dilemma revolving around the concern for the client's readiness and her confidentiality in the first place and duty to report in the second. Consider also a situation in which one learns from a client about an affair the client's friend is having with her therapist who is also one's associate or a case in which one becomes aware of boundary transgressions by a colleague who is currently being sued for one of these transgressions. In both these situations, the impulse to confront, based on a conviction about holding ourselves collectively accountable to ethical standards of practice, may lead to unexpected disempowering effects on clients and undesirable disruption of legal proceedings already in progress. The point is clear that impulsive action in this territory is inevitably in error. Hill, Glaser, and Harden's model for ethical decision making offers a particularly valuable approach to managing these difficult choices in that it acknowledges that no simple answer exists to problems that require the protection of many people's rights and safety. Their model allows for the fact that good decisions about strategy with clients and colleagues most likely evolve over time, are best made collaboratively, are dependent on many idiosyncratic factors such as the feelings and history of the therapist, and recognize the degree of difficulty one experiences in confronting a colleague.

Clearly, decision making about the confrontation of one's colleague involves a complicated and necessarily collaborative sorting through of options. It will be necessary to reckon with many questions. What are the parameters of one's role? What are the boundaries of one's colleague group, and to whom is one accountable? Is the therapeutic process enhanced or undermined by outside advocacy and confrontation of offending therapists? Feminists do not always agree on these matters as is clear from the differences in emphasis among respondents. Much discussion and debate are needed in order to become more familiar with the complexities intrinsic to overlapping responsibilities as ethical practitioners. Brown (1990) urges feminist therapists to accept colleague confrontation as an important professional responsibility, as a means of monitoring professional impact, and as a way of supporting one another in the extremely challenging work with survivors of abuse and other forms of violence.

RESPONDENTS

Gayle Civish, PhD, is a clinical psychologist in private practice in Lakewood, CO, who specializes in women's issues and works with adolescents and children.

Mary Hayden, PhD, is a clinical psychologist in private practice in Pasadena, CA, who works with survivors of childhood abuse and with lesbian issues, particularly relationship enhancement.

Nayyar S. Javed, MEd, born and raised in Pakistan, works as a psychologist in the Saskatoon Mental Health Clinic, Saskatoon, Saskatchewan, and is a feminist therapist who works with racialized populations and women with eating disorders.

Yvonne M. Jenkins, PhD, is a counseling and clinical psychologist on the staff of the Harvard University Health Services and is a coauthor of *Diversity in Psychotherapy: The Politics of Race, Ethnicity, and Gender* (1993).

Jacqueline Mattis, MA, Jamaican-American, is a candidate in clinical psychology at the University of Michigan, teaches psychology and women's studies, and does research on the narratives of women of color and themes of resistance and survival.

Barbara McCandlish, PhD, received her degree from Harvard University in 1976, was one of the founders of the Somerville Women's Mental Health Clinic and the Bay Area Women's Center, and is currently in private practice in Santa Fe, NM.

Lynn Bravo Rosewater, PhD, a clinical psychologist in private practice in Cleveland, OH, works with and on behalf of survivors of violence and battered women as a therapist, consultant, and expert witness.

Janis Sanchez-Hucles, PhD, an African-American feminist with Cuban roots, is currently Associate Professor of Psychology and Director of Clinical Training at Old Dominion University and serves on two national APA task forces, Urban Initiatives and Violence and the Family.

Joan Zald, MSW, is a clinical social worker in private practice in Ann Arbor, MI, who works with survivors of violence and as a consultant to agencies on the subject of boundary violations in therapy.

REFERENCES

Bart, P., & Moran, E. G. (Eds.). (1993). *Violence against women: The bloody footprints.* Thousand Oaks, CA: Sage.

Bograd, M. (1992). Values in conflict: Challenges to family therapists' thinking. *Journal of Marriage and Family Therapy, 18*(3), 245–256.

Brodsky, A. M. (1986). The distressed psychologist: Sexual intimacies and exploitation. In R. R. Kilburg, P. E. Nathan, & R. W. Thorson (Eds.), *Professionals in distress* (pp. 153–171). Washington, DC: American Psychological Association.

Brown, L. (1985). Ethics and business practice in feminist therapy. In L. B. Rosewater & L. E. A. Walker (Eds.), *Handbook of feminist therapy: Women's issues in psychotherapy* (pp. 297–304). New York: Springer.

Brown, L. (1990). Confronting ethically problematic behaviors in feminist therapist colleagues. In H. Lerman & N. Porter (Eds.), *Feminist ethics in psychotherapy* (pp. 147–159). New York: Springer.

Brown, L. (1991). Not outside the range: One feminist perspective on psychic trauma. *American Imago, 48*(1), 119–133.

Brownmiller, S. (1975). *Against our will.* New York: Simon & Schuster.

Butler, S. (1978). *Conspiracy of silence: The trauma of incest.* San Francisco: Volcano Press.

Chan, C. (1988). Asian-American women: Psychological responses to sexual exploitation and cultural stereotypes. In L. Fulani (Ed.), *The psychopathology of everyday racism and sexism.* New York: Harrington Press.

Cole, E., & Rothblum, E. (Eds.), & Espin, O. (Guest Ed.). (1992). Refugee women and their mental health: Shattered societies, shattered lives [Special issue]. *Women and Therapy, 13*(1, 2).

Fairstein, L. (1993). *Sexual Violence: Our war against rape.* New York: Morrow.

Feminist Therapy Institute. (1987). *Feminist therapy code of ethics.* Denver: Author.

Gartrell, N., Herman, J., Olarte, S., Feldstein, M., & Localio, R. (1986). Psychiatrist–patient sexual contact: Results of a national survey. *American Journal of Psychiatry, 143,* 112–131.

Hall, J. D. (1983). The mind that burns in each body: Women, rape, and racial violence. In A. Snitnow, C. Stansell, & S. Thompson (Eds.), *Powers of desire: The politics of sexuality.* New York: Monthly Review Press.

Herman, J. L. (1981). *Father–daughter incest.* Cambridge: Harvard University Press.

Herman, J. L. (1992). *Trauma and recovery.* New York: Basic Books.

Herman, J. L., & Harvey, M. (1993). The false memory debate: Social science or social backlash? *The Harvard Mental Health Newsletter, 9*(10), 4–6.

Higginbotham, E. (1990). Designing an inclusive curriculum: Bringing all women into the core. *Women's Studies Quarterly, 18,* (1, 2), 7–23.

Janoff-Bulman, R. (1992). *Shattered assumptions: Towards a new psychology of trauma.* New York: Free Press.

Javed, N. (1992). *Homeless and abused: Reflections and observations on racialized women's experience of abuse.* Paper presented to the Blue Ribbon Panel on Violence against Women, Saskatoon, SA.

Lederer, L. (Ed.). (1980). *Take back the night: Women on pornography.* New York: Morrow.

Loftus, E. (1993). Repressed memories of childhood trauma: Are they genuine? *The Harvard Mental Health Newsletter, 9*(9), 4–5.

Masson, J. M. (1984). *Assault on the truth: Freud's suppression of the seduction theory.* New York: Farrar, Strauss & Giroux.

McGrath, E., Keita, P., Strickland, B., & Russo, N. (Eds.). (1990). *Women and depression: Risk factors and treatment issues.* Washington, DC: American Psychological Association.

McIntosh, P. (1986). *Unpacking the invisible knapsack.* Wellesley, MA: Stone Center Working Papers.

Miles, R. (1989). *Racism.* London: Routledge.

Ochberg, F., & Willis, D. (Eds.). (1991). Psychotherapy with victims [Special issue]. *Psychotherapy, 28*(1).

Phillips, J. (1993). Review of Roiphe, K. The morning after: Sex, fear, and feminism on campus. *The Women's Review of Books, 11*(2), 6.

Pollit, K. (1993, October 4). Not just bad sex. *The New Yorker,* pp. 220–224.

Pope, K. S., & Bouhoutsos, J. (1986). *Sexual intimacy between therapists and patients.* New York: Praeger.

Psychology in the public forum. (1993). *American Psychologist, 48*(10), 105–107.

Roiphe, K. (1993). *The morning after: Sex, fear, and feminism on campus.* Boston: Little, Brown.

Rosewater, L. B. (1990). Public advocacy. In H. Lerman & N. Porter (Eds.), *Feminist ethics in psychotherapy.* New York: Springer.

Rush, F. (1980). *The best kept secret: Sexual abuse of children.* Englewood Cliffs, NJ: Prentice-Hall.

Said, E. (1979). *Orientalism.* New York: Vintage Books.

Schechter, S. (1982). *Women and male violence.* New York: Macmillan.

van der Kolk, B. A., & Greenberg, M. S. (1987). The psychobiology of the trauma response: Hyperarousal, constriction, and addiction to traumatic reexposure. In B. A. van der Kolk (Ed.), *Psychological trauma* (pp. 63–87). Washington, DC: American Psychiatric Association.

Walker, L. (1979). *The battered woman.* New York: Harper & Row.

Walker, L. (1984). *Women and mental health policy.* Beverly Hills: Sage.

Walker, L. (1987). *Terrifying love: Why battered women kill and how society responds.* New York: Harper & Row.

Walker, L. (1991). Post-traumatic stress disorder in women: Diagnosis and treatment of battered women syndrome. *Psychotherapy, 28*(1), 21–29.

Williams, J. (1993). *Legislative hearings on incest/sexual abuse.* Reported on Women's Studies electronic list, May 10, 1993.

Women's Action Coalition. (1993). *WAC Stats: The facts about women.* New York: The New Press.

Wright, L. (1993, May 17 and May 24). Remembering satan, *The New Yorker,* pp. 60–66; 54–66.

EIGHT

Reproduction/ Health Issues

Denise C. Webster

The development in the United States of the National Agenda on Women's Health during the early 1990s has been only the most recent result of centuries of struggle for Western women to honor the differences between the sexes and not use those differences to justify oppression and exploitation. The Cartesian separation of mind and body, which has dominated the view of Western medicine since the Middle Ages, relegated the "mind" to men and the "body" to women. Historically, then, the term "women's health" has been a euphemism for "women's illness," and the particular illnesses were assumed to be peculiarly "women's" because of women's reproductive capacities. Consequently, most of these definitions have tended to reflect a view that "women's health problems" invariably involve too much or too little reproducing (Webster & Lipetz, 1986). This clearly subjective perception has always been based on variables such as the culture, class, and ethnicity of women themselves and of those who have been in the position of diagnosing or legitimizing "problems" and perpetuating "solutions."

Often in parallel with women's movements, the women's health movement has also been around for centuries. With almost cyclic regularity, periods of oppression are eventually followed by resurgences of expression as new generations recycle woman-centered values to address women's needs in changing societies (Ruzek, 1978). The witch hunts of Western Europe and New England spanning the 12th to the 17th centuries represented an organized assault on women who dared to treat other, often poor, women and to interfere with the will of Providence, as defined by the reigning triumvirate of religious, legal, and medical men (Achterberg, 1991). This historical tragedy vividly highlights the inherently intertwined fates of women as both consumers and providers of health care. It is likely that as long as women are denied legitimate access to information with which to empower their lives, there will be a women's health movement.

During the 19th century in the United States, the "Popular Health Movement" was organized to provide women with information about their bodies. This social movement coincided with the growth of women's medical schools and the beginning of the "modern" period of nursing (Ehrenreich & English, 1978). During the recent women's movement of the later 20th century, increasing knowledge about reproduction has resulted in an "improved technology" that has the potential of forever changing the biological imperatives defining women as primarily childbearers and childrearers. As with any powerful "discovery," this "improvement" has carried with it the potential for abuse. Many women have been exposed to health risks that were disproportionately weighed against financial profits of large pharmaceutical companies. Concern about "overpopulation" in Third World countries has resulted in coercive pressure to force women to be sterilized, have abortions, or use contraceptives in return for financial aid that would allow them to feed the children they already had (Committee on Women, Population, and the Environment, 1992; Holmes, Hoskins, & Gross, 1980). The centrality of the feminist belief in a woman's right to control her reproductive capacity has made access to abortion (either surgical or with abortifacients such as RU-486) among the most explosive political issues of the current century. At the other end of the spectrum are concerns about the ethical, religious, moral, political, and economic feasibility and advisability of "genetic engineering," fertility treatments, and high-risk perinatal interventions.

Although women continue to be the victims of overmedicalization, particularly for caesarean sections, hysterectomies, and psychotropic drug prescriptions, they have, paradoxically, been greatly underrepresented in research that might identify important differences based on the physiology of sex differences. After years of lobbying in the United States, in 1990 the National Institutes of Health established an Office of Research on Women's Health. Both reproductive and nonreproductive health issues are targeted by this office in an attempt to develop information about sexual difference or similarity in the incidence, etiology, and treatment of a wide variety of health problems (Clancy & Massion, 1992; Dan & Hemphill, 1992).

The ongoing controversies about the origins and solutions to problems of "women's health" reflect the same underlying philosophical tensions that appear in the current women's movement. The differences between liberal, socialist, and radical positions tend to blur when applied to real-life situations. The growing number of "feminisms" listed in the Dictionary of Feminist Theory (Humm, 1990) also attests to the difficulty of simplistic solutions to complex issues. Nevertheless, it is still useful to recognize some of these differences, albeit simplified, in assumptions that fuel both the work of the current women's health movement and the tensions that prevail within it.

Fee (1975) described the liberal view as questioning why women do not have more power in the power structures, rather than questioning the power structures themselves. From this perspective, there should be more women physicians and scientists to study and treat women's health problems. Legal assurances of nondiscrimination, such as the protection of women's right to choose abortion, would also be seen as valuable. The socialist feminist, however, would question the elitism of physicians in the power hierarchy and the role of the power elite in supporting hierarchies within the health care provider system. From this perspective, legitimizing "professionalism" and resenting the considerable pay differences between specialists and generalists or between physician and nonphysician workers serve to funnel energies away from recognizing the profit motives in interlocking corporate relationships among government agencies, insurance industries, pharmaceutical companies, and health care "corporations."

Within the radical feminist groups described by Fee (1975), most would identify several major strains. One thrust is toward acting on the beliefs that "the personal is the political" and "knowledge is power." The Boston Women's Health Book Collective compiled and made the book *Our New Bodies, Ourselves* (1992) available to millions of women who were able to obtain information about their bodies that empowered them to undertake self-care, to question health care providers, and to open alternative health care clinics, such as the Feminist Women's Health Centers throughout the country. Within this group are those who see separatism, lesbian or otherwise, as the most reasonable course of action to protect women from the dominant culture and to provide viable alternatives to the power structures within that culture. Some radical feminists like Shulamith Firestone (1970) have advocated rejection of the female biological imperative through the development of reproductive cybernetic technologies. Others celebrate the reproductive capacities of women and see the differences between the genders as of central importance (Gaskin, 1990). For some, the Wiccan and other Goddess-oriented practices create a spiritual impetus for rituals developed around the wonder of women's reproductive abilities (Adler,1986; Carson, 1992; Guiley, 1991; Noble, 1983; Walker, 1983).

The Feminist Therapy Code of Ethics reflects all of these positions, most apparently in those principles related to hierarchy/power and the right to choose. In addition, the principles of respect for cultural differences, involvement in social change, and therapist accountability take on very real dimensions in the following cases. The feminist therapist whose work encompasses a knowledge and practice of women's health has some additional ethical concerns. Cultural differences (I) profoundly affect even what is defined as health or illness. These differences may be obvious or subtle. For example, greater body weight may be considered healthy in some cultural groups. Among contemporary North Americans "fitness" often is a euphemism for "attractive," which is, in turn, a euphemism for "very thin," and possibly unhealthy (Iazzeto, 1992). Power differentials (II) and concerns about overlapping relationships (III) become even more crucial when physical boundaries are lowered as is the case when therapists use "body therapies" in treating long-standing emotional difficulties. Several of the contributors to this section are nurses, as well as feminist therapists. The "license to touch" (e.g., give a backrub, as a nurse), may at times be at odds with the prohibitions against touch among psychotherapists in general.

Therapist accountability (IV) is crucial when dealing with issues around women's health because the rapidly changing information base can have important consequences for clients. Although "overmedicalization" is always to be avoided, it may be at least as important to avoid missing important physical clues to apparently psychosocial presentations. In the cases to follow, reactors are acutely aware that "knowing what you don't know" is a primary concern. In addition to the obvious health concerns related to protecting women's reproductive choice and prevention of physical and sexual abuse, the feminist therapist involved in women's health may have to stay alert to the implications of a particular and ever-changing social change (V) in the form of multiple and varied "health care agendas." Proposals by competing groups of health care providers, insurers, and populations at risk represent very different views about which health care needs are rights, and which are privileges, as well as who should be eligible for any kind of health care (Norsigian, 1993).

Despite the apparent focus on ethical situations involving women's reproductive capabilities, the case respondents make abundantly clear that the mind and body are not separate and that the social and psychological dimensions of health cannot be arbitrarily designated as isolated sources of problems or their solutions. Accordingly, all issues around health are potentially "women's health issues." Therapist accountability becomes increasingly difficult in this period of social change, politicalization of health care, and growing multicultural awareness. The responses to these six dilemmas reflect beautifully the range of differences in emphasis and interpretation that each therapist brings to practice and invite therapists to consider each case from multiple perspectives.

DILEMMA A

Lee is a high school counselor who strongly believes in the right to choose abortion. The state where she works recently passed a law requiring parental notification in cases of teenage pregnancy when the teenager is considering abortion. Judy is a 14-year-old whose parents belong to a fundamentalist religion. After a long, tearful session, Judy tells Lee she is 10 weeks pregnant and is terrified about telling either of her parents. Her father has made it clear that no daughter of his would be allowed back in the home if she became pregnant. Judy does not want to have a baby and recognizes that she is still a child herself. She believes that abortion is "murder" and asks Lee for direction.

RESPONDENT 1

There are many complex ethical issues involved in counseling a pregnant 14-year-old. Helping Judy resolve her ambivalence about her choices is of primary importance. To do so, the client will need accurate information about the health, educational, legal, psychological, cultural, and familial consequences of adoption, abortion, and teenage parenting. The counselor's goal is to increase the client's power and capacity for effective decision making (IIA, B). Once Judy has identified the most appropriate and least traumatic path for herself, other issues arise at each decision-making turn.

Lee has an ethical responsibility to be familiar with relevant community resources (IA). If she has not had experience helping a young woman through the decisions related to pregnancy, she should consider referral to someone who has (IVA). In the area of pregnancy counseling, the responsibility is to assure an experience for the client that will not increase the potential trauma. For instance, Lee and Judy each need to know if Planned Parenthood, Problem Pregnancy Referral services, or clergy representatives are biased in their approaches (IIB).

Lee also has an ethical responsibility to stay aware of her own prochoice biases (IC) and to monitor any subtle means by which she might communicate these to the client (IIA). Additionally, in some cultures adoption and/or abortion are value-laden. It is the responsibility of the counselor to be sensitive and thoughtful in helping the client explore these areas (IB), taking into consideration her unique set of ethnic, religious, and family circumstances.

There are potential threats to confidentiality in this case. Many states have complex procedures for parental notifications, consent, and/or judicial bypass. If the legal system or medical system become involved, the potential increases for Judy's problem being exposed to someone she knows. In a small community the counselor may have overlapping relationships with Judy's parents. If Judy's parents become suspicious and question the school about Judy's conversations with her counselor, Lee needs to be aware of exactly what Judy's parents have a legal right to know. Any rights or legal responsibilities of the putative father need to be discussed. If Judy continues the pregnancy, her parents will probably have financial responsibilities for the child. Lee, the counselor, needs to inform the client as to potential problems in these complex and conflicting relationships (IIIA).

A feminist therapist will be particularly concerned for her client's safety. She will listen closely for any history of violence or abuse in Judy's family. What is the meaning of Judy's father's threats? What if her father is the father of the baby? Judy needs to know her responsibilities for reporting child abuse, if uncovered, and inform Lee if action needs to be taken.

Lastly, if Judy and Lee do live in a state requiring parental consent, which forces a confrontation in a family such as Judy's, political behavior is ethical behavior. Participation in lobbying or public education against forced parental consent would be appropriate if she believes it to be consistent with her prochoice stance (VB). (Sandra Coffman, Dorsey Green, Carol Henry, and Susan Raab-Cohen)

RESPONDENT 2

Essential to this situation are two factors: (1) time and (2) Judy's own moral code. She will have to choose within one week's time which path she will take: abortion with parental notification, abortion without parental notification (perhaps in another state), or completing a full-term pregnancy with or without adoption. Either way, she will need to deal with her own internal moral issues, and the familial, religious, and social ramifications of her choice. Her well-being is first; the well-being of the fetus is part of her own well-being (IIA).

Crucial to this counseling relationship is the counselor's need to keep her own biases and her own personal experiences out of the content. Yet she will need to know where her own political/personal stance is in this matter so that she is aware of when she is intervening appropriately or not (IB, C). Is it in Lee's own professional code to inform Judy of the alternative to leave the state and proceed with an abortion in a state where it is not mandatory for parental notification? If she is committed to having Judy informed of all options, she must (IA).

Again, Judy must make her own choice based on her own internal codes and based on what the options are. Judy is young, impressionable, and in intense crisis. She may want someone to make her decision for her. If the counselor discusses outcomes she has read about or known about from other teens or young women in the same situation, this knowledge might cloud Judy's own sense of what will be right for her (IIA). Her particular religious background, her seemingly authoritative father, and her own sense of her present and future needs conflict, potentially leaving her with a sense of helplessness and a loss of power. She must regain her sense of power through this process of "options" and "choosing." She must be intelligently informed of her rights as an individual, perhaps not a concept she is used to. She must process each option thoroughly, knowing that whatever choice she makes, the counselor will be there to support her in accomplishing it in such a way that Judy restores her power and can go on with her life, knowing she has made the best choice for *herself* (IIA).

Judy will need tremendous help in dealing with the outcomes of either choice. Intervention on behalf of Judy with her family and religious community will be essential, though it might not be directly possible. Would the family be willing to work with the counselor? Would the family allow the counselor to mediate? Would the family wish secrecy within the religious community? Or would the family opt for a cold and impenetrable stone wall (IIIB)?

If Judy chooses abortion and is ostracized by her family, the religious community will know, and the family will experience repercussions. If Judy chooses pregnancy and is ostracized by her family, the religious community will know, and the family will experience repercussions. Will it be possible to empower the family to respect Judy's personal needs and worth, as well as that of the fetus, and can they come together as a family to support each other through this difficult situation?

Eventually follow-up for prevention of repeating an unplanned pregnancy is necessary. Birth control will need to be addressed whether abortion or adoption is the choice at this time. Optimally, in the follow-up, it would be in Judy's best interest for her to look at what circumstances existed and what choices she made that got her into this predicament in the first place. Either way, Judy's life must be positively impacted by all of the trauma and ordeal she will go through. (Nancy Wang)

DILEMMA B

Joan works in a hospital as a social worker and has been assigned a client from Cambodia whom the physician, a white male, has labeled "uncooperative." Mekala has come in for prenatal care but will not let the physician do an internal examination. She has also expressed a fear of "needles" and has indicated she will not allow any stitches after the birth. Joan's task, according to the physician, is to make the patient understand what is necessary for her to allow the hospital to do for healthy delivery.

RESPONDENT 1

What undergirds an ethical response is caring with integrity. Out of this care Joan will get to know the story of Mekala, the story of the white male physician, and will become aware of her own story (IB, C).

Joan must first find out about Mekala's ease in using English and whether it is sufficient for comprehension. If there are no family members with whom Mekala feels comfortable, Joan will be sensitive in reassuring Mekala that she will try to locate a woman translator, because the situation involves intimate female issues. The translator will inform Mekala about confidentiality and give assurances that gossip about her will not be bandied about in the Cambodian community (IIIB).

The obligation to learn a client's story permits the counselor to provide culture-sensitive care (IC) and to confront her own unexamined assumptions about those from different cultures. Similarly, in learning about the physician's story, Joan may become more aware of her unexamined assumptions about gender and professional cultures (IB). For example, Mekala may have no experience with Western medicine and find the idea of an internal examination by a male a serious personal invasion. She may have no understanding of Western medicine's inclinations to using fetal monitoring, anesthesia, or episiotomies for the birth experience. On the other hand, she may be highly educated and fluent in several languages, including English. Her reticence to submit to usual Western medical practices may represent her previous experiences with the medical system, personal preferences for a more natural childbirth, or religious taboos.

When Joan learns more about the physician's story she may find he has a sense of inadequacy in working with someone from another culture or that his concern is to maintain his status with a supervising physician. Another possibility is that there are observable reasons he is worried for the client, such as sudden blood loss or evidence of extremely high blood pressure with risk of seizures. Of course Joan has her own story, and any of these "stories" may challenge Joan's previous experiences with physicians, with clients, and with her own beliefs and values related to birth, life, and death. To receive a person's story with care and integrity and then out of that story act to advocate for a client who may have beliefs very different from her own is surely the essence of feminist ethics (IC, IIA, D). (Christine M. Chao)

RESPONDENT 2

Clients unwilling to accept standard procedures or practitioner's advice are often labeled as "uncooperative." The physician, who was educated from a single-view perspective, believes that his way is prudent, correct, and practical. For clients who are enculturated in the American society, the procedures and advice advocated by the physician may be acceptable. However, in this case, the physician has encountered a woman of another culture. Culture defines reality and meaning and therefore must be considered in all therapeutic interventions (IB).

In this case, Joan's first priority should be to gain an understanding of Mekala's beliefs regarding childbirth, prenatal care, and roles of others in childbirth. In order to do so, Joan may need an interpreter (if language barriers exist) and a culturally competent consultant (one who understands the client's culture) who can help to clarify what the client values in her health care and what she considers the normal process of childbirth. In addition, the interpreter and consultant (who may be the same person) should be used to inform Mekala of what is available to her in the American health care system including routine and emergency care. The client may require detailed explanations of certain services and should be free to choose from available options (IA, IIA).

Caution must be exercised that this client's culture is not used against her. Specifically, one could argue that because she does not seem to want anything that the system has to offer, she therefore does not need to receive any services or can be allowed to receive inadequate services. Joan needs to know about possible alternative resources that may be more acceptable to Mekala. Joan's primary role is to assist the client in obtaining the services that the client finds most helpful and useful. For some people, the appropriate choice might include not using a hospital for the birth or employment of nonphysicians during the birth (IA, IID).

Joan's ability to help Mekala feel accepted, valued, and cared for are critical elements in providing appropriate services to this client. The purpose of the search for meaning within the client's culture is understanding, which leads to identification of options for care and serves to let the client know that her experiences and beliefs are valued (IIA). Joan's role might include speaking to the client's physician regarding the client's wishes and sharing cultural views that must be understood in order to provide services to this client (IIC).

Joan must monitor her own views (IB) regarding clients of Asian descent and health care practices for women so that she does not unconsciously intimidate the client into acceptance or nonacceptance of options (IC). Joan may identify the need to formalize services in her community that meet the needs of women from various cultures. (Ruby J. Martinez)

RESPONDENT 3

Joan has been placed in a difficult position by the physician with whom she is working. She has been put in the middle between her own professional code of ethics and the needs of the physician and hospital to operate from their common stance that there is only one way to practice medicine, and that is their allopathic theory and technique. In addition, the theory and practice of childbirth in the allopathic tradition is usually male based. Thus women are often placed in the position of dealing with inflexible beliefs based on the AMA (allopathic) system and on male dominance (VA).

Joan, as a social worker, has been trained to respect and work with "where the client is." In this case there may be a personal situation and also a cultural mandate that governs Mekala's responses (IB). Joan must research the cultural practices of the Cambodian culture, if she has not already done so. Then, ethically, she must inform the physician, for he may not know them and therefore may not be taking this aspect into consideration in his treatment of Mekala. However, he may already know, or may even, after being informed, not care.

Depending on what the physician's response to Mekala's cultural practices are, Joan will need to make some decisions for outcome. If the physician and the client are willing to learn from each other, there might be a winning experience for both. However, if they are not willing to learn and adjust from each other's points of view, what are the possible directions to take?

1. To force Mekala to submit to the physician's technology against her will, causing her to endure any added hardship that is not necessary, would be unethical. Joan should not take part in this option if this is the physician's request (VA).

2. If Mekala's fears are based on her personal history and not on the Cambodian practice of childbirth, it would be useful to address her fears therapeutically, if she is willing. However, if she is not, it is important to respect her preference, to give her what she needs to make her experience of childbirth a positive one. There are many childbirth practitioners who do not use needles, stitch, or even have a need to stitch after childbirth (IA).

3. If her fear of needles and her request to not receive stitching after childbirth are cultural, her request must be respected. It is unethical to disregard another's cultural beliefs and practices. To treat each person as a whole and complete human being with dignity is an ethical responsibility. It is all too common that the Western world treats people of color or of different cultures as superstitious children (IIA).

4. Therefore, whether because of personal fears or cultural practices, Joan needs to find a birthing practitioner, male or female, doctor, nurse, or midwife, within the same or within another institution who will respect Mekala's needs. This option is her right to choose, and she must be informed of such an option.

Joan may need to empower Mekala to make choices that at first seem to go against her own cultural mandate "to please the authority." When working with Mekala, it is important not to divide her "be-ingness" by separating her "pregnancy" from herself as a whole person. Here again, the social worker must stand for the ethics of empowerment to the individual (and her environment) (IIA). Mekala is not a child-birthing practice; she is an entire entity who is impacted by her culture in every way. It behooves the social worker to know as much about the Cambodian culture as possible if she is going to work with any individual or family system from that culture.

Finally, Joan will need to get the support of her superiors in dealing with this issue. The physician and his colleagues may or may not appreciate her choices. It will be more and more essential that a hospital policy be adopted when such an interdepartmental/interprofessional conflict such as this arises. More and more, hospitals will need to acknowledge that their clientele will include people of many other cultures of the world. They must adjust their own attitudes and therefore their own practices to be inclusive. As a woman and practitioner, Joan has an ethical responsibility to fight for the rights of her clients, those whom she represents. By fighting for clients' rights, she is also fighting for all women's rights. Through her own actions of informing and educating, she will hopefully find the partners she will need in this fight (IIB). (Nancy Wang)

DILEMMA C

Maria is a Hispanic woman in her late 20s who has spent many years in and out of various institutions for drug abuse and attempted suicides. Based on testing, she has been labeled as having "borderline intelligence." Because she has a history of crack cocaine use, contact with multiple sexual partners, and has demonstrated limited ability to maintain herself outside an institutional setting, many staff members believe Maria should be sterilized. Other staff believe that such a decision would be an abuse of institutional power. Her mother has indicated she will take care of any grandchildren; however her ability to support her other children, still at home, is dependent on her maintaining her job. Rita's role is to work with staff to help them help Maria come to some decision about the matter.

RESPONDENT 1

The critical examination of current practices and beliefs in relation to women's health and reproduction are vital in assuring the health, dignity, and rights of all women. Good decisions are made, even in the most difficult situations, when minds and hearts remain open to the diverse and unique needs and values of each individual. Feminists must assertively act to influence prochoice and other political views that do not dictate options to women, but instead help women articulate their own views, feelings, and options. Therapists need to be willing to raise complex issues and to push against "the system" (if need be) in order to mobilize the resources needed in the suggested cases.

In helping staff to help Maria come to a decision, Rita's first goal would be to help staff become more aware of their own beliefs and feelings so that their role in the process may become clearer. Assuming Maria is capable of making a decision, though she may be limited in regard to intelligence and mental stability, Rita would ask them to have an open mind in the interest of helping the client. Remaining united and supportive to each other as well as toward Maria despite confronting such a controversial issue will provide the best opportunity for allowing Maria to come to a decision. Staff would be encouraged to voice their concerns. While respecting their views, Rita's role is to continually reinforce that the decision is complex and ultimately belongs to the client. In fact, the client should be informed that the decision is hers and be assured that she will be respected whatever decision she makes (IID).

In assisting staff to become clearer about their roles, Rita should ask them to consider what their own values are in relation to the issues raised and what they identify as the sources of these beliefs? They and Rita will have to understand what Maria's beliefs are about sexuality, children, and sterilization, and how these may differ from their own beliefs about these subjects. These differences may be based on informational understanding, religious or cultural beliefs, and family and community values (IB, C). In addition, it will be important to protect Maria's confidentiality in any discussions with her family (IIIA).

Power differences between staff and client must be acknowledged and reduced to prevent the client from being intimidated into a decision, particularly given her history of dependence upon institutions (IIA). Establishing too-short a time frame within which a decision from Maria would be expected could be considered coercive. The client must be afforded adequate time to consider alternatives carefully.

Staff members would need to decide whether they could remain open and supportive in Maria's interest. People who are highly conflicted by being asked to remain open to Maria's needs could opt to not work with this particular client. Staff and their views should be respected at all times throughout the process (IB).

As the person in charge of helping staff to help Maria, Rita may have a leadership role in the institution that would make her want to question why this issue is even being raised for this client. If the client had raised the issue of her own sterilization, there would be no conflict of interest, as long as the client received full disclosure regarding the procedure and informed consent was obtained. However, if the issue has surfaced in the interest of the institution, the question of whether all women in similar situations are asked to consider sterilization must be raised, or is Maria being treated differently? Maria, an ethnic minority woman of lower socioeconomic status and having personal limitations, is at risk for abuse of institutional power. Even if all women in similar situations were treated in this fashion, ethical issues would need to be raised regarding the morality of involuntary sterilization. One option might be to assist the client in accessing other health care services; however, it is not always realistic to find such resources (IA). Rita can role model respect for all ways of being and set the expectation that personal choice is highly valued.

Maria's situation is interesting because one can argue that the sterilization is necessary based upon her borderline intelligence, previous high-risk behavior with drugs and multiple sex partners, and limited capacity to care for herself (or a child). Where it may appear that staff are acting with the client's best interest in mind by recommending sterilization, such a recommendation is both paternalistic and may, in fact, simply preclude the necessity to provide other services to this client. Specifically, even the prevention of pregnancy would not diminish the need for staff to help Maria clarify her views about desirable relationships with others, learn to value her sexuality, and alert her to the risk associated with sexually transmitted diseases. (Ruby Martinez)

DILEMMA D

Jenny is a lesbian in her mid 30s, who has been trying to get pregnant, through artificial insemination, for the past 18 months. She and her partner are both professional women and have been active in a support group for lesbians wanting to become pregnant. Jenny and her partner (who is older and has had a hysterectomy) are intermittently active in AA; both have been sober for more than two years and feel ready to make this commitment to each other and to a child. Jenny has a history of sexual abuse and finds the invasive procedures required for insemination very difficult. She is considering having an in vitro fertilization (IVF) procedure and has come to Theresa seeking hypnosis to help her deal more effectively with her responses to the physical procedures associated with IVF.

RESPONDENT 1

The ability of a lesbian couple to bear a child via IVF is a controversial matter in North American society. Theresa, the therapist, will want to examine her values (IB, C) and expertise (IVB) regarding this matter in order neither consciously nor unconsciously to adversely impact her client's therapy. A therapist uncomfortable with a lesbian couple bearing children may rationalize that this family is "unnatural" and that these particular women, based on their past experiences, cannot be adequate parents (i.e., these individuals happen to have substance-abuse problems in their history, and Jenny, having been abused by her parents, may be at risk for abusing her own child). Heterosexual parents having similar histories would not necessarily be discouraged from having a child. Neither is there evidence that homosexual couples are irresponsible or unfit parents, nor is the fear of "spreading of homosexuality" valid. The homophobic concern that homosexual role models encourage homosexuality in children carries as much credibility as the thought that heterosexual parents will produce heterosexual children.

Theresa will need to examine not only her own views but the negative cultural views held against lesbians (IB, C). This lesbian family may experience prejudiced behavior in the health care system (pre- and postnatally), the school system, from the media, and from the community in general as they embark upon bearing a child. Theresa, as a member of the health care network, can address homophobic reactions with colleagues and other health providers (VA), as well as help the couple select a hospital, physician, or midwife likely to be open-minded and sensitive to their needs (IA).

Ethical issues that relate to the unborn child include wanting a caring, loving, healthy environment for the child. Ideally, the couple would be happy to have either a boy or girl. In this particular case, the potential parents have made the commitment to have a child and provide these elements for their child. The parents (this lesbian couple) would need to realize that their child may grow up to be heterosexual, which may or may not be an issue for them. Most children have many questions about their biological parents, and this couple will need to face these issues down the road. (Ruby Martinez)

RESPONDENT 2

The guidelines that seem applicable in this case are related to therapist biases, power differentials, and social change (IC, IIA, VA). These responses are drawn from work as a lesbian therapist, as a registered nurse working as a psychiatric nurse clinical specialist and psychotherapist, and as a substance abuse counselor (IC, IIA). What perspectives Theresa brings to this case are unknown. The concerns about personal bias in the therapist are several. From a lesbian perspective, one concern would be a strong bias about whether lesbians are appropriate candidates to become parents. Since IVF can be even more invasive than artificial insemination, and since attempts to become pregnant have been continuing for 18 months, the questions of primary infertility in Jenny and whether a work-up for primary infertility should be done before further attempts to become pregnant both arise. Continuing an unsuccessful medical process without other assessment is a waste of clients' emotional and financial resources (VA). Theresa might question if the clients know there are other methods of artificial insemination besides the medical model they appear to be using (IIB). These are areas where the therapist needs to be able to educate and facilitate these clients in making knowledgeable choices. Another concern is the high incidence of fetal abnormalities in pregnancies among women in their mid to late 30s and older. How would this couple handle a fetal abnormality?

Assuming she has experience working with clients having sexual abuse histories (IVA), Theresa will have to consider informing Jenny that while hypnosis might relieve the fear of invasive procedures, other major underlying, unresolved issues might well surface to interfere with the pregnancy, the relationship, and the demands of parenting. It would be important that Theresa actively question whether hypnosis is appropriate for these clients at this point and also raise questions about the qualifications of the therapist who might do the hypnosis (IVA, VA).

Finally, if Theresa has a background as a substance abuse counselor, the fact that this couple initially began attempting to become pregnant with just six months of sobriety and has had only intermittent AA involvement, with no indication of utilization of other resources for working with the underlying issues, may be a concern. She will need to monitor her own biases about these issues. Acknowledging that there is a power differential between Jenny and Theresa, it would be important that if Theresa raises questions on the above issues, she does so without mitigating the clients' right and ability to choose (IIA). (Anne H. Napier)

DILEMMA E

Helen is a Caucasian woman in her early 50s, who has spent most of her adult life as a housewife and mother. She is seeking counseling for the first time because for the past three years, since she became menopausal, her husband of 30 years says he has been unable to have sexual feelings for her. He refuses to talk with her about it, but she believes he feels she is "no longer a woman." Helen recently began working as a part-time receptionist for a small accounting firm, and one of the men there has been flirting with her. She feels attracted to him and misses having a sexual relationship. Helen considers herself Catholic, although she no longer attends church regularly, and has indicated that she could not speak to her priest about this problem. Her therapist, Doris, is in her late 20s and has lived all her life in the same small town in which Helen lives.

RESPONDENT 1

One of the primary ethical concerns in this situation is that of overlapping relationships (IIIA). Doris and Helen have lived all of their lives in the same *small* town. They have a history of other relationships and could anticipate the probability of interacting socially and in volunteer situations, which could seriously compromise the therapeutic relationship.

A related therapeutic issue is a difficulty with disclosure within therapy. Many small communities work well with a guardedness that likely interferes with the intimacy required to facilitate therapeutic change. Thus, it is expected that Helen might have great difficulty being completely candid with Doris. There is a significant age difference as well, and it is unlikely that Helen can really believe that Doris can fully understand her dilemmas.

The most ethically desirable solution for this case would be for Doris to refer Helen, and hopefully her husband, to a therapist in a nearby larger community for marital and sexual therapy. At the same time, there could be ongoing support for Helen either in a women's group or with another feminist therapist. If Helen's husband continues to withdraw from the marriage, Helen would need support from a feminist therapist to make decisions in response to that situation such as the decision regarding telling her husband about the other man.

If Doris cannot refer, it is desirable that she assist Helen to fully examine her options. It is also important that her husband be included in therapy and that information about aging, sexuality, and the influence of the social context be part of the consultation and/or supervision. Helen's husband's reactions also need to be set within the social context of active and pervasive conditioning coming from the media and advertising, in which menopausal women are seen as asexual and undesirable, and the prevailing image of sexual desirability is located primarily with nubile adolescents (VA).

Helen identifies the problems she brings to therapy as having to do with marital and sexual issues. If she does not have competency in these areas (IVA), Doris should facilitate Helen's access to a therapist skilled and knowledgeable in sexual and marital therapy. If Doris cannot refer Helen to a more appropriate resource, she needs to receive ongoing supervision and consultation (IVB).

In addition, Doris would need to closely examine herself for evidence of bias or of discriminatory attitudes (IC). If Doris is not Roman

Catholic and/or given the age difference, it may be difficult for her to understand both the compelling nature of Helen's commitment to her marriage and her guilt over an attraction to another man. If so, Doris might have a tendency to impose her values on Helen, or have difficulty hearing, supporting, and understanding Helen's need to stay in what appears to be an unfulfilling marriage. As well as examining the problems inherent in this situation, hopefully Doris can celebrate Helen's response to life: that she *can* still have these exciting feelings about another man; and that, after all these years at home, she can find joy and fulfillment in work. (Kathy Ingraham)

RESPONDENT 2

The ethical guidelines that appear most applicable in this case are those associated with awareness of cultural diversities and oppressions, power differentials, and overlapping relationships (IB, C, IIA, IIIA, B). Doris will need to monitor for possible therapist bias for several issues. As a feminist therapist, Doris may have a strong reaction to perceptions of a husband valuing his wife only if she is able to bear children, or his seeing his wife as "old" or "unwomanly" if she is menopausal. Such reactions, as biases, might skew the therapeutic process. Given the cultural, generational, and experiential differences between how Helen and Doris might view menopause, and how each might view the possibility of an affair, Doris will need to be self-aware about her own biases and demonstrate respect for Helen's perspective.

Without abusing the inherent power differential between therapist and client, Doris could be very supportive of Helen's pursuing more dialogue with her husband, perhaps even suggest couples' therapy. She could also teach assertiveness skills to Helen. At the same time, Doris will need to be careful not to impose her views, attempt to control or push Helen in any direction she would not choose for herself (IIA).

From the perspective of a therapist who has practiced in a small town for many years, the ethical issues of overlapping relationships, boundaries, and confidentiality are many (IIIA, B). In an urban setting, anonymity and very limited contacts with clients are possible. In a small community, they are not. Contacts and boundaries are very different in a small community. By even parking in front of the therapist's office, a person is assumed by others to be in therapy. Intakes and assessments have to include a question by the therapist: "How do you want me to act toward you if we meet in the grocery store?" Doris, as an active community member, may end up on committees or in events and/or social situations with Helen. Doris may also have knowledge from the community that the client herself may not know, that is, that Helen's husband in this case is having an affair. Another ethical issue arises if

Doris is the only therapist for many miles, which is often the case in a small town. Is the man who is flirting with Helen also seeing Doris? Is Helen's husband a client of hers? If either is true and there are no referral alternatives, is it more ethical to refuse to see this client, or to work with this client, being very careful of boundary and confidentiality issues, including not divulging who other clients might be? Therapist access, productivity, and scheduling are also issues in a small town, where back-to-back clients may well know each other, even be related, or perhaps be in a relationship, unknown to the therapist. The differences in boundaries, overlapping roles, and confidentiality for a psychotherapist practicing in a small town or rural area, versus those for a therapist practicing in an urban area, are seldom addressed when ethical guidelines are taught, and stringent application of such guidelines is not always possible in a small town. The Feminist Therapist Ethical Guidelines lend themselves to issues of overlapping roles and relationships such as those found in small or rural communities. (Anne Napier)

DILEMMA F

Gina has been working with women and specializing in issues of sexuality for 10 years. She has given several professional presentations about her work with women who experience severe premenstrual symptoms. She has a private practice and also provides consultation for several local agencies. Gina has been asked by the courts to do an evaluation of a 34-year-old woman, Clara, to determine her fitness as a mother as part of a custody evaluation. Clara's former husband claims that she is prone to fits of rage premenstrually and would be too unpredictable to have custody of their children.

RESPONDENT 1

In this case there could be a conflict as to whether the actual client is Clara or the courts. Gina must be very clear with both parties about her role. Her ethical obligation is to empower Clara, but it is possible her assessment and testimony could be used against Clara. Gina also has an ethical obligation to Clara to advise her about her rights regarding the assessment, confidentiality, and Gina's role in the court (IIID).

Gina is an expert on premenstrual syndrome (PMS), and she has been asked to do an assessment of Clara "to determine her fitness as a mother." Gina must be clear about her own level of expertise and what she is assessing (IVA). Is she qualified in the area of PMS only, or is she qualified to assess maternal competency? The case outline suggests she adheres to IVC because she is actively involved in teaching and lecturing, which implies she is keeping up to date with her area.

If Gina provides an assessment of Clara for the courts, she has an opportunity to adhere to guideline V, social change. The presentation of the case suggests Clara's situation may be trivialized as a "female problem." It may be that her anger has more to do with her husband than her PMS. The assessment gives Gina an opportunity to educate the court about women and PMS. (Margaret McLeod)

RESPONDENT 2

Scientifically, "premenstrual distress," by whatever name,[1] remains a puzzle with potential for being used unfairly against women (Bart & Moran, 1993). A court battle over custody of children is a particularly difficult ethical dilemma for a feminist therapist, inasmuch as she is being asked to do an "objective" evaluation for the court, rather than to represent or advocate for Clara. This dilemma clearly raises questions in the realms of therapist accountability (IV), social change (V), and power differentials (II). A legitimate stance for Gina to take is that of the "reasonable woman" standard of judgment, developed in relation to legal battles over violence against women and pornography (MacKinnon, 1987).

Part of Gina's responsibility (IVA) is to consider the scope of her own competency in this area, to make sure that she has the most complete and recent information about this rapidly moving area of expertise, and to inform the court about current diagnostic issues for premenstrual distress. These include, of course, the controversy over inclusion of a premenstrual diagnosis in the fourth edition of the *Diagnostic and Statistical Manual of Mental Disorders* (DSM-IV). Premenstrual dysphoric disorder (PMDD) has been listed as a provisional diagnosis (status unclear; further research needed), under the category of Depressive Disorders, with criteria for the diagnosis appearing only in the Appendix. Paula Caplan suggests that in order to address the social change necessary for eliminating the negative impact of this diagnosis on women (VA, B), feminist therapists can monitor legal use of the diagnosis for actionable cases where it has been used unfairly to the detriment of women (Caplan, 1993).

In the present case, Gina needs to be aware of research demonstrating the difficulty (some say impossibility) of accurately diagnosing PMDD using current accepted criteria (Hamilton & Gallant, 1993). On the other hand, it is a well-replicated finding that premenstrual

---

[1]The variety of names probably reflects the lack of consensus about the nature of premenstrual distress; it has recently been referred to as premenstrual syndrome, premenstrual dysphoric disorder, premenstrual symptoms, or (everybody's favorite) late luteal phase dysphoric disorder (L2PD2).

distress is associated with the level of stress in women's lives (Dan & Lewis, 1992). Such information points to the context of Clara's life as an important determinant of her premenstrual symptoms. It would not be surprising that the extremely stressful time leading up to divorce action would aggravate distress experienced premenstrually; however, this does not necessarily indicate that the postdivorce period would be equally distressing. Premenstrual symptoms can be thought of as an early warning system, or as Sheryle Gallant has suggested, as an indicator of the level of oppression in a woman's life. (Alice J. Dan)

IMPLICATIONS

Nothing would seem more incongruous, following these thoughtful questions, positions, and stories, than to imply that conclusions are possible. The issues raised by the case of Judy and Lee pose ethical dilemmas between the individual's rights and autonomy in this society in possible contrast to the rights of the families in which members (or some members) retain other cultural beliefs. The principles of nonmaleficence and beneficence must be considered in the context of possible rejection by family and community. In a situation with clear parameters for some options (i.e., abortion), any consultant would have to be aware of such time limitations. Both respondents addressed the importance of understanding existing laws and policies that may be brought to the definition of the problems and to the range of possible solutions. The rights of "putative fathers" will become increasingly important from a legal standpoint. What ethical positions will feminist therapists take? The possibility of a domestic violence problem, which is also raised in this situation, is becoming a highly controversial concern within the women's health and domestic violence communities. Although many domestic violence groups support laws that mandate an arrest in cases of domestic violence, the National Women's Health Network (1992) has taken the position that the "medicalization" of a social problem will displace responsibility from batterers and serve primarily to provide another reimbursable medical diagnosis for physicians at the cost of a woman's right to decide if and when she chooses to press charges. What positions should a feminist therapist take with respect to legislating "safety" that others may construe as intrusive?

The case of Joan and Mekala illustrated graphically the several interrelated difficulties described. The need to consider interprofessional tensions reflects not only differences in hierarchy and power, but also the need to consider the dominance of the allopathic medical paradigm of Western medicine. The possibility that cultural "translation" problems extend beyond, and must include, ethnic differences is poignantly raised by the possible stories each person brings to a single moment of decision. Even the choice of translator could have an important influence on what becomes defined as "the problem" and who is ultimately responsible for choosing among the several solutions that may need to be weighed. Professional, theoretical, and life-experience factors mingle with the social, cultural, and gender issues. Even when some cultural characteristics are shared with clients, as in the case of Helen and Doris, one set of problems is traded for another. When "all the players" are known, as in a small, homogeneous community, feminist therapists may be culturally congruent and become blind to other areas of incongruence, such as age and religion. The ethical choices the rural, isolated therapist faces are many. Even though these guidelines are sensitive to the potential problems of overlapping relationships, it may take considerable feminist creativity to procure either supervision or other community resources suggested. Perhaps the image of the circuit preacher/teacher will offer some alternatives, as may use of telephone and computer networking (which bring their own confidentiality concerns).

The role of the feminist therapist as existing within social institutions is implicit in all the cases and perhaps most explicit in the case of Maria. The questions raised must consider not only the rights of the individual client with respect to autonomy and nonmaleficence and the rights of the individual therapist, but those of staff, family, and, often, legal and institutional concerns whose intentions may be beneficent. When the latter are in conflict with the rights of the client and/or the ethics of the therapist, the questions become even more difficult. If feminist therapists are both obligated to know the laws and resources in their states and jurisdictions, does that mean they are bound to uphold them when feminist therapists believe they are ethically wrong? Political action to change laws is one action that may be untenable. What are the ethical positions regarding passive resistance or outright obstruction? How many, if the right to abortion is removed, would risk becoming involved with groups such as JANE, the underground abortion group that functioned in Chicago prior to *Roe v. Wade* (Boston Women's Health Book Collective, 1992)?

The issues raised in these cases do not fully reflect the range of issues that encompass the vast terrain of women's health. For example, if a woman's right to make her own decisions about her body is respected, does that mean her right to get silicone breast implants to increase her self-esteem by changing her body image must also be given support? Without universal health insurance, how can lesbian couples, like Jenny and her partner, in committed relationships, obtain adequate insurance coverage without jeopardizing their employment in the wake of Colorado's Amendment 2 vote? For now, the federal courts appear unlikely to uphold this proposed law that would effectively legalize discrimination in housing and jobs and leave those discriminated against without recourse to the courts. In a country purportedly founded on freedom of religion, increasingly opposing values, often based on "religious" insights, are being battled in the courts. How much do feminist therapists wish to be involved in custody evaluations, such as that described in the case of Gina and Clara? By participating, are therapists supporting the growing litigious tendencies in the United States, an adversarial strategy that may actually contribute to greater polarization of the winning and losing parties? If feminist therapists either become or refuse to be involved in such cases, do they compromise their ethical position as advocates?

How are personal and social costs in a faltering economy balanced? Women disproportionately experience chronic illnesses and live longer than men. It is expensive to provide high-technology care to the elderly. This observation, along with the growing legislation about the "right to die," have led to some concern that active euthanasia might become an "acceptable" alternative. Women have always been the primary caregivers in families for themselves, partners, children, and aging parents and in-laws. With increasing numbers of women supporting themselves and families by working outside the home, the continued assumption that "somebody" will be home to care for the acute or chronic illnesses in the family creates personal and financial dilemmas. The probable "rationing" of health care will bring these life and death and quality-of-life issues to the doorstep of all North Americans.

RESPONDENTS

Christine M. Chao, PhD, Eurasian, is a clinical psychologist in Denver with a long-standing interest in Asian mental health and cross-cultural issues.
Sandra Coffman, PhD, Dorsey Green, PhD, Carol Henry, PhD, and Susan Raab-Cohen, PhD, are members of a Seattle consultation group that has been meeting for about 10 years.
Alice J. Dan, PhD, is Director of the Center for Research on Women and Gender and Professor at the College of Nursing, University of Illinois at Chicago.
Kathy Ingraham, MSc, is a psychologist in private practice in Calgary and in the mountains at Banff.
Ruby J. Martinez, RN, PhC, Hispanic, practices nursing administration at the Colorado Mental Health Institute at Fort Logan and is pursuing doctoral studies regarding culturally congruent care.

Margaret McLeod, BA, MEd, Canadian, is a psychologist in private practice in Calgary, Alberta.

Anne Napier, EdD, RN, CS, is a psychiatric clinical specialist in private practice for 25 years.

Nancy Wang, MSW, LCSW, Chinese-American, is a psychotherapist using eclectic modalities and working with children, young adults, families, and couples, with a speciality in biculturalism in San Francisco.

REFERENCES

Achterberg, J. (1991). *Woman as healer*. Boston: Shambhala.

Adler, M. (1986). *Drawing down the moon*. Boston: Beacon Press.

American Psychiatric Association. (1994). *Diagnostic and statistical manual of mental disorders* (4th ed.). Washington, DC: Author.

Bart, P., & Moran, E. (1993). *Violence against women: The bloody footprints*. Newbury Park, CA: Sage.

Boston Women's Health Book Collective. (1992). *The new our bodies, ourselves*. New York: Touchstone.

Caplan, P. (1993). Premenstrual syndrome DSM-IV diagnosis: The coalition for a scientific and responsible DSM-IV. *Psychology of Women: Newsletter of Division 35, American Psychological Association, 20*(3), 4–5, 13.

Carson, A. (1992). *Goddesses and wise women: The literature of feminist spirituality 1980–1992*. Freedom, CA: Crossing Press.

Clancy, C., & Massion, C. (1992). American women's health care: A patchwork quilt with gaps. *Journal of the American Medical Association, 268*(14), 1918–1920.

Committee on Women, Population and the Environment. (1992). Women, population and the environment: Call for a new approach. *Network News, 17*(6), 3.

Dan, A., & Hemphill, S. (1992). *Women's health: 1993 medical and health annual* (pp. 405–410). Chicago: Encyclopedia Britannica.

Dan, A., & Lewis, L. (1992). *Menstrual health in women's lives*. Champaign, IL: University of Illinois Press.

Ehrenreich, B., & English, D. (1978). *For her own good: 150 years of the experts' advice to women*. Garden City, NY: Anchor Press.

Fee, E. (1975). Women and health care: A comparison of theories. *International Journal of Health Services, 5*, 397–415.

Firestone, S. (1970). *The dialectic of sex: The case for feminist revolution*. New York: William Morrow.

Gaskin, I. (1990). *Spiritual midwifery* (3rd ed.). Summertown, TN: Book Publishing Co.

Guiley, R. (1991). *Harper's encyclopedia of mystical and paranormal experience*. San Francisco: Harper.

Hamilton, J., & Gallant, S. (1993). Premenstrual syndrome: A health psychology critique of biomedically oriented research. In R. Gatchel & E.

Blanchard (Eds.), *Psychophysiological disorders: Research and clinical applications* (pp. 383–438). Washington, DC: American Psychological Association.

Holmes, H., Hoskins, B., & Gross, M. (1980). *Birth control and controlling birth: Women-centered perspectives*. Clifton, NJ: Humana Press.

Humm, M. (1990). *The dictionary of feminist theory*. Columbus: Ohio State University Press.

Iazzeto, D. (1992). What's happening with women and body image? *Network News, 17*(3), 1, 4–8.

MacKinnon, C. (1987). *Feminism unmodified: Discourses on life and law*. Cambridge, MA: Harvard University Press.

National Women's Health Network. (March/April, 1992). Warning: AMA family violence campaign may be hazardous to women's health. *Network News, 17*(2), 7.

Noble, V. (1983). *Motherpeace*. New York: Harper & Row.

Norsigian, J. (1993). Women and national health care reform: A progressive feminist agenda. *Journal of Women's Health, 2*(1), 91–94.

Ruzek, S. (1978). *The women's health movement: Feminist alternative to medical control*. New York: Praeger.

Walker, B. (1983). *The woman's encyclopedia of myths and secrets*. New York: Harper & Row.

Webster, D., & Lipetz, M. (1986). Changing definitions; changing times. *Nursing Clinics of North America, 21*(1), 87–97.

NINE

The Medical Model

Rosemary Liburd
Esther Rothblum

Ideas about what is "normal" come from the consciousness
of those with the power to define. . . . The power to define
. . . is an effective means of social control.
— PENFOLD AND WALKER (1983, p. 41)

The problems for which women are treated in the
medical system cover a wide range. They include
those related to reproductive function—men-
struation, menopause, childbirth, abortion, premenstrual syndrome
(PMS). They encompass sexuality and violence issues, and, more recently, acquired immunodeficiency syndrome (AIDS). They also involve the so-called women's psychological disorders such as anorexia,
bulimia, agoraphobia, and depression. How these problems are perceived and approached from traditional and feminist perspectives differ.
The differences and contradictions between the traditional medical
model of treatment and feminist treatment models present ethical
questions for those who identify themselves as feminist therapists and
follow the Feminist Therapy Code of Ethics.

Feminists have engaged in an ongoing critique of the medical
model of treatment for women. By definition, this model is individualistic, disease-oriented, and views diseases as belonging to the
individual (Sherwin, 1992). Traditional mental health systems have
adopted this model and, along with it, its focus on pathology and
inherent power relationships. The connection of psychology (and
therapy in particular) to the medical model is affirmed by the
historical and contemporary assumptions about the relationship
between mind and body, the interplay between emotions and physical health or disease. These assumptions have a clear impact on the
role that health issues play in psychological treatment and on the

relationship between mental health and medical professionals who frequently treat the same patient.

Feminist criticism of the medical model moves beyond its individualistic, pathological focus. The medical model has been criticized not only for minimizing or ignoring sociological factors but for medicalizing social problems in general and women's experience in particular. The pathologizing of a single mother on welfare experiencing depression or of the midlife woman with multiple-role responsibilities who is concerned with anxiety and forgetfulness are examples of this tendency. Beyond this, feminist criticism has been directed toward the medical model of treatment for its paternalistic approach to both treatment and the physician–patient relationship. Some observations suggest that "physicians have a large and growing interest in asserting their authority over women's health" (Sherwin, 1992, p. 150), a pattern that has a long history in the medical treatment of women.

Two characteristics of the medical model that have particular relevance for women are (1) the focus on the individual as the sole or primary source of the problem, ignoring both the realities of women's lives and the broader notion of social construction of gender; and (2) the power and authority embedded in the medical model, which is of particular relevance to the physician–client relationship. These two factors will be discussed in relation to their implications for the treatment of women as exemplified through a discussion of women and depression and the social control of body weight.

"REST CURES": WOMEN AND DEPRESSION

In the 1880s, Charlotte Perkins Gilman got married and had a child. Soon afterwards, she became so depressed that she consulted a neurologist who specialized in women's disorders. He recommended a "rest cure" that prohibited Charlotte from writing and limited her reading time. The treatment almost drove her mad and resulted in her fictionalized account, "The Yellow Wallpaper" (Lane, 1980). When she left her husband and child, the depression lifted.

There is an enormous amount of medical and psychological literature on the symptoms, etiology, and treatment of depression. Yet none of the traditional theories of depression even consider the fact that women are twice as likely as men to become depressed. Nor do the theories incorporate the reality of women's socialization and the consequences of sexism. In the last two decades, feminists have begun to examine the relationship between depression and women's roles (McGrath, Keita, Strickland, & Russo, 1990). Traditional gender role stereotypes encourage women to be passive and helpless during times of stress. Demographic factors that place women at risk for depression include being married. In men, being single is more of a risk for depression (Rothblum, 1983). Childrearing and lack of full-time paid employment are also risk factors for depression in women. The association of violence against women and depression has been generally ignored by theorists and researchers until recently. Yet women are severely depressed as the result of childhood sexual or physical abuse, battering, sexual harassment, rape, and sexual abuse by a therapist, to mention some examples (Cutler & Nolen-Hoeksema, 1991; Russo, 1990).

Enormous medical, psychopharmaceutical, and psychotherapy industries profit from the prevalence of depression among women. These industries focus on cognitive, behavioral, affective, or physiological understandings and interventions for depression. What would happen if more contemporary women avoided the societal risk factors of marriage and childbearing, as modeled by Charlotte Perkins Gilman in the last century? What if depression were not viewed as a medical disorder, but as the result of sociopolitical factors that keep women oppressed? Societal institutions would fall apart, as women ceased to be caretakers and victims of relationship-induced violence. Women would rely less on psychotherapy and would no longer be the primary consumers of psychopharmaceutical agents.

THE SOCIAL CONTROL OF BODY WEIGHT

Throughout history and across cultures, societies have had strict norms about women's permissible appearance. Usually, what was permissible for women was to accentuate a body part that was already smaller than the corresponding body part in men (Brownmiller, 1984). Women's feet were bound in China, women in Europe were required to wear corsets to restrict the size of their waist, and the clitoris of women in Africa was removed (Rothblum, 1994). These practices caused distinct health problems in women. For example, wearing corsets weakened women's muscles, placed pressure on women's lungs, and caused women to faint if overexerted. The medical profession colluded in these oppressions of women, usually endorsing the practice as health-promoting. An example occurs in Africa, where both traditional healers and Western-trained medical professionals are involved in performing clitoridectomies on women, and yet large numbers of women are being treated for medical complications from the practice (Brownmiller, 1984).

In the United States, the current "fad" for women's appearance is a low body weight. Other European and Western nations, such as Canada and Australia, favor low body weight in women, but not to the extreme extent of the United States (Tiggemann & Rothblum, 1988). The medical profession equates being fat with being unhealthy. The mental health professions, along with medicine and life insurance companies, have narrowly defined the "ideal" weight: to be 15% "below expected weight" is defined as displaying anorexia (American Psychiatric Association, 1994, p. 540); to be over 20% above expected weight is considered obesity (Rothblum, 1990).

The medicalization of body weight denies the reality that women diet not for health reasons but for sexual and social appeal (Brown & Rothblum, 1989; Rothblum, 1992). In fact, the association between obesity and health risks is so taken for granted that even feminist mental health professionals are unaware of the methodological confounds in this research (Garner & Wooley, 1991; Rothblum, 1990). For example, Rothblum (1994) states:

> Studies often fail to control for income and may suffer from a number of confounding variables, since in Western nations fat people are poorer than thin people. These studies compare the rich and poor on health risks, and poor people do not have the same access to health insurance and preventive care. Fat people diet more than thin people, and dieting itself can result in a number of health risks, including the very health risks often associated with obesity, such as hypertension, high cholesterol, and diabetes (Polivy & Herman, 1983). A recent article in the *New England Journal of Medicine* (Lissner et al., 1991) reported that people who have dieted and regained weight had higher mortality rates than those who had not dieted and stayed at the same (high) weight. In addition, fat people are subjected to stigmatization and discrimination, and the stress of such oppression can result in stress-related health problems. (p. 55)

The economy, especially the medical industry, in Western nations profits from women's obsession with weight. In adhering to the medical model view of weight and weight loss, each year in the United States alone, people, mostly women, spend $33 billion on diets and diet products such as low calorie food, and $300 million on cosmetic surgery mostly to look thinner and younger. If women stopped caring about their weight, a significant percentage of the medical profession would be affected; yet the economic necessity of this spending is kept hidden.

Along with the medical profession, the media focuses on maintaining women's preoccupation with weight. Low body weight for women is idealized in all aspects of the media, including advertisements, with no association made of this body weight with anorexia. The feminist movement is often associated with ugly and "unfeminine" women, and many women fear joining the feminist movement precisely because of this association.

The medical model and the media serve as institutions of social control for maintaining women's appearance norms. As Rothblum

(1994) has stated, "Women's appearance norms are not created by women, and they are not healthy for women. Rather, the norms profit men, define the erotic, pump money into the economy, and restrict women's power" (p. 72). Thus, trying to determine the actual link between obesity and health problems, such as diabetes and coronary risks, becomes very problematic for feminist therapists.

GENDER AND HEALTH CARE

Feminists place a strong emphasis on the social construction of gender that assumes that society, not biology, dictates how gender is understood. Gender affects how illness is defined and diagnosed, how and when symptoms are expressed, how they are explained, and what treatment strategies are formulated (Travis, 1988). More precisely, women's lower status results in a lower standard of health care for them. It is crucial, however, to note that gender is not the only significant variable that impacts the treatment of women in the health care system. Although women, as a group, are vulnerable to poor health care, this difficulty is compounded by factors such as race, economic class, age, body size, disabilities, intelligence, and a history of mental illness (Sherwin, 1992).

Medicine constructs a medicalized view of women's experiences in which normal aspects of these experiences, such as menstruation, menopause, body size, or feminine behavior, are viewed as unhealthy and as requiring medical management (Sherwin, 1992). This view disregards the social construction of gender and has dramatic implications for society as a whole and for women in particular. If social problems, such as racism, violence against women, poverty, or compulsive heterosexuality are medicalized, the solution to these problems is left in the hands of the medical establishment, and society at large does not have to be accountable for them (Penfold & Walker, 1983). If acts of violence against women, for example, are viewed as problems of an individual woman, the social context and the prevalence of these acts in society become irrelevant. The scene is then set for locating the source of that problem within that individual woman and for pathologizing her experience.

Feminists have not only addressed the importance of a sociopolitical understanding of experience but have also identified power as a significant factor in this regard. The traditional medical model is a hierarchical one that reflects the "maintenance of a male power advantage through withholding and reconstructing information" (Albino, Tedesco, & Shenkle, 1990, p. 233). The paternalism associated with this model assumes that patients are not only incapable of making appropriate medical decisions but that the authority of the physician is an integral part of the patients' healing (Sherwin, 1992). This model is not just sustained through the manner in which information is constructed and used. It is also embedded in the roles and relationship of the (male) physician and (female) patient. These roles are a reflection, if not an exaggeration, of the dominant/subordinate relationships between men and women that persist in the larger culture. Miller's (1983) description of dominant group behavior (in relation to subordinates) fits the description of the traditional physician–client patterns of relationship. For example, it restricts the subordinate group's range of action, does not encourage subordinates' full and free expression of their experiences, characterizes the subordinates falsely, and describes this situation as the norm. This situation effectively restricts women from playing an active role in their own health care and makes it difficult, if not impossible, to collaborate with their physicians on their own behalf.

Not only is the medical model a hierarchical one, but it clearly reflects the negative stereotypic notions about women that are consistent with the way dominants view subordinates in the culture at large. Stereotypic views about women have a far-reaching effect on women's health and impact the manner in which women are viewed, diagnosed, and treated within the system. Health care practitioners have also fostered views of women as weak and incompetent and have devalued and trivialized women's health problems (Albino et al., 1990). For example, when complaints associated with a woman's reproductive system (i.e., menopause, menstruation) are discounted or regarded as psychological in origin, the health care women receive is clearly influenced in a negative direction. When women's genuine physiological symptoms are minimized, characterized as psychosomatic or devalued, misdiagnosis can occur. Misdiagnosis, along with overmedication, are two major problems experienced by women today (Mowbray, Lanir, & Hulce, 1985).

GENDER AND MENTAL HEALTH

Misdiagnosis occurs in the realms of mental as well as physical health. Since the Broverman, Broverman, Clarkson, Rosenkrantz, and Vogel (1970) study described the existence of a double standard of mental health for men and women, the question of how the double standard affects women has remained in the forefront of feminist inquiry. An ongoing focus in this regard has been the *Diagnostic and Statistical Manual of Mental Disorders* (DSM) classification system. Caplan (1992) has highlighted two DSM categories with particular relevance for women, self-defeating personality disorder (SDPD) and late luteal phase dysphoric disorder (LLPDD). Her criticisms of the SDPD are based in the facts that it (1) pathologizes women for having learned and displayed the roles that culture has prescribed, (2) is descriptive of the "typically battered or severely emotionally abused woman" (p. 74), and (3) postulates that women have a pathological need to be hurt and humiliated. LLPDD, another term for premenstrual syndrome, places a psychiatric diagnosis on problems associated with the menstrual cycle. In both instances there are no equivalent male categories, and Caplan concludes, "The variety of gender biases in diagnosis. . . . reflects the power and pervasiveness of sexism in the realm of diagnosis" (p. 78).

Although overmedication of women can occur in any sphere of medicine, one of the most visible examples is the prescription of psychotropic drugs for women (Caffetera, Kasper, & Bernstein, 1983). In a review of prescription drug use by women, Cooperstock (1981) indicated that women receive more prescriptions than men in all classes of drugs but the greatest difference is in psychotropics. Women are also more likely to use psychotropics frequently and consistently. This tendency is interpreted in several ways. The maladaptive, stressful nature of the traditional female roles, which goes unrecognized in the medical system, is seen as a strong, mitigating factor (Penfold & Walker, 1983). Since the function of psychotropic medication is, reportedly, to reduce symptomatology, the cause of the stress is not addressed. The status quo is, thereby, sustained and supports the notion that overprescription of psychotropic medication for women reflects a move in society to maintain the second-class status of women and to support those behaviors associated with traditional stereotypes (Mowbray et al., 1985).

In general terms, feminist ethics views oppression as morally wrong, is committed to eliminating subordination, and is interested in the relationship between subordination and specific practices (Sherwin, 1992). The Feminist Therapy Code of Ethics is consistent with these premises, defines the personal as political, assumes a proactive stance, and advocates social change activities (Preamble). In this context, the relationship of feminist therapists to the medical treatment model presents a variety of ethical considerations. It also presents potential dilemmas in which the medical model, traditional professional ethics, and feminist therapy ethics conflict.

In addressing professional relationships, the American Psychological Association's (1990) Ethical Principles of Psychologists state, "Psychologists act with due regard for the needs, special competencies and obligations of their colleagues in psychology and other professions. . . . and take into account the traditions and practices of other professional groups with whom they work and cooperate fully" (p. 393). Since the medical model represents a form of institutionalized sexism, the question of when and how oppression is confronted in this system is a crucial one. The feminist therapist may, in fact, be employed by the system that is the object of her social change efforts. Although working within the system does not necessarily place her in a position of conflict, the difference between aspects of the traditional and feminist ethical codes can create an ethical dilemma. Traditional ethics, as indicated, calls for full cooperation with other professional groups within the context of that group's traditions and practices. If the "traditions and practices" reflect sexist ideology and reinforce the oppression of women, feminist principles of working toward social change and the traditional principle of cooperation are in clear conflict.

The feminist therapy principle of working toward eradicating oppression is concomitant with that of working toward empowering women (Preamble). This goal is in direct conflict with the medical model stance that is hierarchical, assumes "expert" status, and is disempowering of women. The interface between the values and practices of feminist therapists and medical model practitioners will continue to present ethical dilemmas as feminist therapists work toward social change. These dilemmas speak to the belief that "ethics must be revised if it is to get at the patterns of dominance and oppression as they affect women" (Sherwin, 1992, p. 42).

DILEMMA A

Sally is a 50-year-old woman who has recently been laid off from a 25-year job. In the midst of the recession, she has had considerable difficulty finding other employment. She went to her physician who placed her on hormones for menopause and medication for depression. She also is seeing a therapist, Ellen, at the local mental health center. Ellen does not think Sally is inappropriately depressed and is concerned that the medication may interfere with Sally's job hunting. Ellen is in her 50s and has rejected the idea that all females need to be on hormone replacement therapy for the rest of their lives. Because of her concerns about "undercutting" another professional, Ellen decides not to say anything about her views to Sally.

RESPONDENT 1

It would be wrong for Sally's psychotherapist, Ellen, to influence Sally's decision to take or not take hormone replacement therapy (HRT) and antidepressive medication (IIA). It would be wrong, first, because hormone replacement is a controversial therapy that makes sense for some women and not for others. Antidepressive medication, too, has its advantages and drawbacks. Second, a goal of psychotherapy is to help a client make her own decisions based on good information. Presumably the physician has already informed Sally about the most significant pros and cons of medication. Ellen might help her evaluate the importance of these pros and cons *if*—but only if—Sally is questioning them herself. If Sally understands the consequences and side effects and is entirely comfortable taking HRT and antidepressive medication, and the psychotherapist is not, then the problem is Ellen's, not Sally's.

At the same time, Ellen ought to ensure that Sally is well-informed and not passive in the decision-making process (IIB). Ellen should ask Sally what she knows about the prescribed medications and obtain a signed release to confer with the prescribing physician. Doing so avoids "undercutting" another professional and collaborates on Sally's behalf.

Ellen might express her reservations about the medications to the physician and ask what Sally has been told about their advantages and disadvantages. Sally needs to know, for instance, that antidepressive medication might have negative consequences related to her job search. For instance, an interviewer might ask for a medical history. If she answers truthfully she might be seen as having a mental illness. In addition, antidepressants can make people lethargic and give them the appearance of looking dull. If the physician did not disclose these possibilities to Sally, Ellen and the physician in consultation would hopefully agree that she needs to be informed.

If Sally is ambivalent, Ellen can recommend unbiased reading material to her to help her be proactive in her health-care decision making. In addition, it would be appropriate for Ellen to disclose that she herself has decided not to take HRT, if that is the case, and that she does not believe all women need to be on hormone replacement for the rest of their lives. This disclosure might provide balance to the prevailing medical position on HRT and allow Sally an option. However, Ellen needs to be clear with Sally that current research is contradictory, that each woman must make her own decision, and that Ellen will respect and support Sally's decision no matter what (IIB).

Few psychotherapists have expert knowledge about HRT and psychotropic medication. Ellen needs to recognize her limitations, share them with Sally, and at the same time educate herself to gain at least a minimal understanding of the medications that have been prescribed (IVA). (Ellen Cole)

RESPONDENT 2

Although the therapist focuses on whether the client should have been given medications at all, the important issue may have more to do with the degree to which the client was involved in this decision and given the information she needed to participate fully in decision making (IIA,

D). This question is raised by the use of the term "placed on" when discussing medication being prescribed for depression and for menopausal symptoms.

In this regard several further questions need to be answered. How depressed is Sally? How long has she felt this way? Does she feel that something needs to be done immediately to alleviate her level of distress? Were different medication and treatment options explained to her, and were the risk–benefit factors and possible side effects discussed? It may make a great deal of sense, and in fact be ethically responsible, for someone with all of the symptoms of a clinical depression to be offered medication and even to be encouraged to accept a medication trial. However, the client needs to be an informed participant in the decision. The treatment issues are not whether she is appropriately or inappropriately depressed, but whether she has the kind of depression that is responsive to medication and whether *she* feels sufficiently distressed or uncomfortable about hormonal replacement therapy or her menopausal symptoms.

There are also problems in Sally's care with regard to the relationship between the professionals involved and in the relationship between the therapist and the client. Ellen's ability to communicate both with her client and with the other service provider seems to be hindered by preconceived ideas and by her overidentification with Sally. She is biased against the use of medications and identifies with her client because of their similar ages, despite the fact that their symptoms, feelings, and experiences may be quite different. A feminist therapist should be involved in ongoing consultation, supervision, and continuing education, all of which might well be beneficial to the therapist in this case (IVB). Because of Ellen's preconceived opinions, she is not able to be open and honest with her client and consequently does not find out what the client knows or wants, and so she cannot support her in getting any additional information she may need. These preconceptions interfere with Ellen's ability to educate her client regarding her rights as a consumer (IID). Ellen could also have modeled effective use of personal power (IIA) by discussing the medication decision directly with the physician (with Sally's permission). An opportunity for the therapist and another service provider to work as partners in the best interest of the client has been lost; and the therapist's silence has almost certainly been perceived by Sally as disapproval about her simultaneous seeking of assistance.

Overmedication of women clients who are dealing with societal stressors is certainly a source of serious concern, but it is one that needs to be confronted from an informed and open perspective, which does not seem to be the case here. Consequently the therapist's relationship with the client and her ability to help her client make choices about her own care and to take charge of her relationship with other powerful care providers is paralyzed. (Mary E. Willmuth)

DILEMMA B

Olga is a 30-year-old English-speaking Latina who is a law student. She is a highly acculturated, third-generation Mexican-American woman with professional status. Her clinical picture includes symptoms of depression and anxiety. After an initial evaluation, the therapist, Ruth, referred her for a psychopharmacological consultation. Olga was diagnosed as having both depression and panic attacks and placed on a monoamine oxidase (MAO) inhibitor. However, after a week on this medication trial, Olga complained of not being able to eat cheese while on that medication and, thus, stopped the medication on her own. Instead, she began taking a home remedy that her aunt from Mexico had sent her for her symptoms. When Ruth asked her about this decision, Olga stated that it is common practice among Latinos to share medications among relatives and, additionally, pharmacists prescribe medications in Mexico. Olga stated that she was feeling better using such a remedy. Ruth recommended that Olga inform her psychopharmacologist of her decision, and she agreed to do so. One month later she received a call from an emergency room saying that Olga had had an adverse drug reaction caused by a combination of clomiprimine with cold medication. (Lillian Comas-Díaz)

RESPONDENT 1

The ethical dilemma faced by Ruth is how to maintain the feminist principle of not taking control or power, which rightfully belongs to Olga (IIA), while also ensuring that Olga receives appropriate services and is not harmed by the therapeutic process. In Olga's case, maintaining this balance is especially complex because another service provider (the doctor prescribing medication) is involved, and the therapist is not familiar with Olga's cultural and ethnic background. Although certain aspects of Ruth's behavior, such as not interfering with Olga's decision to stop taking the MAO inhibitor, were acceptable, she violated a number of the FTI Guidelines and in doing so put Olga's health and well-being at risk.

By continuing to see Olga after referring her for medication, Ruth may have been operating beyond her competencies (IVA). Olga brought up the fact that she was dissatisfied with not being able to eat cheese while on the MAO inhibitor, but Ruth apparently did not explore the issue and instead referred Olga back to the psychopharmacologist. A therapist who works with clients on medications must have a minimum amount of knowledge regarding the efficacy and side effects of medications as well as possible alternative medications and must be willing to engage in discussions of these issues with the client. It is also possible that Ruth possessed adequate knowledge about medications, but in an attempt not to usurp power that belonged to Olga, she chose not to share it with her. If so, poor judgment was used, and Ruth was remiss in not disclosing to Olga any information she had about pertinent medications, including possible adverse drug interactions (IIB). Such educational information may have assisted Olga in accessing the psychopharmacologist's services so that the medications she received were appropriate and palatable to her.

The other component of Ruth's behavior that appeared ethically problematic was that she did not seek out information and knowledge about Olga's cultural background from sources other than from Olga herself (IB). Despite the fact that Olga is a professional who appears to be well assimilated into mainstream American culture, her Latina culture and familial ties seemed strong. As soon as these issues became apparent in therapy, Ruth had a responsibility to become familiar with elements of the Latina culture from additional sources and, as Olga was on medication, in particular how the culture views and deals with medication and mental illness. By relying only on Olga for information, Ruth was unable to support Olga effectively in her decision-making process regarding continuing or changing her medications. Without such understanding, Ruth's referral for medication was premature and, ultimately, damaging to Olga.

To address these ethical issues, Ruth must first recognize the limitations of her competencies and work to learn more about medications and the Latina culture through formal education, consultation, and ongoing supervision. Second, she needs to be more vigilant about sharing information with Olga about medications and perhaps other issues that will facilitate the therapeutic process. Finally, Ruth and Olga need to work together to understand how their interaction contributed to Olga's adverse drug reaction and, if necessary, to reevaluate their relationship so that further damaging incidents are averted. (Jessica Morris and Miriam Frankel Stoll)

RESPONDENT 2

The therapist's ethical dilemma in this case arises out of her following conflicting responsibilities: respect for Olga's right to use a cultural-bound medicine and commitment to her client's overall well-being. Following the ethical guidelines for feminist therapists (IB), the therapist has demonstrated respect for Olga's culture and right to choose her treatment (IIA). By recommending consultation with a psychopharmacologist, the therapist has taken an appropriate action for ensuring

Olga's safety from a potential risk. This step is also an acknowledgment by the therapist of her limits in her competency with regard to knowing the risk inherent in the cultural-bound medicine (VA).

According to Rack (1982), "cultural-bound medicine"/healing is a common practice among individuals of diverse cultural backgrounds. Meanings attached to culture and its traditional healing practices are central to the effectiveness of the healing process. Treating these practices as equal to other modalities of intervention is significant in affirming an individual's cultural identity. However, many traditional medicines, though often effective, lack a research base. Their chemical composition is generally not known and in some cases they have serious health implications. In England, individuals of South Asian origin have developed brain damage and other complications of lead poisoning because some of these remedies contain lead and other metals. Guiding Olga to consult her psychopharmacologist is an appropriate measure to ensure that Olga becomes aware of the risk. However, with Olga's permission, the therapist could have consulted the pharmacologist to check the possibilities of a risk and brought it up with Olga in her discussion.

In addition, Olga is third-generation Mexican-American. Using a culture-bound medicine indicates the possibility of pressure to continue Mexican cultural practices. A discussion on the issue could have revealed valuable data for intervention. (Nayyar S. Javed)

DILEMMA C

Janie has some minor mood changes during the three days preceding the onset of menstruation. She has been seeing Mary as a therapist for about 12 weeks. Janie has talked about her distress over the mood changes and how much her husband, Charles, is upset with her for not controlling them. Charles does not take her seriously in discussions most of the time and frequently uses as an excuse that "it's just the wrong time of the month" when he does not agree with Janie. Janie is tired of these reactions and is becoming convinced that if she took some medication for PMS, she would be able to control her mood changes, and Charles would take her more seriously. She insists that Mary refer her to a medical doctor for a prescription.

RESPONDENT 1

Two guidelines seem very relevant in this case (IA, IVC). Mary must ask if the request by Janie is appropriate. Janie is requesting medication for PMS as a way to change her moods to please her husband, Charles. Her request does not seem to be based on self-knowledge, empirical data about PMS, or medical facts. Janie seems to be reacting to life scripts, cultural conditioning, and the stereotyped role expectations of women in relation to men. She has not fully explored her options or the consequences of her request.

The other critical ethical issue (IVC) is that Mary must be aware of and use research in feminist knowledge in her work. By using fundamental feminist knowledge, the therapist knows that medication alone will not make Janie feel self-empowered nor make her be heard and taken seriously by Charles or enable her to find her own voice. Jack, in recent research on women and depression (Jack, 1991), reports on several cases of women in marriages who lose their voices and then become seriously depressed. It is as likely that Janie is having mood changes as a result of her relationship as it is that her mood changes result from PMS. A more appropriate referral may be family therapy.

Mary needs to discuss her concerns about the appropriateness of the referral with Janie, encourage her to explore more fully her request for medication, and handle with care the treatment issues as she deals with the ethical issues. If she does not, she will be violating another ethical guideline (IVB). An ethical solution as well as a good treatment solution would be to ask for a consultation with an expert in PMS and depression who is also knowledgeable about feminist issues. In addition, a referral for family therapy is appropriate. (Pauline Rose Clance)

RESPONDENT 2

The ethical dilemma here involves a conflict between what the client wishes to do and what the feminist therapist believes to be the appropriate thing to do. The Feminist Therapy Code of Ethics (IIA) states the therapist "does not take control or power which rightfully belongs to the client." On the other hand, the code also requires therapists "assume a proactive stance toward the eradication of oppression" and "challenge oppressive aspects of both their own and their client's value systems" (Preamble). In this particular instance, Mary should begin by letting her client, Janie, know that she respects her right to choose medication for her PMS symptoms, but that she would like to ask her permission to explore another perspective on the situation before Janie commits to the medication course. She may negotiate a specific number of sessions for exploring the problem and generating alternative approaches to it.

During this time Mary can introduce Janie to nutritional or other holistic resources for PMS symptoms. Mary can address Janie's fears that therapy may further threaten her already strained relationship with her husband. She can begin teaching Janie to view the feelings that are arising premenstrually as a source of information about herself and her relationship with Charles. And she can start discussing the ways she and Charles are caught up in oppressive sex roles hindering their ability to communicate and understand each other.

If Janie still wants to pursue the medication course, or if she is so adamant about it that she will not enter into this exploration of alternatives, Mary will need to decide whether she can continue to work with her. If Mary cannot in good conscience continue her treatment while Janie also receives drug treatment for PMS, she will need to explore whether Janie might be more comfortable with a therapist of a different orientation or with a medication-centered form of treatment conducted by a psychiatrist. (Mary Hayden)

DILEMMA D

A 54-year-old eminent scientific researcher, Catherine, who has been dieting since the age of 13, entered therapy with Nancy to learn why she had never been able to maintain her weight loss. One of Catherine's stated goals of therapy is to uncover and deal with the unconscious feelings that cause her to remain fat. Currently, at 5' 3" and 275 pounds, she decided to undergo vertical-banded gastroplasty (commonly referred to as "stomach stapling"), which limits the size of the stomach so that it can hold only about two ounces. Eating anything more than a small amount causes nausea and vomiting; thus, it is impossible to get proper nutrition. This procedure, which involves major surgery with general anesthesia, is regarded as permanent. Because of the vomiting overextension induces, there is a possibility of the staples releasing, thereby returning the stomach to presurgery size and potentially causing future digestive problems from adhesion. Catherine seems aware of the drawbacks and risks of the procedure but has decided it is absolutely essential for her to be thinner, and this surgical procedure is the only route left. Aside from the many different kinds of diets she has tried, there is no history of abnormal eating behavior. (Phyllis Bronstein)

RESPONDENT 1

The main ethical dilemma in this case concerns whether a feminist therapist should be working with a client whose stated goal is "to learn why she had never been able to maintain her weight loss." The Preamble to the Feminist Therapy Code of Ethics emphasizes the importance of the "impact of society in creating and maintaining the problems and issues brought into therapy" and states that "each individual's personal experiences and situations are reflective of and an influence on society's institutionalized attitudes and values." Catherine provides a clear example of the impact of society's attitudes on an individual's experience

(Preamble). This intelligent, successful woman has been personally unhappy for 41 years because the shape of her body does not fit the current beauty ideal!

For the therapist, Nancy, to accept Catherine for weight loss therapy is to accept society's insistence that women can and should control their body's weight and shape. The Feminist Therapy Code of Ethics states that it is the therapist's responsibility to evaluate her interactions with clients for evidence of discriminatory attitudes or behaviors (IC). Nancy should consider whether her willingness to help Catherine blame herself for her weight and to continue to strive for an unrealistic ideal is evidence of Nancy's own fear of fat. Will the therapy liberate Catherine from years of unhappiness or collude in her oppression and perpetuate sizeism?

Catherine states that one of her goals in therapy is "to uncover and deal with the unconscious feelings which caused her to remain fat." Is Nancy sufficiently knowledgeable about the physiology of weight to evaluate the appropriateness of this stated goal? The Feminist Theray Code of Ethics (IVA) states feminist therapists should only work with issues with which they are competent. If Nancy chooses to work with Catherine on her weight issue, she needs to educate herself about the latest research on weight and dieting.

It may, of course, be possible for Nancy to provide benefits to Catherine by assisting her to explore the reasons she believes "it is absolutely essential for her to be thin" and working on increasing self-esteem and self-acceptance. Nancy might attempt to renegotiate the goals of therapy (IIC), but she must be careful in doing so to respect Catherine's experience (IB) and not to usurp her right to control her body (IIA) through surgery. It may be necessary for Nancy to self-disclose (IIB) something about her own struggles with sizeism and fat phobia in order to work effectively with Catherine. Finally, if Nancy wants to work with Catherine in relation to her weight or other body-image issues, she should not only educate herself about these issues but also work for social change through public education and lobbying for laws that will diminish fat oppression (VB). (Joan C. Chrisler)

RESPONDENT 2

The first ethical imperative of the feminist therapist is empowerment of the client. The issues presented by Catherine challenge Nancy to attend to ways in which she may inadvertently disempower Catherine by imposing her own values (IC, IIA, IVB). Nancy may find the nature of vertical-banded gastroplasty distasteful and be unwilling to participate in Catherine's self-blame for her weight. However, Nancy needs to respect Catherine's right to define her own value base (IB, C). Although the therapeutic process often results in clarification and revision of old values, too early explicit exposure to Nancy's differing value system may interfere with Catherine's need to work through to her own authentic value system (IIA). Nancy needs to be aware of her values and make them explicit in the therapeutic process for Catherine's benefit but must first "do no harm" (IIB). It makes sense for Catherine, living in U.S. culture, to want to be thin. This culture rewards and punishes women for their degree of conformity to the socially accepted standards of beauty. Good feminist practice honors women for their struggle for survival on whatever terms they can manage, at whatever point they may be in that struggle (IC).

Although Nancy might disagree with Catherine's decision to have the gastroplasty, her right to make this decision must also be respected. Empowerment means the right to make even poor decisions that might be regretted later. Catherine, a scientific researcher, seems to be aware of the risks and appears able to give informed consent. Meeting her at her own entry point in the therapeutic process means allowing her to have the dignity of surviving on her own terms and in her own context. Nancy's ability to dissuade Catherine represents a potential abuse of therapist power. For Nancy to impose her values on Catherine's decision-making process is to substitute another external standard of authority by which Catherine defines herself (IIA). An ethical therapist, however, can be honest in expressing her discomfort with the serious health risks of this procedure, while still respecting Catherine's right to set her own life agenda (IIB).

The feminist ethical task of sharing power within the therapy process requires that the task of setting treatment goals be a mutual one (IIC). Nancy must respect Catherine's assessment of her life experiences and needs while also relying on her own training and understanding of psychological and sociocultural processes of human development, growth, change, and healing (IVC).

As an ethical therapist, Nancy also has the responsibility to provide treatment within her realm of competencies (IVA). She must be prepared to acknowledge whether or not she has the training or skill to work psychodynamically with Catherine on food and body-image issues. If she does not, a referral to another therapist may be appropriate.

The last ethical concern involves therapist self-care (IVD). Weight and body-image issues are potent ones for most women in this culture. Nancy needs to be aware of her own oppression as well as how her biases and values may impact on the therapeutic process (IB, C). Strong views regarding this degree of surgical intervention require that Nancy consider whether she can work with Catherine without running the risk of interfering in her process. Alternatives range from Nancy seeking appropriate supervision and consultation to referring Catherine to another therapist. (Karen M. Lodl)

DILEMMA E

Frances is a feminist therapist in a small rural town. She specializes in dealing with women who have addictions and is the only one in her area who does so. Because of her excellent reputation as a very giving therapist, she has been very busy in her practice. She comes from an addictive family background but thinks she has worked through the personal issues that arose from substance abuse in her own family. She believes that the multiple workshops she attended on addictions accomplished her goal of looking at her own problems. She derives a great deal of pleasure from her practice, the focus of her life, and is especially pleased to help clients who have been unsuccessfully treated in the past. She is surprised to find herself feeling somewhat depressed, especially in the morning when she dreads the very busy day ahead. As she gets busy, she forgets her depression, and at night she is too tired to consider dealing with her depression. At the end of one long day of seeing clients, she received a call from a prospective client, Alice. Although very tired, fatigue left Frances as she listened to this client's story and realized Alice was at a point where her denial had been breached. Frances realized therapy for Alice would be very helpful, even to the point of being life saving. Alice was suicidal in her despair over the destructiveness of her alcoholism. As Frances looked through her appointment book, she was hard pressed to find an opening for the initial interview. Seeing Alice would require Frances to add an extra hour to her already overcrowded schedule. The only therapist she could refer Alice to was 250 miles away, and Alice did not have insurance to cover inpatient treatment and could not afford to pay for it herself.

RESPONDENT 1

Therapist self-care and isolation are the two main issues in this dilemma. Part of a therapist's responsibility in caring for a group of clients consists of regularly monitoring her own needs and general well-being (IVB, D). In this account, Frances's sense of self is derived primarily from her work, potentially leaving her vulnerable to the "ups and downs" of therapeutic process. In such situations, perceptions of client progress are required for the therapist to feel competent, and inevitable difficulties in the work can interfere with a therapist's clinical judgment. In this case, Frances is ignoring the status of her own well-being, affecting the quality of her work if it remains unaddressed.

This dilemma is further compounded by her rural isolation. Frances's reliance on her work is likely to be less obvious to her than if she were able to view herself alongside respected peers with whom she collaborates. In addition, Frances is vulnerable to taking on too much not only because her work is so vital to her but also because the need for her expertise exceeds her community's resources.

Frances is within the large category of women who become depressed but continue to function in activities that "support or enhance someone else" (Kaplan, 1984). Even though she possesses important skills that others do not offer, Frances may be acting unwisely for herself and irresponsibly for her clients and herself by taking on more hours than she can comfortably handle (particularly when clients like Alice initiate therapy in life-or-death crises). As Kaplan (1984) indicates, women who are depressed often experience an absence of connection as a failure of the self, and so, seek out experiences that will enhance the sense of self through supporting others. In low moments Frances would likely find relief from her feelings of disconnection and unimportance during her clients' crises and when she experiences the promise of new interpersonal connection as a new client seeks out her help.

Certainly, Frances is not at fault for the dearth of trained clinicians in her area. However, it is possible that her role as lone supporter for some clients may indirectly discourage them from advocating for additional supports in their community. Frances may do well to invest some of her professional efforts in educating her community about the need for additional providers, resources in the area of substance abuse and crises interventions, and supports (VB).

Finally, although Frances actively engages in continued education through workshops and remains up-to-date in her field, she does not have a more active professional peer group. She is not regularly engaging in supervision or peer consultation in order to more directly monitor and energize her work. As Kaplan (1984) reiterates Belle's finding, the presence of a confidante is a major barrier against depression under stressful circumstances. From this case description, it is unclear to what extent Frances experiences supportive personal relationships outside of her work. The image from this reading is of a woman who works long hours and interacts little with people who are not coming to her for help. Frances might network with other types of providers, such as nurses or physicians, who deal with similar clients. Computer communication through e-mail or Internet, telephone calls, or letters might broaden access to ongoing support and decrease her isolation. (Janice Berman)

RESPONDENT 2

There is an ethical dilemma between Frances's obligation as a feminist therapist to increase her accessibility "through flexible delivery of services" (IA) and self-nurturing and acknowledging her own emotional problems (IV). Frances, by not addressing the issues of her own depression, may be jeopardizing her emotional health and in turn be incapable of modeling "the ability and willingness to self-nurture in appropriate and self-empowering ways" (IVD). She believes that by attending "multiple workshops" on addiction she has worked through her issues of growing up in a family who abused drugs and/or alcohol. Workshops tend to be a passive form of education, are not usually individualized, and are only useful as an introduction to in-depth issues. There is evidence that Frances is exhibiting typical adult child of an alcoholic (ACOA) behaviors and could probably use supervision, peer support, and/or personal therapy to improve her potential to work effectively with Alice and other clients and increase her emotional well-being (IVB).

Part of Frances's ethical obligation is to "assist . . clients in accessing other services" (IA). It is difficult to believe that Frances thinks the only resource to whom she could refer Alice lives 250 miles away. Frances might consider referring Alice to an AA meeting within the next 24 hours, suggesting she call the nearest crisis clinic or suicide prevention hotline. Frances could remain accessible by suggesting to Alice she might have an opening in the future.

It is important for Frances to make an appointment with a therapist so she can deal with her own depression and possible ACOA issues. She also needs to seek supervision (IVB), be more honest with her present supervisor, or find another one who will confront Frances on her tendency to overwork and to act as if she is indispensable. (Carol E. Cohen)

IMPLICATIONS

She strode out proudly. "Not normal." And what do they consider a normal girl? One with beaten eyes who walks with closely-bound legs, obedient and submissive, with amputated sexual organs? One who drips with perfumed powders and paints, saturated day and night with sad songs and sex films? One who knows romantic stories by heart and can't really experience anything? The virtuous and pure virgin preoccupied with removing body hair and enticing men? (el-Saadwi, 1985, p. 112)

Ever since 1972, when Phyllis Chesler's book *Women and Madness* described the ways that women were oppressed by the mental health establishment, feminists began to examine the ways in which the patriarchy labeled women "mad." In 1985, the *Handbook of Feminist*

Therapy was edited as a result of the first Feminist Therapy Institute conference. The editors, Lynne Bravo Rosewater and Lenore Walker, focused on four issues: (1) an understanding of the therapist's power, (2) the growth in psychotherapy, (3) feminists' contributions to new areas never before covered by traditional systems, and (4) the importance of training and supervision for new feminist therapists.

When feminist therapists and their clients interface with the medical system, power differentials occur between therapist and client and between the therapist–client relationship and the medical establishment. All respondents in this medical model section referred to power differentials (IIA) and discussed them at some length. They stressed the issue of power, the importance of understanding power in the context of feminist therapy, and empowerment of the client as she needed to make decisions about her life. Feminist therapists can assist clients in accessing other systems, including the medical system. "Knowledge equals power," and educating the client about medical issues empowers her.

Most respondents also incorporated the ethical principle of ongoing self-evaluation and supervision (IVB) to resolve these ethical dilemmas and brought up other ethical principles on therapist accountability. Therapists need to educate themselves about the issues, especially about different cultures, and communicate with the client's physician. Therapists' isolation and therapists' limitations of knowledge and competency put clients at risk.

Most case respondents followed the steps of the "rational–evaluative process" in the order described by Hill, Glaser, and Harden (Section 2, this volume) with an emphasis on recognition and definition of the problem. A number of respondents also focused on development and choice of a solution, although most played the role of case reactor by remaining in the "consultant" role and brainstormed several possible solutions rather than selecting solutions to the ethical dilemmas.

Feminist therapists are sophisticated in their analyses of the issues concerning use of medication and the medical model in Western society. They can identify the problems and make decisions using the ethical principles of the Feminist Therapy Code of Ethics. However, respondents rarely initiated discussion of ethical principle V (social change). The preamble of the Code of Ethics, as well as feminist theory (e.g., Brown & Root, 1990; Rosewater & Walker, 1985), places a strong emphasis on social change in feminist practice.

Ever since the beginning of the feminist therapy movement, a major focus has been sociopolitical change. Butler (1985) presented guidelines for feminist therapy. Her final guideline consisted of encouraging women to pursue areas of growth outside of the therapy experience. Larsen and Cammaert (1985) described grassroots feminist programs. Caplan (1992) critiqued the DSM by developing her own criteria for macho behavior, which she labeled "delusional dominating personality disorder." Authors focus on the theme "the personal is political" (e.g., Faunce, 1985, p. 313). Have feminist therapists incorporated sociopolitical change as a major focus of their work? As the case dilemmas illustrate, there is need for social change in affecting the power structure of the medical system.

Feminist therapists today are profoundly affected by the medical model. They use the DSM to label clients in order for health insurance firms to reimburse their care. Training has been in traditional mental health professional programs. Most clinical placements, particularly if therapists were trained as psychiatrists, clinical psychologists, or psychiatric nurses, were in medical settings. Most clinical psychology internships in the United States are in Veterans Administration hospitals, pointing to the close connection between psychology and the military.

Yet medical model issues readily lend themselves to social change. Feminist therapists can play a role in reeducating society about the ways in which women have been overmedicalized or inappropriately medicalized. They can serve as community resources about substance abuse and medications, including medications for reproductive issues. They can play a pivotal role in changing fat-oppressive attitudes and emphasizing the dangers of many weight-reduction techniques.

As Hannah Lerman said, "Just as individuals brought up in a two-dimensional spatial world cannot imagine or comprehend three-dimensional space, we probably have not yet recovered sufficiently from the mental set associated with second-class status to develop .. a comprehensive view of total human functioning" (1985, p. 8). More writing and discussion are needed to detail ways in which feminist therapists can interact with feminist activism and social change in order to change the mental health system so that future generations of women are allowed to "stride out proudly."

RESPONDENTS

Janice Berman, PhD, does clinical work in areas of trauma and adolescence in the Boston area.

Phyllis Bronstein, PhD, is Associate Professor of Clinical Psychology at the University of Vermont and specializes in family therapy with research interests in parenting, early adolescent development, and gender role socialization.

Joan C. Chrisler, PhD, is Associate Professor at Connecticut College and has written extensively on women's health issues, particularly on weight and eating and on the psychosocial aspects of the menstrual cycle.

Pauline Rose Clance, PhD, is Professor of Psychology at Georgia State University and author of *The Imposter Phenomenon: Overcoming the Fears that Haunt your Success* (1985).

Carol E. Cohen, CSW, social worker and feminist therapist in private practice in Burlington, VT, is a political activist focusing on lesbian and gay liberation, Middle East peace from a Jewish feminist perspective, and the creation of a women's land project.

Ellen Cole, PhD, a psychologist specializing in sex therapy, directs the Master of Arts program at Prescott College in Arizona and coedits the journal *Women and Therapy.*

Lillian Comas-Díaz, PhD, Executive Director of the Transcultural Mental Health Institute, is a clinical psychologist in private practice and Associate Professor at the George Washington University Department of Psychiatry and Behavioral Sciences.

Miriam Frankel Stoll, MBA, is a graduate student and Research Fellow in clinical psychology at the University of Vermont.

Mary Hayden, PhD, a psychologist, has a private practice as a feminist therapist in Pasadena, CA.

Nayyar S. Javed, MEd, a feminist therapist, works with the racialized population at the Saskatoon Mental Health Clinic, Saskatoon, Saskatchewan.

Karen M. Lodl, MSc, a psychologist in private practice in Calgary, Alberta, teaches Women's Studies at the University of Calgary.

Jessica Morris, AB, is a graduate student and Research Fellow in Clinical Psychology at the University of Vermont.

Mary E. Willmuth, PhD, is Clinical Associate Professor at the University of Vermont, works in health psychology at the Medical Center Hospital of Vermont, and has a private psychotherapy practice.

REFERENCES

Albino, J. E., Tedesco, L. A., & Shenkle, C. L. (1990). Images of women: Reflections from the medical care system. In M. A. Paludi & G. A. Steurnagel (Eds.), *Foundations for a feminist restructuring of the academic disciplines* (pp. 225–253). Binghamton, NY: Harrington Park Press.

American Psychiatric Association. (1994). *Diagnostic and statistical manual of mental disorders* (4th ed.). Washington, DC: Author.

American Psychological Association. (1990). Ethical principles of psychologists. *American Psychologist, 45*(3), 390–395.

Broverman, I., Broverman, D. M., Clarkson, F. E., Rosenkrantz, P. S., & Vogel, S. R. (1970). Sex role stereotypes and clinical judgments of mental health. *Journal of Consulting and Clinical Psychology, 34*(1), 1–7.

Brown, L. S., & Rothblum, E. D. (1989). *Overcoming fear of fat.* Binghamton, NY: Harrington Park Press.

Brown, L. S., & Root, M. P. P. (1990). *Diversity and complexity in feminist therapy.* Binghamton, NY: Harrington Park Press.

Brownmiller, S. (1984). *Femininity.* New York: Fawcett Columbine.

Butler, M. (1985). Guidelines for feminist therapy. In L. B. Rosewater & L. E. A. Walker (Eds.), *Handbook of feminist therapy: Women's issues in psychotherapy* (pp. 32–37). New York: Springer.

Caffetera, G. L., Kasper, J., & Bernstein, A. (1983). Family roles, structure, and stressors in relation to sex differences in obtaining psychotropic drugs. *Journal of Health and Social Behavior, 24*, 132–143.

Caplan, P. J. (1992). Gender issues in the diagnosis of mental disorder. *Women and Therapy, 12*(4), 71–79.

Chesler, P. (1972). *Women and madness.* New York: Avon.

Cooperstock, R. (1981). A review of women's psychotropic drug use. In E. Howell & M. Bayes (Eds.), *Women and mental health* (pp. 131–140). New York: Basic Books.

Cutler, S. E., & Nolen-Hoeksema, S. (1991). Accounting for sex differences in depression through female victimization. *Sex Roles, 24*(7, 8), 425–438.

el-Saadwi, N. (1985). *Two women in one* (O. Nusairi & J. Gough, Trans.). Seattle, WA: Seal Press.

Faunce, P. S. (1985). Teaching feminist therapies: Integrating feminist therapy, pedagogy and scholarship. In L. B. Rosewater & L. E. A. Walker (Eds.), *Handbook of feminist therapy: Women's issues in psychotherapy* (pp. 309–330). New York: Springer.

Garner, D. M., & Wooley, S. C. (1991). Confronting the failure of behavioral and dietary treatments for obesity. *Clinical Psychology Review, 11*, 729–780.

Jack, D. C. (1991). *Silencing the self: Women and depression.* Boston: Harvard University Press.

Kaplan, A. G. (1984). *The "self-in-relation": Implications for depression in women* (Work in Progress, No. 14). Wellesley, MA: Stone Center.

Lane, A. J. (1980). The fictional world of Charlotte Perkins Gilman. In A. J. Lane (Ed.), *The Charlotte Perkins Gilman reader* (pp. ix–xiii). New York: Pantheon Books.

Larsen, C. C., & Cammaert, L. P. (1985). Introduction to feminist psychotherapeutic techniques and practices. In L. B. Rosewater & L. E. A. Walker (Eds.), *Handbook of feminist therapy: Women's issues in psychotherapy* (pp. 47–50). New York: Springer.

Lerman, H. (1985). Some barriers to the development of a feminist theory of personality. In L. B. Rosewater & L. E. A. Walker (Eds.), *Handbook of feminist therapy: Women's issues in psychotherapy* (pp. 5–12). New York: Springer.

Lissner, L., Odell, P. M., D'Agostino, R. B., Stokes, J., Kreger, B. E., Belanger, A. J., & Brownell, K. D. (1991). Variability of body weight. *Journal of Medicine, 324*, 1839–1844.

McGrath, E., Keita, G. P., Strickland, B. R., & Russo, N. F. (1990). *Women and depression: Risk factors and treatment issues.* Washington, DC: American Psychological Association.

Miller, J. B. (1983). *The construction of anger in women and men* (Work in Progress, No. 83-01). Wellesley, MA: Stone Center.

Mowbray, C. T., Lanir, S., & Hulce, M. (Eds.). (1985). *Women and mental health: New directions for change.* Binghamton, NY: Harrington Park Press.

Penfold, S. P., & Walker, G. A. (1983). *Women and the psychiatric paradox.* Montreal: Eden Press.

Polivy, J., & Herman, C. P. (1983). *Breaking the diet habit.* New York: Basic Books.

Rack, P. (1982). *Race, culture and mental disorder.* London: Tavistock.

Rosewater, L. B., & Walker, L. E. A. (Eds.). (1985). *Handbook of feminist therapy: Women's issues in psychotherapy.* New York: Springer.

Rothblum, E. D. (1983). Sex-role stereotypes and depression in women. In V. Franks & E. D. Rothblum (Eds.), *The stereotyping of women: Its effects on mental health* (pp. 83–111). New York: Springer.

Rothblum, E. D. (1990). Women and weight: Fad and fiction. *Journal of Psychology, 124,* 5–24.

Rothblum, E. D. (1992). The stigma of women's weight: Social and economic realities. *Feminism and Psychology, 2,* 61–73.

Rothblum, E. D. (1994). I'll die for the revolution but don't ask me not to diet: Feminism and the continuing stigmatization of obesity. In P. Fallon, M. A. Katzman, & S. C. Wooley (Eds.), *Feminist perspectives on eating disorders* (pp. 53–75). New York: Guilford Press.

Russo, N. F. (1990). Overview: Forging research priorities in women's mental health. *American Psychologist, 45,* 368–373.

Sherwin, S. (1992). *No longer patient: Feminist ethics and health care.* Philadelphia: Temple University Press.

Tiggemann, M., & Rothblum, E. D. (1988). Gender differences in social consequences of perceived overweight in the United States and Australia. *Sex Roles, 18,* 75–86.

Travis, C. B. (1988). *Women and mental health psychology: Mental health issues.* Hillsdale, NJ: Erlbaum.

TEN

Conflicts in Care: Early Years of the Lifespan

Jane Close Conoley
Paula Larson

There are many parallels between women's issues and those of children and youth. Children, like women, have historically been viewed as property, most often of a husband or father. Women and children have traditionally been perceived in most societies as dependent, intellectually inferior, physically weak, and with limited role potentials. This obvious connection compels feminists to pay particular attention to child treatment.

Children have less control over themselves, less ownership of and access to information, and to other important aspects of their lives than do most adults. The basis for these limitations lies in the assessment of their physical, cognitive, social, and moral development as immature.

Challenges to ethical decision making around child and adolescent clients comes from many sources: (1) current beliefs about and assessment of the young person's knowledge and thinking skills; (2) the legal/judicial/ethical codes that identify rights of young persons with certain chronological ages; (3) the assumption that children are surrounded by protective and nurturing guardians who have young people's best interests at heart; and (4) the role of the family unit in nurturing, protecting, and making decisions regarding the young person.

Each of these forces bears some scrutiny when actual decisions are being made about particular clients. A special knowledge of child development and assessment as well as knowledge about the law in various jurisdictions is critical for practitioners who work with young people. Further, an intimate understanding of the contexts in which the child or adolescent is living is a prerequisite for ethical therapeutic work.

HISTORICAL CONTEXT

Children have been regarded as property in all but a few societies (Fraad, 1993). The child's role has often been "to be seen and not heard" and to do whatever the adults deemed necessary in order to preserve the family unit. Historically, parenting was seen as "breaking the will of the child" so she or he would adjust to societal expectations (Miller, 1983). The writings of John Locke (1693/1964) and Jean-Jacques Rousseau (1763) were influential in changing the view of children as animalistic sinners in need of control to a view of children as integrated human beings who are to be valued and understood for what they are rather than what they will become (Maccoby, 1980).

Children have traditionally been at the bottom of the hierarchy in terms of status, power, control, and/or decision making. The concept of children as property has allowed parents and guardians invasive powers over children. Children can be hit or have their movements severely restricted without their consent and with little rationale or explanation. Many of the commonly accepted protections guaranteed by the U.S. Constitution are not automatically available to children. Even in modern codes of ethics, children have no rights to confidentiality or the right to seek treatment independent of the permission of their guardians. It is only recently that children have been granted even minimal status, respect, and privacy. In Western societies, rights guaranteed to children deal mainly with their physical welfare. It was not until early in this century that child labor laws and child protection laws were passed in the United States (Nardinelli, 1990). Mandatory schooling is also a rather recent historical development (Ensign, 1921/1969). When considering the challenges to the ethical treatment of children, it is important to remember the continuing impact of early cultural beliefs regarding the nature of children, the rights of parents, and the purposes of parenting.

THERAPEUTIC CONTEXT

The rather recent and seemingly cursory attention to children from both legal and social systems is analogous to the attention given by the therapeutic community. Although there are notable exceptions, most diagnostic categories and therapeutic approaches used with children were designed for use with adults.

Children have been viewed as unfinished adults in primitive stages of development and so were thought to be unable to engage in the therapeutic process. Further, despite overwhelming evidence to the contrary (e.g., Solomon, 1992), childhood was seen as a rather protected, idyllic time for most children. For those children who, for whatever reason, failed to fit this mold, harsh discipline was often viewed as the solution. Therapists were unlikely to view young people as potential clients. Intrusion of a therapist into the family where the father held absolute power was rare. Fathers may not have known best, but their authority was supported by law and custom in most cultural contexts.

The practice of child therapy has been further hindered by a paucity of accurate diagnostic tools for use with children and adolescents. Many behaviors that may be considered as maladaptive at one age are considered less problematic or even normal at another age. It is difficult to pinpoint the frequency and intensity of problem behaviors across settings and across developmental stages. Thus depression in a 10-year-old may be exhibited very differently than depression in a 14-year-old. Given the number of developmental stages of childhood, as well as the variability within each stage, accurate assessment of a young person can be far more complex than assessment of an adult and is more dependent on one's knowledge of and ability to assess relevant developmental characteristics such as cognitive, physiological, social, and emotional factors.

Many, if not most, forms of psychotherapy for children have been developed from therapies designed for use with adults. The earliest forms of psychotherapy relied heavily on verbal skills and abilities to conceptualize at symbolic levels and so severely limited children's active involvement. Their dreams might have been interpreted using adult metaphors. The formats used by most early therapists were not consistent with age-appropriate engagement with a child. Even play therapy was not interactive with a therapist but rather considered a projection of the child's inner life.

Although Anna Freud (1927) and Melanie Klein (1975) were early pioneers in child treatment, it is noteworthy that their approaches relied on interpretations of unconscious material from children's dreams and play using only internal psychodynamic structures for explanations. This procedure circumvented the political and social realities of children's lives and called forth pathological interpretations. Because fantasy, projection, and transference were such powerful constructs in these systems, the reality of a child's plight, for example sexual abuse, might not be recognized in spite of years of intervention or therapy.

The focus of child treatment also raises many issues. Children rarely seek professional help themselves. Thus, the nature of presenting problems is most often defined not by the child but by the parent or guardian.

In fact, they are most often the complaintants. It is their language that represents the child's problem, at least in the early stages of therapy. Many significant problem behaviors may go unnoticed because parents or guardians may not consider them seriously maladaptive or, perhaps more critically, parents or guardians may conceal or deny maladaptive behaviors in an effort to protect themselves.

Practitioners who work in public practice, especially schools, may have greater access to children than do many private practitioners. The conflict that can arise between a school psychologist's perceptions of what a child may need and both the school's and the parents' willingness to support such service is an everyday dilemma.

More recently, the focus of child therapy has shifted from an emphasis on internal psychodynamic processes to developmental status, social reinforcement, learning, and interactional patterns as foundations of both adaptive and maladaptive behaviors (Patterson, 1990). Although children continue to precipitate many referrals, the focus of treatment is often the family context (Kazdin, 1988). Treatment is more cognizant of the everyday accumulated stresses faced by the child that predict maladjustment, such as impaired intelligence, substance-abusing parents, poverty, and racism (Borocas et al., 1991).

IMPORTANCE TO FEMINISTS

Feminists give special attention to social context, power relationships, and the recognition and integration of diversity and difference. These priorities suggest that children and young people are especially important to feminists because of their structurally based powerlessness.

Children and young people are targets of abuse and neglect due to their relative powerlessness and the lingering perspective of them as property. Children and young people who bear the double or triple oppressions of being from ethnic minority groups or being gay or lesbian are clearly at great risk from the societal pathologies that surround them. Girls are vulnerable to sexual exploitation in addition to being raised in societies that devalue their voices and their contributions (Haugaard & Reppucci, 1988).

Psychology theorists and practitioners in developmental and clinical psychology know very little about the cognitive, social, sexual, and moral experiences of young people of color growing up in Western societies (Brown, 1991a). Attachment, separation, or individuation are rarely considered from multiple ethnic or racial vantage points, but they are critical to understanding children's development.

Heterosexist constructs are still considered the desirable norm. New avenues of research suggest that preference for same-sex partners or for partners of either sex is (and has been) evidenced in well over 10% of the population (Worell & Remer, 1992). Psychosexual development is not well understood, and the unique and shared experiences of heterosexual and homosexual youth are only recent areas of serious research (Kitzinger, 1992). Most available research continues a tradition of pathologizing homosexuality and fails to offer a normal developmental framework for gay and lesbian youth (Kitzinger, 1992). Currently almost no information is given to future practitioners and practicing psychologists relating to the developmental, social, and societal milestones faced by gay and lesbian youth. It is clear, however, that such youth are at increased risk for abuse from peers and from family members (D'Augelli, 1989; D'Augelli & Rose, 1990).

Sexual abuse of female children is an epidemic. Estimates suggest that before the age of 18 more than 37% of American women experience sexual abuse, and 20% are sexually abused by a family member (Badgley et al., 1984; Russell, 1986).

The U.S. Advisory Board on Child Abuse and Neglect (1990) reported that 2.5% of American children are abused and/or neglected every year. Consider also the numbing statistic that among murder victims, women are more than four times as likely as men to have been killed by a spouse or other intimate partner (Reiss & Roth, 1993). Often these murders are committed in front of children and have been preceded by years of physical, sexual, and emotional abuse within a family system (Jaffe, Wolfe, & Wilson, 1990). It is likely that up to four million women are battered annually (Straus, 1994; Straus, Gelles, & Steinmetz, 1980).

No longer can it be assumed that the adults who care for children will inevitably have their best interests at heart. Although the majority of parents remain committed to protecting their children's welfare, it is becoming increasingly clear that a sizable minority of parents and other predatory adults either lack the necessary skills or basic moral standards to be entrusted with caring for and making decisions for children and adolescents.

Children are affected by violence as its direct and indirect casualties. Being victimized and observing victimization have devastating effects on children. It puts them at risk for physical and emotional disorders, school failure, substance abuse, legal difficulties, and the likelihood, especially for boys, they will cope with problems by using aggression themselves (Fantuzzo, DePaola, Lambert, & Martino, 1991; Pynoos & Nader, 1990; Reid, 1993). Girls who are witnesses and victims of abuse are at life-long risk for depression, dysfunctional relationship issues, and revictimization (Haugaard & Reppucci, 1988).

Despite the magnitude of the risk to children, in the United States in particular, raising children is a very private enterprise. There is very little state intrusion into parental rights (Coleman, 1992). The misdeeds of adults toward children are shrouded in legally supported secrecy under the guise of individual and family rights to privacy. Unlike other Western nations, there is no regular "window" into the homes that receive infants, no universal health system to monitor physical status of children and youth, and limited resources to support prevention or investigation of abusive situations. Feminists will recognize this situation as analogous to the one faced by women who live in threatening and/or abusive environments.

TREATMENT APPROACHES

Feminist approaches to treatment seek to emphasize the equal status of the therapist and client (Brown, 1991b). Although this egalitarian stance may not be possible for clients at every age, it is certainly the vision that guides feminist treatment. A special consequence of this stance toward egalitarianism is the need to determine the skills children possess to make decisions regarding their own futures. Recent analyses (Melton, 1983; Moshman, 1993) of children's cognitive development suggest their ability to make rationale decisions is present earlier than their so-called age of majority. Such pronouncements are noteworthy, but the translation of them into real-case situations is difficult.

Traditional approaches to child and adolescent treatment have relied on intraindividual or intrapsychic causes of pathology that tend to place the blame on the victim and emphasize a rather fixed developmental sequence. Theories that minimize the influence of the situational variables or environmental stressors also maximize the responsibility of the individual in "fixing" his or her situation. In the case of almost all children and young persons, many solutions to problems lie outside of their control or influence.

Also inherent in many approaches to child development and treatment have been assumptions that adversely affect a practitioner's ability to recognize and respond to all children's needs. Worell and Remer (1992) group these theories into several categories.

First, developmental constructs tend to be androcentric, using men as a standard. Accordingly, women are viewed as not only different from men, but as inferior to men. For example, Freud's (1965) and Erikson's (1963) androcentric constructs of personality and identity development explained development from a male perspective, generalized the theory to women and explained differences as deficiencies in women's development.

Kohlberg's (1981, 1984) theory of moral development was based almost entirely on a young, white male sample. He too generalized findings to females, concluding that females were inferior to males in terms of moral development. These few examples suggest why therapists tended to see even healthy adult women as childlike while they equate mental health with male characteristics.

Second, female researchers such as Gilligan (1982; Brown & Gilligan, 1992) gave women's development a new perspective, one that suggests differences rather than deficiencies. She is an example of a "gendercentric" theorist. Gendercentric constructs continue to view women and men as following two separate paths of development. These paths are considered separate but equal. The limitation of this approach is that differences rather than similarities are emphasized. Little attention is given to areas in which male and female development intersect.

The theories of Chodorow (1978) and Miller (1976) exemplify gendercentric constructs suggesting that differences between women and men are related to early mother–child relationships. Although an improvement over traditional dynamic theorizing, the role of societal demands or cultural values in the development of male and female sex roles is given only narrow attention.

Third, ethnocentric constructs base their observations on primarily Anglo-European populations and assume very little variability across races, cultures and/or nations. For example, concepts defining normal family functioning are inherently tied to traditional Anglo-European values that emphasize a hierarchical structure, unequal power differentiation between women and men, and lower status and power of children within the family structure (Worell & Remer, 1992).

Of special concern for therapists who work with young girls is the developmental progression in women's lives, from an acceptance of the conventions of female goodness to a critical feminist consciousness (Brown, 1991b). Adolescent girls often lose their voices and their self-confidence as they enter adolescence (Rogers, 1993). Therapists and researchers are faced with helping girls speak their minds truthfully in a social context that conspires to silence them. Therapists have little support from traditional theories to guide their work with children.

Family Therapy Issues

Traditional family systems approaches have been faulted for failing to take into account the social, political and economic context in which the family exists. Family system therapy, in attempting to maintain neutrality, often fails to recognize the power differentials inherent in most families (Avis, 1992). Stereotypic gender roles are frequently reinforced. Because women are traditionally more involved in the care of children, they all too often become the scapegoat for relationship or parenting problems (Enns, 1993; Dutton-Douglas & Walker, 1988).

Therapists who treat children and youth must be particularly expert in forging therapeutic alliances with entire families. Such alliances allow children to be offered many of the traditional safeguards of therapy as appropriate to their capacities (Terry, 1992). For example, the limits of confidentiality for the child client must be negotiated within the framework of the parents' goodwill, as there is no legal support for confidential treatment of children and adolescents except in matters of abuse or potential for harming self or others.

Psychologists who work in schools are often faced with this dilemma as they are caught between requirements of laws enabling service to handicapped children and youth, the needs of the children, ethical codes, perceived rights of the parents, and constraints of the school organization. A common conflict is that of protecting as much of a young person's information as possible so as to avoid adverse actions from school officials and/or parents while meeting the letter of the law. It is especially difficult to work with adolescent girls and not encounter situations where their information regarding incest, pregnancy, abortion, sexual activities and/or orientation, or drug use does not create some conflicts in their care.

Keeping clear the identity of the client may be the most basic of the ethical issues surrounding child work. The issue of client identification is of utmost importance because it defines limits of confidentiality, management of overlapping relationships, duty to warn, and other issues of loyalty as they relate to client welfare vis-à-vis existing laws and regulations.

Social Change

Another issue that may be particularly relevant to the treatment of children and youth is the feminist therapist's commitment to promoting social awareness and change. The feminist therapist works to change oppressive social conditions. Given children's lack of power, therapist involvement in community programming, educational events, and preventive interventions is particularly important. Children have suffered from not having powerful voices to support them.

Awareness of the family's role in the socialization process can be useful as well. Families and parental interactional styles/roles are models of traditional or flexible gender-specific behavior. Parents also contingently reinforce certain desirable patterns of behavior that may be gender specific. As an egalitarian role model, the feminist therapist provides modeling, information, and direct instruction in how to develop these flexible or more egalitarian roles within the family (Enns, 1993; Dutton-Douglas & Walker, 1988; Worell & Remer, 1992).

The following dilemmas deal with some of the issues raised in the preceding paragraphs. In particular, therapists are put into situations that test their understandings of who is the client, their expertise in certain matters, the complexities of multiple and overlapping relationships, and the possible effects of diversity on their decision making.

DILEMMA A

Judy is a 12-year-old girl who lives with her mother and her mother's lesbian companion. After three years of no contact, Judy's father has decided he wants custody of her. He has recently remarried and believes that he and his new wife can provide a healthier home for Judy than his ex-wife can. Sandra has been Judy's counselor at her school for the last three years and sees Judy as a very well-adjusted preadolescent. Judy's mother asks Sandra to be a "character" witness at the custody hearing. Sandra is willing but her principal informed her that she must decline. He does not want one of his counselors involved in a highly publicized and "controversial" court case, fearing publicity will detract from the positive things that happen at the school.

RESPONDENT 1

The therapist is obligated to assist in the social change process (VB) by educating the court about issues regarding homosexuals as parents. Not only should she provide information about the efficacy of this minority group as parents, she should also advocate for her client's own best interest (IA). The court must consider the disruption caused by removing the client from the home she has known and to which she apparently has made good adjustment. The counselor is in a good position to advocate for her client as well as to make her expertise about child development available to the court. These concerns are of much higher priority than the principal's concerns about negative publicity. Indeed, he cannot prevent the counselor from testifying.

As the counselor gives testimony, she needs to be aware of confidentiality issues (IIIB). She must place her client's interests above those of the client's mother as well as ahead of court efforts to gain information that she may deem a breach of confidentiality toward her client. She must be prepared to go to great lengths to protect this privileged relationship.

Finally, it would serve the therapist and her clients well to consult with other professionals (IVB). Such professionals can help broaden the therapist's perspective, uncover blind spots, prepare her for giving court testimony, clarify ethical questions, and, in general, assist in interacting with a system (school) that is exceedingly political and slow to change. (Mary Coady-Leeper)

RESPONDENT 2

The ethical dilemma that may arguably take precedence over all other issues in this scenario is immediately apparent: Who is the client? Although Sandra may think that support to the mother is appropriate or even necessary in this situation, Sandra must be careful to accord appropriate status to Judy as her client. Sandra has an obligation to determine and act on the child client's wishes, guided also by the principle of what is in the best interests of a child. The need is evident to recognize the numerous overlapping relationships (IIIA) in this case: child–therapist, mother–therapist, therapist–principal. However, Sandra can be guided by "recognizing that her client's concerns and general well-being are primary" and by monitoring both public and private statements (IIIB) in accordance with the needs and wishes expressed by Judy.

Further, Sandra must take care that she has adequate first-hand information about the father's opposition to the mother having custody before being guided by feminist principles regarding social change (VB). Unless she can be certain the father's opposition is based on his exwife's sexual preference, she could act on erroneous assumptions. Should Sandra determine with reliable first-hand information that the father's opposition is based primarily on sexual preference, she then would "seek . . . avenues for impacting change" (VB).

However, testifying would be an acceptable avenue for such change only if it is in accordance with the child client's wishes. Further, even if Judy wanted Sandra to testify, Sandra would still be faced with the dilemma presented by her employer's opposition (VB). Finally, if testifying were not compatible with the child client's wishes, Sandra might resolve this ethical double-bind by finding other means of promoting social change that are not client-specific, such as education and advocacy. (Maureen Kitchur)

DILEMMA B

Lori is a therapist in a small rural community. She has been seeing her client Martha, a single mother, for five months. Martha has expressed concerns about her six-year-old daughter's lack of discipline. Lori agrees to see the girl, Tammie, in play therapy while still seeing Martha individually. During the

third session, Tammie is playing with dolls and acts out the mother's hitting
the daughter for being a "bad girl." Lori asks Tammie if her mother has hit her
and Tammie replies in the affirmative. Lori reports Martha to the police for
child abuse.

RESPONDENT 1

This scenario raises ethical dilemmas in two areas. Questions exist about what considerations Lori made when she agreed to see Tammie and what options she considered when reporting Martha.

When Lori and Martha agreed that Lori would see Tammie for play therapy, a concern is raised regarding therapist accountability (IVA). Is Lori competent in play therapy? Assuming Lori is competent in play therapy, and given the fact that she is seeing Martha, a second concern is raised regarding overlapping relationships (IIIA). As Martha is Lori's client, how did Lori set the stage so that she could act in the best interests of both Martha and Tammie if these interests should conflict? Given Lori's responsibility to monitor the relationship between herself and Martha to prevent potential abuse of or harm to Martha, she was obliged to discuss with Martha the issues of confidentiality regarding Lori's relationship with Tammie and to explain to Martha the limits of confidentiality and Lori's duty to inform regarding disclosures of child abuse.

It is important to remember this scenario occurred in a rural community. It is fair to assume that services are limited and therefore special considerations may be warranted in this setting. In all probability, Lori was obliged to be flexible in her delivery of services because of the setting and therefore considered the ethical guideline related to cultural diversities and oppressions (IA).

Lori may have been more empowering to Martha, however, had she worked with Martha to help her manage Tammie's behavior rather than seeing Martha and Tammie separately, and thereby, perhaps communicate a bias that Martha was not able to help Tammie, and therapy was needed to "fix" Tammie (IC). Once Tammie disclosed child abuse, concerns are raised regarding power differentials (IIA). The power differential exists in view of the fact that Lori had knowledge of Martha, which she did not learn from Martha, but which she was obliged to disclose. To address the power differentials, Lori could have considered empowering Martha by encouraging Martha to make the disclosure herself. However, this solution only appears to empower Martha. Although Martha may have a choice regarding who makes the call to the police, Lori is still obliged to ensure that the call was made by both monitoring Martha while she calls and following up with her own call. Thus the power differential still exists.

A secondary problem of informing Martha of the call to the police concerns the power differential between Tammie and her mother. Lori is obliged to consider Tammie's best interests. If Lori is concerned about Tammie's safety in her home, telling Martha of the disclosure before telling the police may bring potential danger to Tammie. Clear agreements and guidelines before seeing Tammie would have avoided these ethical dilemmas. (Roslyn Mendelson)

RESPONDENT 2

Given feminist's historical interest in children's issues as an extension of women's issues and mandatory reporting of child abuse laws, the omission of a specific feminist ethical guideline regarding the reporting of child abuse is curious. Nonetheless, there are principles (I, II, III) that offer appropriate guidance in this situation.

Lori is bound by state and federal law to report suspected child abuse. However, Lori is also bound to educate her clients on their rights and the consequences of the therapeutic process (IID). This is the only point upon which Lori appears to have been ethically remiss. Counselors must educate clients about the limits counselors face in maintaining confidentiality. Most clients are unaware that some matters may not be kept confidential if the welfare of another is threatened. If this is done in the spirit of educating the client so that he or she is able to work with the counselor in disclosing abuse, then it is feminist and empowering.

The other two issues that enter into this situation have to do with cultural diversity and overlapping relationships. Lori's responsibility is to "prevent potential abuse of or harm to the client" (IIIA). Although involvement with a child protection agency may not be abusive, Lori's reporting of the abuse may be damaging to the therapeutic relationship. In addition, Lori is responsible for "monitoring" overlapping relationships. By choosing to see Martha and Tammie separately, rather than together, Lori is accountable to two clients whose interests may be in conflict.

Lori's goal as a feminist therapist is to serve those that she can and to refer when appropriate (IA, B). She needs to be open to cultural diversities and continue to work toward a better understanding of those cultures she does not understand. Small rural communities constitute a different culture with different values compared to the mainstream urban culture. Resources are limited and overlapping relationships are common. Therapists in such situations must take extraordinary measures to be sure their overlapping/dual relationships are not exploitative. Because such situations happen fairly frequently in rural communities, they deserve special attention and care.

In this context, Lori's interaction with Martha and Tammie was not unusual. As a result, her monitoring of the overlapping relationships was appropriate based on an assumption there were no other qualified child therapists available in the community. (Peg M. Miller)

DILEMMA C

Peg is a therapist in a mental health agency working with adolescents and their families who are referred by Juvenile Court through a diversion program for juvenile offenders. Sarah was reported as a run-away and was found in possession of alcohol. Sarah is seeking permission to move from the family home, saying she will continue to run away if she has to stay there. Her mother, with her stepfather's passive agreement, says she cannot leave. After discussing Sarah's complaints and the parents' complaints, which do not include abuse, Peg asks Sarah what she would want from her mother that would make it acceptable to continue to live at home. Sarah replies that she would like her mother to spend some time—maybe an hour—talking to her after school a few times a week. Peg, expecting the mother to say "yes" or reply with an alternative suggestion, asks if Mom is willing to do that. Mom looks directly at Sarah and tells her that she is not willing to do that.

RESPONDENT 1

Working in the context of feminist analysis, the therapist recognizes the effects of sexism on development and the relationship of sexism to other forms of oppression based on gender, class, sexual orientation, and culture (IB). In this scenario, as Peg is met with the stepfather's passive agreement with the mother and the mother's refusal to respond to her daughter's legitimate request for parental care, Peg must question the power differentials in this family system (IIA). Recognizing the mother may be responding from a powerless place within the marriage, it is incumbent on Peg to provide a safe therapeutic environment, such as individual time with the mother, to fully assess from a cultural and experiential viewpoint the mother's sense of oppression and/or freedom to make decisions within the family. If the hypothesis is confirmed regarding the mother's sense of powerlessness in her relationship, this power differential may also be part of Sarah's issues regarding her own socialization as a young woman attempting to challenge a future of giving power to others based solely on gender.

When working with adolescents and their families an important ethical question becomes who is the primary client? In this case, Sarah has been referred by Juvenile Court, thus making her the primary client. Peg should acknowledge the inherent power differential between client and therapist and also therapist and parents. This acknowledgment provides her with an opportunity to model respectful use of power with Sarah and her family. Peg has the power to act in the child's best interest, and the parents must be aware of this (IIA). The therapist can and at times must act on behalf of the children's best interest even when this is contradictory to the child's or the parents' wishes. It is a fine line the therapist must walk, not to take control of power that rightfully belongs to the client and to model effective and respectful use of power as necessary for the child's safety. Walking this line respectfully is also crucial for continuation of a therapeutic relationship with the family.

Based on the mother's refusal to accept her daughter's request for positive child care or to suggest alternatives, Peg must question at what point this situation becomes a concern for the child welfare authorities based on the child being at risk for emotional abuse. Advocating for the child with the parents and child welfare authorities may become the role of the therapist at this time (IVA).

Peg's ethical responsibility in working with adolescent girls and their families would be to keep current in the field of research pertaining to girls' developmental needs and the impact of patriarchal norms in this development (IVC). Knowing the research findings would allow Peg to use this knowledge in making her assessment of Sarah's psychological needs. Peg also must assess how to use this knowledge in such a way as to empower Sarah and support her developmental need for meaningful relationships at this time in her life.

Peg may add to her work with Sarah and her family by choosing other avenues available to her for impacting change (V). Peg can use her power and knowledge to challenge societal beliefs regarding power imbalances in male–female relationships and advocate for equality, teaching about the damage done to everyone when anyone is denied access to her own voice. Social change has many faces and is a necessary piece of a feminist practice that challenges the society that continues to create and maintain the problems brought into the therapy room. (Lois Sapsford)

RESPONDENT 2

Although the race/ethnicity of the characters in this case is not specified, it would certainly behoove any therapist to do a careful self-analysis before starting this work with an African-American family. This scenario could happen with a family of color, but there would be powerful traditions and forces at work. Many women of color would be uneasy and unwilling for their children to be seen in therapy at all but certainly unwilling for them to be seen alone. The legitimate need to be self-protective and protective of family matters in a racist society works against easy self-disclosure among people of color.

Issues of power are clearly evident in this scenario. There are obvious misuses and obvious misperceptions. For example, a family's ability to keep a child from running away is quite limited. The mother and stepfather imagine they have more power in this situation than they do. On the other hand, they do not seem to recognize the invitation to have influence they have been given by Sarah. Their refusal to be involved with their child, except to demand that she remain in what appears to be an oppressive environment, suggests either skill/informational deficits or a destructive commitment to rigid power relationships (IIA).

It is true, however, that in many minority families the suggestion that parents negotiate with their children will appear incongruent. A therapist hoping to facilitate positive change in a minority family system may have to see the mother or parents alone and give them information and directive comments about what is likely to happen to their daughter if they do not lead the family toward more harmonious interactions. While modeling egalitarian interactions, the culturally sensitive therapist might do well to use existing understandings of power relationships and give the parents a sense of purpose and responsibility rather than an ultimatum.

In some minority families, the position of the stepfather in this matter would be quite peripheral. His ability or right to influence Sarah would be seen by her and by most others as quite minimal. This situation would be affected, of course, by the current and past marital and parental histories of the family. The biological link between Sarah and her mother puts the decision making squarely in the mother's purview. Sensitivity to cultural differences might suggest the therapist make a special effort to see the mother and daughter together. Peg might need consultation to support her in this matter (Dolores Simpson-Kirkland)

IMPLICATIONS

School counselors and school psychologists may be caught by conflicting loyalties to a child client, parent, political issue, and job security. Their daily access to children requires frequent clarification of who the client is, the credibility of their information, and their duty to inform the courts of current psychological research.

Kitchur's special note that duty to the client's wishes outweighs political and social agendas is of extreme importance. There is such a need for valid information in courts about parental fitness that being so involved can have great saliency. As she so expertly points out, however, the ethical counselor weighs client individual good over social action.

The responses to Dilemma A highlight the need for careful weighing of whose political agenda is being followed. It is probable that members of varying cultural groups will have markedly diverse reactions to homosexuality. A therapist always straddles the line of being forthright about personal values while attempting to remain helpful to those who seek her services. Many therapists work in compromised public systems. Help for children most often must come from within these systems. A dedication to feminist ethics must not artificially constrain the population that benefits from service. Although a private practitioner may legitimately limit her practice, those in public practice (schools, mental health centers, child guidance centers) must reflect on how to stay helpful to the greatest array of people while remaining congruent with personal feminist values.

Child abuse is pervasive in North America, and society's responsiveness to it is often ineffective. Practitioners must be skilled in identifying abuse and working toward positive resolutions. These are difficult goals. There is often tension among the law, personal ethics, and experience with the child protective service. It would be most useful to explore if a therapist's mandatory duty to report is ever superceded by her duty to protect the client. Although other standards provide guides for action, the problems of child abuse are so common and complex that even more distinct standards might be helpful. In particular, therapists find themselves in situations where the mandatory report of abuse does not guarantee service and safety for the child but does lead to a loss of therapeutic relationship or even contact with the young person. Injury and death are immediate dangers from abuse. Long-lasting physical, cognitive and emotional effects are possible as well (Wyatt & Powell, 1988). The decisions made around the care of children who are in abusive situations are of extreme importance. Personal and professional ethics exist as a supplement to jurisdictional laws.

Abuse of children, especially girls, within families is a staggering problem and is compounded by the violence in the communities where children live. Everyday dozens of children suffer gunshot wounds (Novella, 1991), hundreds witness someone being stabbed or shot (Roper, 1991), and thousands are victimized by violence in their schools (Goldstein, Harootunian, & Conoley, 1994). Their experiences are rarely examined, but they are clearly life-endangering and life-changing ones (Garbarino, Kostelney, & Dubrow, 1991). Practitioners, especially those in public practice, such as school psychologists and counselors, have a special ethical responsibility to understand the context of this violence and its effect on the children in their care.

Potential dilemmas raised by overlapping and multiple relationships deserve special attention as well. Rural environments promote these relationships. Although not necessarily problematic, such overlapping relationships always have the potential for difficulty. As such, the ethical therapist must invest extra effort in educating clients about the potential problems that may occur because of the overlapping relationships. It is not uncommon for therapists to avoid raising the specter of potential difficulties with clients. Prior information in writing is, however, a great investment in clarity and later security. It frees the client to make better decisions regarding treatment and protects the therapist when conflicts in care do arise.

A cutting-edge issue is how to be respectful of different cultural definitions of important constructs, such as what is appropriate discipline and how families should be organized, without losing critical elements of the feminist perspective. An overarching feminist value may be the self-determination of the client. This is easy to say and difficult to live.

The final scenario presents a somewhat more ambiguous situation. The therapist is attempting a therapeutic manuever with a mother and adolescent. A request for positive time between a parent and child is a common strategy to increase a young person's likelihood of obtaining attention through positive means. Most therapists would be thrilled to hear that a former runaway wanted a conversation with a parent. The parent's refusal presents a therapeutic challenge that may or may not be an ethical dilemma.

Every suggested strategy is merely a hypothesis. The refusal from one member to carry it out suggests a lack of readiness. What does the mother need from her daughter to feel more confident in their relationship, more ready to risk emotional connections? Perhaps a more reasonable approach relies on a reciprocal strategy that requires both mother and daughter to change in some small way in order to show investment in the relationship.

Although the feminist focus is often on the patriarchal nature of family life, healthy expressions of power needs are a legitimate goal of therapy. Every family member wants influence with other members. Is the mother's reluctance based on a need to placate the stepfather? If this were the case, how else could the stepfather be involved with the situation? The overriding issue here is that therapists must not attempt to rigidly control families just as family members must not attempt to rigidly control each other. Alternative strategies, attempting to reframe behaviors for their adaptive elements and attempting solutions that allow all the family members to feel heard and valued, may be the most important contributions a therapist can make to family well-being.

Violence in families is extremely hurtful to children. How do feminist family therapists maintain a systemic understanding of family difficulties while calling oppressive or abusive situations by their real names, that is, predictable outcomes of patriarchy that are reprehensible? The analysis of the stepfather's psychology in Dilemma C might raise some critical concern if the scenario had contained elements of child or wife abuse. Should feminists look for the adaptive functions of family actions? When this tack is taken, there are no villians or victims. There is a dance of interactions that maintain even the most dysfunctional systems. Women stay with abusive men thereby putting their children in danger not only because they lack alternatives. Some stay because their relationships are sticky with negative and positive elements that defy simple solutions.

Therapists find themselves balancing attempts to help families change with legal requirements for reporting dangerous situations in a world that offers few options to children. Liability concerns become a companion to efforts to behave in ethically responsible ways. For example, is a school psychologist liable for responding to a child who approaches her with a report of maltreatment that is not clearly abusive? Will the parents sue the psychologist for seeing the child without permission? Will the attorney general of the jurisdiction prosecute if injury occurs as the child's requests for help are diverted while parent cooperation is sought? What if the child has fabricated the story?

Therapeutic work with children is done through a layer of other adults, some of whom are not working in a child's best interests. Not only can children be harmed by such people, but professionals can be caught in the myriad of laws regulating work with children and find themselves with a dizzying array of conflicting loyalties. Therapists are allowed independent action on the behalf of children only in extreme situations. Careful consultation with others, painstaking care in keeping therapeutic targets clear, and expertise in relevant laws are essential for successful work. In spite of all these difficulties, working in therapy, prevention, and gender-fair educational opportunities for young people is an important commitment for feminists because the girl becomes the women.

RESPONDENTS

Mary Coady Leeper, PhD, a clinically certified psychologist trained in Counseling Psychology at the University of Nebraska–Lincoln, is in private practice in Omaha, NE, where she does evaluations, individual therapy, and therapy groups for youths and adults.

Maureen Kitchur, MSW, RSW, a social worker in private practice in Calgary, Alberta, provides therapy, consultation, and training with specialties in sexual abuse and working with aboriginal clients.

Roslyn Mendelson, PhD, a white, middle-class, Jewish psychologist in private practice in Calgary, Alberta, specializes in child psychology.

Peg M. Miller, MSW, a doctoral candidate in counseling psychology, is currently an intern at the Father Flanagan's Home for Boys and Girls in Omaha, NE.

Lois Sapsford, MSW, RSW, a clinical social worker in private practice in Calgary, Alberta, specializes in adolescents and their families, sexual abuse, grief, and loss.

Dolores Simpson-Kirkland, PhD, an African-American counseling psychologist, is the Administrative Assistant for Student Services for Lincoln, NE public schools and works with very troubled and troubling youth and their families in matters regarding discipline.

REFERENCES

Avis, J. M. (1992). Where are all the family therapists? Abuse and violence within families and family therapy's response. *Journal of Marital and Family Therapy, 18,* 225–232.

Badgley, R., Allard, H., McCormick, N., Proudfoot, P., Fortin, D., Oglivie, D., Rae-Grant, Q., Gelinas, P., Penin, L., & Sutherland, S. [Committee on Sexual Offences Against Children and Youth]. (1984). *Sexual offences against children* (Vol. 1). Ottawa: Canadian Government Publishing Centre.

Brown, L. M., & Gilligan, C. (1992). *Meeting at the crossroads: Women's psychology and girls' development.* Cambridge, MA: Harvard University Press.

Brown, L. S. (1991a). Antiracism as an ethical imperative: An example from feminist therapy. *Ethics and Behavior, 1,* 113–127.

Brown, L. S. (1991b). Ethical issues in feminist therapy: Selected topics. *Psychology of Women Quarterly, 15,* 323–336.

Borocas, R., Seifer, R., Sameroff, A. J., Andrews, T. A., Croft, R. T., & Ostrow, E. (1991). Social and interpersonal determinants of developmental risk. *Developmental Psychology, 27,* 479–489.

Chodorow, N. J. (1978). *The reproduction of mothering: Psychoanalysis and the sociology of gender.* Berkeley: University of California Press.

Coleman, H. (1992). "Good families don't" (and other family myths). *Journal of Child and Youth Care, 7,* 59–68.

D'Augelli, A. R. (1989). Lesbian's and gay men's experiences of discrimination and harassment in a university community. *American Journal of Community Psychology, 17,* 317–321.

D'Augelli, A. R., & Rose, M. L. (1990). Homophobia in a university community: Attitudes and experiences of heterosexual freshman. *Journal of College Student Development, 31,* 484–491.

Dutton-Douglas, M. A., & Walker, L. E. (1988). *Feminist psychotherapies: Integration of therapeutic and feminist systems.* Norwood, NJ: Ablex.

Enns, C. Z. (1993). Twenty years of feminist counseling and therapy: From naming biases to implementing multifaceted practice. *The Counseling Psychologist, 21,* 3–81.

Ensign, F. C. (1969). *Compulsory school attendance and child labor.* New York: Arno Press. (Original work published 1921)

Erikson, E. (1963). *Childhood and society* (2nd ed.). New York: Norton.

Fantuzzo, J. W., DePaola, L. M., Lambert, L., & Martino, T. (1991). Effects of interparental violence on the psychological adjustment and competencies of young children. *Journal of Consulting and Clinical Psychology, 59,* 258–265.

Fraad, H. (1993). Children as an exploited class. *Journal of Psychohistory, 21,* 37–51.

Freud, A. (1927). *The psychoanalytical treatment of children.* London: Imago.

Freud, S. (1965). *New introductory lectures on psychoanalysis.* New York: Norton.

Gabarino, J., Kostelny, K., & Dubrow, N. (1991). What children can tell us about living in danger. *American Psychologist, 46,* 376–383.

Gilligan, C. (1982). *In a different voice: Psychological theory and women's development.* Cambridge, MA: Harvard University Press.

Goldstein, A. P., Harootunian, B., & Conoley, J. C. (1994). *Student aggression: Prevention, management, and replacement training.* New York: Guilford Press.

Haugaard, J. J., & Reppucci, N. D. (1988). *The sexual abuse of children.* San Francisco: Jossey-Bass.

Jaffe, P., Wolfe, D. A., & Wilson, S. K. (1990). *Children of battered women.* Newbury Park, CA: Sage.

Kazdin, A. E. (1988). *Child psychotherapy: Developing and identifying effective treatments.* New York: Pergamon Press.

Kitzinger, J. (1992). Sexual violence and compulsory heterosexuality. *Feminism and Psychology, 2,* 399–418.

Klein, M. (1975). *The psychoanalysis of children.* New York: Dell.

Kohlberg, L. (1981). *The meaning and measurement of moral development.* Worcester, MA: Clark University Press.

Kohlberg, L. (1984). *The psychology of moral development: The nature and validity of moral stages.* San Francisco: Harper & Row.

Locke, J. (1964). *John Locke on education* (edited with an introduction and notes by Peter Gray). New York: Teachers College, Columbia University. (Original work published 1693)

Maccoby, E. E. (1980). *Social development.* New York: Harcourt Brace Jovanovich.

Melton, G. B. (1983). Toward personhood for adolescents: Autonomy and privacy as values in public policy. *American Psychologist, 38,* 99–103.

Miller, A. (1983). *Am Anfang war Erziehung [For your own good: Hidden cruelty in child-rearing and the roots of violence]* (H. Hannun & H. Hannun, trans.). New York: Farrar, Straus & Giroux.

Miller, J. B. (1976). *Toward a new psychology of women.* Boston: Beacon Press.

Moshman, D. (1993). Adolescent reasoning and adolescent rights. *Human Development, 36,* 27–40.

Nardinelli, C. (1990). *Child labor and the industrial revolution.* Bloomington, IN: Indiana University Press.

Novella, A. C. (1991). Violence is a greater threat to children than disease. *Public Health Report, 106,* 231–232.

Patterson, G. R. (Ed.). (1990). *Depression and aggression in family interaction.* Hillsdale, NJ: Erlbaum.

Pynoos, R. S., & Nader, K. (1990). Children's exposure to violence and traumatic death. *Psychiatric Annals, 20,* 334–344.

Reid, J. (1993). Prevention of conduct disorder before and after school entry: Relating interventions to developmental findings. *Development and Psychopathology, 5,* 243–262.

Reiss, A. J., & Roth, J. A. (Eds.). (1993). *Understanding and preventing violence.* Washington, DC: National Academy Press.

Rogers, A. G. (1993). Voice, play, and a practice of ordinary courage in girls' and women's lives. *Harvard Educational Review, 63,* 265–295.

Roper, W. L. (1991). The prevention of minority youth violence must begin despite risks and imperfect understanding. *Public Health Report, 106,* 229–231.

Rousseau, J. J. (1763). *Emilius and Sophia: A new system of education.* London: T. Becket and P. A. de Hondt.

Russell, D. (1986). *The secret trauma: Incest in the lives of girls and women.* New York: Basic Books.

Solomon, J. C. (1992). Child sexual abuse by family members: A radical feminist perspective. *Sex Roles, 27,* 473–485

Straus, M. A. (1994). State-to-state differences in social inequality and social bonds in relation to assaults on wives in the United States. *Journal of Comparative Family Studies, 25*(1).

Straus, M. A., Gelles, R., & Steinmetz, S. K. (1980). *Behind closed doors: A survey of family violence in America.* New York: Doubleday.

Terry. L. L. (1992). I want my old wife back: A case illustration of a four-stage approach to a feminist informed strategic/systemic therapy. *Journal of Strategic and Systemic Therapies, 11*(4), 27–41.

U.S. Advisory Board on Child Abuse and Neglect. (1990). *Child abuse and neglect: Critical first steps in response to a national emergency.* Washington, DC: Author.

Worell, J., & Remer, P. (1992). *Feminist perspectives in therapy.* New York: Wiley.

Wyatt, G., & Powell, G. (1988). *Lasting effects of child sexual abuse.* Newbury Park, CA: Sage.

ELEVEN

Conflicts in Care: Later Years of the Lifespan

Theo B. Sonderegger
Rachel Josefowitz Siegel

Psychotherapy with the middle-aged or older adult requires that the therapist understand the process of aging and the ways society discriminates against old people—especially old women—and makes fun of them. Myths and misconceptions about older individuals abound and are generally unquestioned. The therapist needs to understand that these myths often translate into stereotypical beliefs about older people and can result in discrimination against older people. Discrimination because of age, known as "ageism," is one of many forms of oppression that a feminist therapist is committed to oppose (Preamble). (The Ethical Principles of Psychologists also forbids discrimination because of age [American Psychological Association, 1992, 1.08, 1.09].)

Although it may be a particular incident of traumatic age-related oppression that brings an older woman to psychotherapy, the cumulative effect of age-phobic, age-rejecting, and youth-worshiping society can be just as damaging and is not as easily perceived as a precipitating factor. These more subtle, cumulative experiences with ageism may compound other difficulties facing an older client seeking therapeutic help.

Ageism as a form of oppression causes suffering for all people at midlife and beyond but is especially harmful for older women. Society often stands by amused when an older man dates a young woman but looks askance when an older woman dates a young man. Ageism can enter the therapeutic process in various ways even if the therapist has been educated about changes that occur during the aging process. Therapists who are aware of other biases may not be aware of the extent of their age-related biases and misconceptions.

AGEISM AND THE USEFULNESS OF PSYCHOTHERAPY FOR OLDER PEOPLE

Prevalence of Ageism

Ageism refers to the overlapping attitudes and behaviors that express society's fear and avoidance of aging, the devaluation of older people, the secrecy and avoidance of death as a normal and expectable part of life, and the accompanying overvaluation of youth. Ageism and age-oppression are as prevalent and as invisible in society as sexism and sexist oppression were before the current women's movement. Ageism is compounded with sexism in the case of older women who are even more consistently devalued and ridiculed than their male counterparts. The emerging political activity of retirees and the new antiageism literature by elder feminists have had, as yet, only minimal impact on the general public, including therapists and older women themselves. Everyone wants "to live to a ripe old age," but how often does an older person express the following sentiment: "I don't want to be like them" or "I'm not like those people," referring to other older people. Clearly, living through an earlier life stage does not make the individual an authority on what will happen at the next stage, although useful coping strategies may be learned.

Ageism prevalent in youth-oriented society extends to those offering psychotherapy to the elderly. The first ethical problem is in the use of the word *old*. Since the word itself has so many negative connotations and associations, its use becomes problematic. Although some clients of advanced age feel validated when their age is referred to with respect, others might be insulted or feel rejected when referred to as *old* when they are trying to imbue the word and the process of aging with more positive meaning. In this section the authors have reluctantly chosen to refer to *older women* rather than *old women*. Although recognizing the ethical and political value of desensitizing selves and readers to the ageist connotations of *old*, the intent is to use a term that would include women at midlife and that would not elicit undue resistance in readers.

Therapists of all ages participate in a multitude of unexamined assumptions, jokes, phrases, and attitudes toward old women that are derogatory, infantilizing, or intended to make the older woman feel better by denying her age. Not so long ago, health care professionals from a variety of disciplines believed that psychotherapy was best invested in younger individuals who would live longer and reap more benefits from treatment (Levy, Derogatis, Gallagher, & Gatz, 1980). Older individuals were often simply given medications and frequently overmedicated (Gutmann, 1977). Fortunately, the view that psychotherapy should not be "wasted" on older individuals has begun to change.

Data have now emerged demonstrating the effectiveness of the therapeutic process with the older client. For instance, once neuropsychological testing has differentiated dementia from depression, psychotherapy may alleviate the depression to restore a better quality of life for the affected individual. A variety of treatment procedures have proven to be effective in working with the elderly (Pollock, 1987).

Demographics of Aging Population

A major reason for altering the view about the importance of psychotherapy for older people is the recognition of changing demographics. Populations of nations throughout the world, including the United States, show increasing numbers of people 65 and older. By the year 2025, it is estimated that one person in five will be 65 or older; the population of 85 and above is now the fastest growing segment of the U.S. population (Park & Cavanaugh, 1993). Data from the National Institute on Aging suggest that by 2040, the number of Americans over 85 could be 30 million, up from the 3.3 million of today (Kirkland, 1994). Moreover, the majority of this older population will be women; although the life expectancies of the entire population of the United States have increased, women continue to live longer than men. Currently, the life expectancy of a woman in this country is 79.6 years compared to the life expectancy of a man, which is 72.7 years. With the size of the older population increasing, so does the need for psychological services.

BRIEF REVIEW OF RELEVANT LIFESPAN
THEORIES OF AGING

People at midlife and beyond not only face different problems but view these problems from different perspectives than their younger contemporaries. Although both older and younger individuals have many comparable mental health problems, the therapist may need to reconceptualize some problems for the effective treatment of her older clients (Pollock, 1987). The feminist therapist who works with older clients needs to be aware of the nature of older clients' problems and of their perceptions of them. She also must have theoretical knowledge about the nature of changes produced by aging. The feminist therapist only provides services in areas in which she is competent and undertakes any educational work that is necessary for her to maintain her competence in a particular area (IVA). Principle A of the Ethical Principles of Psychologists also asserts that psychologists are to provide only those services and use only those techniques for which they are qualified by education, training, or experience (American Psychological Association, 1992).

A wide array of everchanging theories has been promulgated to categorize the biological and psychological transitions that occur with aging. Lifespan theorists view aging as one component of development. One such "stage-based" approach examines individuals as they grow older by grouping concerns in sequential age blocks ranging from early in life until death. Another type of lifespan theory, the "ecological approach," focuses on the ways that people, events, and institutions encountered by a person during a lifetime affect that individual's development (Goldhaber, 1986). It is beyond the scope of this section to review these theories in depth, but a brief examination of two that use lifespan approaches will identify elements of the knowledge needed when working with people of midlife and beyond. Both stage-based and ecological approaches stress that there are individual differences as well as similarities in the passage from youth to old age.

Roger Gould's theory divides the lifespan of an adult into seven stages ranging from four to 11 years in length beginning at age 18, that is, "adulthood" (Gould, 1978). Each is named for, and focuses on, a major problem with additional minor problems mentioned as well. Of interest here are the stages that extend from midlife to old age: Midlife Explosion (ages 35–43); Settling Down (ages 44–55); Mellowing (ages 56–64); and Retirement (age 65+). As an individual solves the problems at one stage, others develop, and the pressures associated with them cause the individual to move to the next stage. For example, the problems associated with the Midlife Explosion Stage according to Gould are (1) search for meaning; (2) reassess marriage; (3) reexamine work; (4) relate to teenage children; (5) relate to aging parents; (6) reassess personal priories and values; (7) adjust to single life; (8) solve problems associated with this stage; and (9) manage the stress accompanying the change to the next stage. During the Midlife Explosion Stage, an individual may make a drastic but successful career change, solve the myriad problems associated with the move, and then enter the next stage, "Settling Down."

In the ecological approach, another type of lifespan theory, the focus is on experiences that an individual faces during a lifetime. Living through the Great Depression and World War II has affected today's

60-, 70-, and 80-year-olds in ways that younger individuals may have trouble comprehending. The unique socialization process and societal expectations manifested during the first half of the century also contribute to the ways older individuals perceive themselves and their ability to cope. Today's older woman, for example, may have grown up with strict mores about permissible sexual behavior, with strong admonitions defining her place in life as a wife and mother, and with messages that her intellectual ability was not as important as that of her husband or brothers. Such a woman, socialized that her role in life is to please a man, husband, or father, who has made the major decisions in her life, may not know how to cope as an autonomous individual. This problem with independence may surface when the older woman becomes a widow or finds her husband having an affair with a younger woman. All of the significant events of a lifetime, societal as well as individual, may affect the nature of the problems experienced by the older woman and must be understood in this broader context when they are dealt with in the therapeutic process.

The perception of time changes as a person passes through the later lifespan stages. It is important that the therapist be aware of and understand this. The older client is cognizant, perhaps only covertly, that she no longer has an infinity of time. She knows that her life is finite and coming to an end, that death is imminent. She often, by this time, has endured the loss of a spouse or other loved ones, and she now may be dealing with her own life-threatening health problems.

These changes in the perception of time and the increased awareness of death through either the actual or anticipated loss of significant others have been demonstrated empirically by Rachel Josefowitz Siegel (1993). Over a period of seven years she conducted taped therapeutic interviews individually or in groups with 56 women between the ages of 60 and 70. In each type of therapeutic setting, the women talked about their preparation for possible infirmities and practical preparations for death. This study demonstrates that other motivational changes may occur in later life. The therapist, therefore, must recognize that the "client's proximity to life's ending also acts as a strong motivator for engaging in activities that had previously been put off; these include a variety of self-selected and often pleasurable learning experiences" (Siegel, 1993, p. 173).

THERAPEUTIC CONCERNS RELATED TO THE AGE OF THE CLIENT

Many of the age-associated issues that occur in the therapeutic process with an individual in midlife and beyond have been described elsewhere

(Siegel & Sonderegger, 1990; Sonderegger & Siegel, 1987) and are reviewed briefly here. Although the ensuing comments are generalized to a span of possibly 50 years, that is, from age 40 to the 90s, the therapist must keep in mind that the issues, attitudes, and life experiences of older women are vastly different in each decade of later life. Older women of every age also differ from each other as much as younger women do in all the psychological, social, and economic variables, as well as in sexual preference. The enormous social and technological changes of the 20th century have left their mark in a variety of ways on women who have lived through 50 or more adult years of such change, adapting and contributing to this process of change in their own individual fashions.

Not all older women have led sheltered lives or continue to maintain the patterns of their early upbringing, though most of them do carry some traces of very traditional values and attitudes. Among the older women who are changing the stereotypical image of old age are the early feminist leaders and theoreticians such as Betty Friedan, Gloria Steinem, Phyllis Chesler, and Jean Baker Miller, as well as lesser known feminists, who are now in their 50s, 60s, and 70s. It is also worth mentioning that many lesbians over 60 continue to live closeted lives, unless they are in large metropolitan centers with openly lesbian communities and support systems. It is the therapist's ethical responsibility to be aware of the full range of differences among older women and to refrain from making generalized assumptions that may be based on an ageist stereotype of old women.

Health-Related Issues

Problems with health are often present and can infiltrate many aspects of therapy with the older client, interacting with social, economic, and emotional stresses and bringing the individual to therapy sessions. Issues range from problems of menopause to concerns about the health of an ailing, older spouse. Ethical dilemmas concerning confidentiality can arise in communicating with family members or other health care providers.

Diagnostic Issues

Some therapy cases require careful diagnostic assessment. When confusion is a presenting problem, for example, a misdiagnosis of dementia can totally disenfranchise an older woman. A careful psychometric assessment may be needed to delineate the nature of the confusion that brings the client in for therapy. Careful therapeutic preparation may be necessary prior to the assessment; that is, the client may need help to understand what will happen and what will be learned in the testing situation. Malnutrition or combinations of over-the-counter and therapeutic drugs may produce confusion. Other difficulties in day-to-day coping may be related to age-related health changes. Impaired vision or hearing, for example, together with decreased opportunities to interact with other people, can produce paranoid-like ideations. Sensory impairment may even lead to a client's decision to "give up."

Medication

Ethical issues may also arise when aged women are perceived as untreatable or when they receive either inappropriate or too much medication. Tranquilizing an older woman tends to make her less demanding and is often easier than giving her information about her own aging. The older body metabolizes some drugs differently than the younger one, so medication dosages may need to be adjusted for the older person. If the client has a short-term memory loss, she may need help in planning how to remember to take various medications at their proper times. Care must be taken, however, not to infantilize her. It is well known that women as compared to men receive much more medication and fewer types of other treatment for certain types of health problems (Russo, 1985). Ageist biases may cause a therapist to assume that frailty and confusion in an older woman is to be expected rather than to search for a cause of the problem, for example, overmedication, as would be explored with a younger client.

Caregiver Role

A health-related problem not already addressed concerns the older client who is also a caregiver. Ethical issues arise when individual needs tangle and conflict with the needs of the person receiving or expecting her care. The caregiver is often a middle-aged or older woman whose needs tend to be overlooked while her services tend to be taken for granted. Her own female upbringing may have taught her to be self-effacing and endlessly giving; the recipient of her care, be it spouse, parent, or other person, may well expect these qualities in her and be endlessly demanding. Here, as in other oppressive situations, the ethical dilemma is between accepting and respecting the client's own value system and giving her the tools for overcoming her own oppression.

The feminist therapist can help her client find and accept a variety of services that fit within the client's values and finances, ranging from a few hours of domestic help or personal care to eventually placing the ailing patient in a nursing facility. The decision to provide care for a loved one by placement away from home can be beneficial to both patient and caregiver, but it is not always acceptable. The feminist therapist must examine carefully her own bias when exploring that option with her client.

A dedicated caregiver can sometimes be helped to make some accommodations for her own needs by having it suggested that helping herself can also be good for her family, since she can be a better caregiver when she herself is more rested and relaxed. There are times, however, when the only ethically therapeutic stance is that of being a respectful and empathic listener without expecting or even suggesting any change, while the client expresses her own feelings.

In some situations, the caregiver may become neglectful or even abusive. The frail elderly living at home or in the community are vulnerable to what has come to be known as "elder abuse" (Moody, 1992). The fact that the term "elder abuse" is widely used is indicative, unfortunately, of the extent of the problem. There are other ways in addition to therapeutic interventions that the therapist can use to help the potentially abusive caregiver deal with her problems. If the cared-for person is suffering from a dementia, for example, the therapist might suggest the caregiver deal with her frustration problems by participating in a support group. Within a group of individuals with shared experiences, it is all right to admit feelings that society at large does not condone and thereby prevent the translation of feelings into actions. Another relief strategy for the caregiver dealing with a person with dementia is the use of regular periods of respite from her work. The literature on caregiving is extensive. The feminist therapist working with caregivers needs to keep herself informed and aware of the resources the community provides for assistance.

Death and Dying

Other difficult ethical questions confronting older women and their therapists, as mentioned previously, deal with death and dying and with the older woman's changed perception of time. Even if she is in good health, but especially if she is critically or chronically ill, an older woman often is actively and realistically involved in thinking or planning for her own death.

Older clients may wish to talk about suicide as an option when the quality of their life makes it no longer worth living. The therapist has an obligation at this point to sort out her own ethical priorities, possibly with the help of a consultant. When assessing the client's competence to make a decision of suicide or elect to refuse treatment, the ethical concept of client self-determination needs to be kept in mind. But, it is also important to recognize that in older as in younger women talk of suicide may be masking a profound yearning for a life worth living.

Financial Concerns

Large numbers of older women are in financially precarious situations, a fact that can lead them into therapy. The therapist, in turn, needs to attend to her own self-care by earning a living and planning for her own retirement years. The therapist who wants to be accessible to clients who are old enough to be on Medicare faces the ethical dilemma of accepting a Medicare-determined fee that is lower than the going rate, even when the older client has the means to pay more.

THERAPIST ISSUES IN PSYCHOTHERAPY WITH OLDER PEOPLE

Therapists need to examine their therapeutic tactics in treating all clients, but some of the following issues in particular emerge in dealing with older clients.

Therapists' Age Bias

If lucky, all people, therapists included, ultimately become old, and some may develop negative attitudes toward the elderly. Therapists who have not dealt with their own aging and deaths may find they have sexist/ageist fears. They may carry some sexist ambivalences toward mothers. Such feelings, when unexamined, may cause female therapists, as well as other women, to avoid and oppress older women and to distort the aging process within themselves. Caring for aging parents or other older relatives or friends while experiencing the problems of one's own aging may add further strains to the life of the therapist (Knight, 1992).

Underlying this age bias are mother-blaming theories and therapeutic attitudes that label old women as "bad-mother" figures, that is, as controlling and intrusive. Such an attitude on the part of the therapist tends to pathologize any behavior that draws attention to the older woman's needs and to ignore providing help that may be warranted. Therapists of any age who assign older women to stereotyped categories prevent equality in the therapeutic interaction.

Empowerment

Empowerment is an important component of feminist psychotherapy, but the therapist may have difficulty in working to empower an older woman who has lived much of her life outside of the power arena. The process of empowerment of her older client may also lead the feminist therapist to fear resumption of her daughter status. Consultation with another therapist about this possibility can be helpful if therapy has reached an impasse.

Communication Styles

Important differences in communication styles exist between a younger therapist and an older client. Generally, women over 60 have not been trained for assertive communication and are not as facile with the language of emotions. They are likely to be more guarded in revealing their real concerns, especially if criticizing loved ones. One consequence may be a slower pace in therapy, which may be difficult for the therapist but which may be very effective for the older client.

Cultural/Generational Differences

Besides different styles of communication, older women also have different beliefs about what they should and should not be concerned with or talk about. It may be difficult for the older woman to talk about sex or her body image not only because it may violate her social mores but also because sexist ageism prohibits her from acknowledging herself as a sexual person or from experiencing her body as sexually desirable. Even if the older woman may have more difficulty expressing her sexual concerns, she is still a sexual person. She very well may be coping with sexual frustration and the need to sort out her options for continued sexual activity and intimacy (Weisbord, 1991). As communication patterns become clearer, the therapist may help the client to deal with her frustrations and to sort out her options.

Independence/Interdependence Conflicts

The younger therapist must recognize that the older woman has been socialized in an era in which she was brought up to appear dependent on her spouse while actually taking care of his emotional and physical dependency needs. She was given contradictory messages about not becoming a burden on others in her old age, especially on her children, while not being permitted to even think of herself as capable of making independent decisions. She may also have been socialized to undervalue the friendships of women and not to depend on them. The therapist needs to remember, however, that many older women have made great strides in overcoming these early messages and have made life decisions that encompass the widest possible range of attitudes toward dependency and independence. She will find older women whose lives have become woman-centered whether or not they have made lesbian choices.

Current feminist literature has made women aware of the importance of "interdependence" and the value of networking and of relational skills. Daughters, not sons, are usually still expected by society to become the caretakers of failing parents, and daughters-in-law, if families lack girls, still become caretakers of the husband's invalid parents. Some of the problems of being a caregiver could be alleviated, perhaps, if both the elderly parent and the caregiver would join forces with others with similar problems and share resources.

Characteristics of the Therapist

In some cases the age gap between the therapist and the older woman client may be too great to allow the therapist to understand and thereby empathize with the older woman's problems. Conversely, the older therapist may herself face self-care problems as she ages. For example, she may face physical impairments, including memory impairment, loss of stamina, and/or family crises that could affect her ability to work adequately with an older client. If there are questions about the effectiveness of the therapeutic process, possibly caused by the age of the therapist, appropriate consultation with colleagues may be needed.

Client's Own Ageism

The client's own internalized ageism may block the therapeutic process. Both the older client and her therapist will find themselves at some point on a continuum ranging from very traditional negative assumptions about aging to radical feminist informed anger at the sexist/ageist treatment of older women in society. The individual older client, however, may present a complex situation. The most militant feminist, for example, may not be aware of her ageist assumptions, and the most conservative antifeminist on the other hand, may have a positive regard and compassion for certain aspects of the aging process and for herself as an old woman. The therapist, moreover, must be aware of her feelings about her own aging process. In turn, she must also recognize and accept the client's priorities and timetable for recognizing *her* process of aging.

CUES FOR RECOGNIZING AND CORRECTING THE THERAPIST'S AGE BIAS

In order to develop more bias-free interactions, the therapist can become more aware of her own age bias by asking herself the following questions:

1. How would I treat this client if the client were under 40?
2. Does this client remind me of my mother?
3. What feelings about my own aging does this client evoke in me?
4. Am I applying a deficit model of aging to this client?
5. Am I looking for client strength as I would with a younger client?
6. Do I assume this client is open to change through therapy?
7. Do I assume this client can absorb information about her condition?
8. Am I respecting this client's world view as if she were younger?

The reader might keep these questions in mind when reading the following five ethical dilemmas involving psychotherapy with individuals in the later part of the life-span.

DILEMMA A

Marie, a white therapist in her early 30s, has been professionally seeing Olive, 48, a white lesbian, for 18 months. Olive was released by her company during a major downsizing. Although Olive received a modest severance package, she lost her insurance benefits. She has requested reduced-fee services from Marie. Marie has used a sliding-scale fee schedule occasionally but thinks Olive will get another position very soon and refuses her request.

RESPONDENT 1

Marie appears unaware of the economic realities possibly confronting a 48-year-old woman out of a job and seeking a new one. Ignoring societal ageism is a form of ageism on the therapist's part (Preamble). She also has refused a fee adjustment for a client, although the therapy has been going on for 18 months (IA, IIC). Renegotiation of formal and/or informal contacts with clients is an ongoing mutual process in feminist psychotherapy (IIC), and use of this ethical guideline could help Marie be more flexible with her client.

For example, how can Marie be sure that even if Olive does get another position "soon," it will have medical benefits covering psychotherapy? Marie may believe she is modeling "effective use of personal power" (IIA), but if so, she is ignoring the inherent power differentials between herself and her client (IIA) at a time when the client is particularly vulnerable as a result of loss of employment, apparent need for new employment, and rational concerns about age-appropriate and perhaps career-appropriate employment prospects.

Marie may also believe she is taking care of herself and modeling self-empowerment (IIA, IVD). Considering, however, that "the well-being of clients is the guiding principle underlying this code" (Preamble), the client and others would have reason to hold Marie to the part of the Preamble that states, "When ethical guidelines are in conflict, the feminist therapist is accountable for how she priori-tizes her choices."

If Marie seeks consultation (IVB), she may recognize that Olive has already taken an important step in requesting a lowered fee; it is seldom easy for a client already vulnerable outside therapy to make herself further vulnerable through such a request. Marie can still im-prove the situation by making sure Olive does not leave therapy prematurely because of this issue. She can tell Olive she has reconsid-ered her position (an excellent form of modeling) and that she would like to discuss further with Olive what is at stake, in principle, for each of them, around the fee issue. (Jeanne Adleman)

RESPONDENT 2

In this situation, there are two ethical issues being addressed. The first is related to power differentials (II). Olive is making less money than she once did, and Marie is using her power as a therapist to make her client continue to pay full fee. Because she has used sliding-scale fees in the past, Marie is making a decision that is unilateral and appears a bit unjust. She is also not including Olive in the decision making (IIC). It seems that she is forcing Olive to do something Olive feels she can not do: pay full fee. Olive is in a less powerful situation in that she has no equality in negotiating the fee; she must pay what Marie asks or curtail therapy. Marie seems to be abusing her power here. In fact she should probably educate her client as to her rights as a consumer of therapy (IID) and provide her with a procedure for resolving this difference; otherwise she is violating one prime ethical feminist therapy edict, which is trying to equalize power and acknowledge the inherent power differentials between therapist and client (IIA).

The second ethical dilemma is related to cultural diversities and oppressions. One can only wonder why it is that Marie will not slide the scale in this situation. Is it because Olive is a lesbian? Does she have some bias or discriminatory attitude that makes her treat this client differently than she has others? An ethical feminist therapist needs to evaluate the ongoing interaction to see if she has any biases that are interfering with her practicing competent therapy (IC). Marie needs to get supervision on this issue or at least ask herself why she has come to this decision (IVC). If her attitude is too hard to overcome, perhaps she should help Olive find another therapist who would slide the fee so that there will be a therapist for Olive who is more flexible (IC). Marie needs to do some self-reflection and then consider dropping her fee or curtailing her service to this client. Marie needs to "evaluate her own bias" (IA) and "acknowledge the power differential" (IIA) with this client. (Elaine Leeder)

DILEMMA B

Hortensia, a 50-year-old Latina, has been caring for her 85-year-old mother in her home. Janet, Hortensia's social worker, is concerned that caring for her mother is interfering with Hortensia's employment search and recommends that Hortensia place her mother in one of the local subsidized nursing homes. Hortensia had promised her mother for years that she would not put her in a home. Janet has also discussed the risk of Hortensia losing her welfare benefits by not looking for employment.

RESPONDENT 1

Being Latina does not mean that Hortensia's value system is similar to that of another Latina. Some Latinos have been born and raised in the United States, which will have some bearing on their value formation. Latino cultures themselves are heterogenous, and even when there are characteristics that bind them together such as family pride, family honor, language, and so forth, the historical base for how those values are formed may be different. A point of departure to help members of individual Latino groups would be awareness of their cultural background by asking the client for the information if the therapist is not bicultural or knowledgeable of the particular culture (IB). In general, honoring elders and showing respect, love, and care for them is culturally mandated for members of a culture that depends on the extended family ties perhaps more than in members of the dominant culture in the United States, where the family relies more on the nuclear family. The threat of having to place an 85-year-old mother in a nursing home, a possible alien surrounding, after promising to personally care for her, may be felt as a violation of values held by both her mother and Hortensia. It will be important to explore with Hortensia her feelings about having to take care of her mother as well as her feelings about placing the mother in a nursing home after she made that promise.

As a poor woman, possibly alienated from the majority culture and dependent on the welfare system, Hortensia is vulnerable to pressure (IIA). The cost of feeling oppressed by a government system that seems to be trying to impose values that may be in contradiction to hers could result in lowering her self-esteem and consequently aggravate her feelings of powerlessness.

A therapist working with poor women needs to take the role of an advocate (VA). In this case, Janet could use her knowledge of the welfare system to help access different resources that may help to simplify Hortensia's decision (IIB, D). Janet could examine with Hortensia all the options and empower her to select the best option for herself. The therapist could also work with Hortensia to empower her to honor her feelings, discuss her issues and frustrations, and in so doing, reinforce the need for her to gain control of her own and her mother's destiny. (Gloria M. Enguídanos)

RESPONDENT 2

The ethical issues in this case are centered around cultural diversities (IA, B, C). Janet's recommendation that Hortensia place her mother in a nursing home is most probably a violation of an important Hispanic value, namely, that of a daughter honoring the wishes of, and caring for, a parent in old age. Indeed, it is possible to postulate that Janet, by suggesting only the option of placing the mother in a nursing home, is acting from a middle-class Caucasian bias.

In order to act in accordance with feminist therapy ethics, Janet might better explore with Hortensia all the options available in order to satisfy as much as possible the conflicts within her client, for example, caring for her mother and also caring for her own financial needs and her need for time for herself. Hortensia might, for example, be able to find low-cost caregivers or neighbors or other relatives who might come into the home so that she could work, at least part-time. There also might be Hispanic, even church-related homes or adult day-care centers that would appeal to her mother and thereby enlist the mother's support for such placement, relieving Hortensia's guilt.

Within feminist therapy ethics, it is feasible for the social worker to explore what other agencies Hortensia might employ to further her ability to care for her mother and still care for herself and then disclose and discuss these with her client (IA, IIB). (Elizabeth Friar Williams)

DILEMMA C

Zak, a 59-year-old chronic schizophrenic, was referred to the mental health clinic by Adult Protective Services at the Department of Social Services. He still lived with his 80-year-old mother, Mrs. Parker. He attended a day program, and his medications were stabilized. There was some concern that he was abusing his mother.

Zak's therapist, Sheila, made a home visit to ascertain the severity of the situation. The house was cold and dark, remarkably unkempt and in ill repair, smelling of the 10 cats and six dogs that lived with them. Mrs. Parker sat on the sofa dressed in a filthy housedress, watching the soaps. There was running water and electricity. The kitchen, though dirty, was well stocked with necessities, paid for by Mrs. Parker's Social Security money and Zak's SSI benefits. On a visit to the neighbors, Sheila was told that they heard screaming arguments coming from the house. Once a neighbor saw Zak slap his mother on the face. There was no other actual evidence of abuse. The neighbors said that the situation had been under control when Zak's father was alive but had deteriorated in the last few years since his death.

RESPONDENT 1

As presented, it is Zak's therapist who is evaluating the possibility that he is abusing his mother. What is the nature of her relationship with Zak? Is she actually a case manager or a therapist and how frequent and intense have her sessions with Zak been? If she actually is the therapist, there are ethical conflicts. In that case, she needs to try to have the abuse evaluation reassigned to someone else (IA), preferably someone she thinks will be fair, objective, and sensitive to these concerns, someone who can evaluate Mrs. Parker's mental and neurological state as well as get some insight into her wishes. If Sheila's social service system is not sensitive to these concerns, this becomes a matter of education and other public advocacy efforts (VA, B).

Regardless of who does the evaluation, the actual living situation for these two individuals needs to be assessed. Based on some knowledge of their wishes, perhaps it would be possible to provide some supervised living arrangement for them, together or separately, depending upon the assessment. That this view is from a different social class perspective and concern about the differing view of the therapist and the assigned client should be taken into account (IB). (Hannah Lerman)

RESPONDENT 2

Sheila acted ethically by going into the home to ascertain whether reports of elder abuse against her client were true and to see whether the mother was in need of help as well as Zak (IA, B). By doing so, the therapist saw that neither Mrs. Parker nor Zak was adequately able to maintain the home in a health-enhancing way, although accusations of elder abuse were not sustained. One recommendation would be for Sheila to try to hire such services as home health aides. If Sheila could go beyond middle-class assumptions (IB, C) that dirt and smelliness constitute abuse in order to make an unbiased assessment of the client's needs and could enlist needed help from other agencies, she would be acting within the code of feminist therapy ethics (IA). (Elizabeth Friar Williams)

DILEMMA D

Cassandra is a 70-year-old white woman who has been placed in a large, publicly run psychiatric facility for the treatment of depression. She is in frail health from injuries incurred from a number of recent automobile accidents when her husband was driving. She is also unhappy over her husband's extramarital affair. Cassandra's husband is primarily responsible for decisions regarding her care. Although she is very angry at her husband, Cassandra is unwilling to question or contest any of his decisions. Cassandra is very wealthy and could afford better care in a more pleasing environment. Cassandra's therapist, Jane, is concerned that the husband's decisions may not be in Cassandra's best interests.

RESPONDENT 1

The major ethical conflict seems to center on Janes's personal opinions on this case. Jane is probably younger than the client and has been socialized differently. She cannot foist her way of dealing upon the client. She would be oppressive should she make the client do something she does not want to do (IC), namely, confront the husband and challenge his decisions. However, it also would be ageist of Jane to assume that the client is either unable or unwilling to make changes in her life, even at this later stage in the life cycle. Two ethical injunctions are at odds here: that of respecting client values (IB) versus the value of providing tools for a client to change. It is hard to determine which should be the priority. Perhaps it is up to the client to decide, with the therapist providing her own observations for the client to chose or ignore (IIB).

Certainly some of the client's depression might be related to being hospitalized, the husband's marital infidelity, and his poor decisions. However, Jane must respect the client's right to decide not to do anything about all of these things, should she chose to ignore Jane's observations about the oppressive and possibly abusive nature of the relationship she has with the husband. She might help the client to see the source of her depression. Beyond that, however, it seems that Jane would be overstepping boundaries if she were to intervene any further. This is a difficult ethical dilemma but one which really gets to the heart of feminist therapy. The heart of the matter is the ultimate respect for the client's viewpoint, even if it is not in the client's best interest in the therapist's judgment. The therapist must always respect the client's right to do nothing. To do otherwise here would be an abuse of the therapeutic relationship. (Elaine Leeder)

RESPONDENT 2

Age is a factor in this case, but the other main issues frequently occur in many therapy circumstances. The therapist may view the situation one way and the client another. The age issue here is this: when a relationship involves a male partner, the older the client is, the less likely she will believe that she can survive, much less make independent decisions if they differ from the views of the man. The therapist's views are often different. Jane needs to provide a safe place for Cassandra to express her opinions about the situation and give her permission to value them. This is a slow process at best. What is necessary is therapeutic sensitivity to the emotional and value situation of the client. It is more a therapeutic than an ethical problem unless the therapist is unaware that a difference in attitudes between the client and the therapist is a political problem (IVC) in which case an ethical concern may arise.

Since Cassandra is hospitalized, it does behoove Jane to express her opinion about the husband's decisions to the remainder of the treatment team. Perhaps, someone could be assigned to discuss the matter of his decisions with him and try to enlist his cooperation in doing more of what would be in his wife's best interest. This is a potential form of advocacy (VA) and would be useful. (Hannah Lerman)

DILEMMA E

Eleanor, a 50-year-old therapist, had decided to give up her private practice of 20 years and was about to cancel her malpractice insurance. She received an entreating call from Imogene, a woman of the same age, who was calling for therapy because of severe depression. She wept and pleaded with Eleanor to see her once, even if they decided not to continue. She was in crisis and said she could not find anyone else who could see her. Because of Imogene's despair, Eleanor decided to make an appointment.

In their first meeting, it was clear that Imogene was suicidal and suffering from a clinical depression. Her husband of 25 years had decided to leave her, and her daughter was moving hundreds of miles away. Imogene, though well educated, employed, and with a large circle of friends, had given up hope for living and saw therapy as her only salvation. Eleanor had decided prior to this first session that it would be a crisis intervention session with immediate referral. However, Imogene reminded her of her own life condition just a few years earlier, and upon seeing her, Eleanor was faced with a number of ethical dilemmas.

RESPONDENT 1

This case raises a number of issues both overt and subtle. On the surface the ethics seem clear. The client has asked for even a single session and the therapist has reluctantly agreed. It is possible to infer from the case outline that Eleanor indicated to the potential client on the telephone that she was not taking new clients. Either way, Eleanor has freedom to make a referral in good conscience (IA) but apparently is tempted to accept Imogene as a client. This is where location can be a critical concern. In a large urban area, a therapist who has been in practice for 20 years and is almost at the point of giving up her practice usually has numerous referral sources. In more isolated circumstances, there might be few if any choices. The reader is not told anything about location.

Because nothing more was promised than a single session, Eleanor has freedom to explore ethical next steps. First, however, she will need intense personal self-evaluation (IVB) to understand how powerfully she is feeling drawn into the possibility of changing her decision, perhaps even questioning the correctness or importance of the decision itself. Imogene seems to be in particular need of a specifically feminist perspective on life and its possibilities (Preamble). Eleanor has had— and presumably has surmounted—a comparable challenge in her past. Would this success lead her to be the uniquely best therapist for Imogene and thus to justify to herself reversing or postponing her decision to end her practice? Or, would it lead to a difficult and painful course of therapy during which Eleanor might reexperience her own past pain, or, in contrast, might Eleanor overidentify with Imogene and intrude on what must necessarily be Imogene's solution? In either instance, Eleanor might want or need ongoing consultation or personal therapy.

It is even possible that Imogene knew something of Eleanor's past history when she placed the entreating call; the private lives of therapists are seldom as private as therapists believe, would like them to be, and strive to keep them. The path toward ethical resolution of Eleanor's dilemma would seem to wend through a garden—perhaps a forest—of Eleanor's own feelings. (Jeanne Adleman)

RESPONDENT 2

The first concerns that come to mind are issues of abandonment. Imogene is obviously dealing with those issues regarding her husband, her daughter, and perhaps friends who, knowingly or unknowingly, are not available to her. Eleanor has made the decision to stop seeing Imogene once the crisis is over (IA). However, an experienced therapist should have been able to tell from the phone conversation that Imogene needed more than crisis intervention and that she will have to work on developmental issues arising from suddenly having to live alone and make decisions concerning her new status. For Eleanor to start therapy with Imogene with prior understanding that she will only help with the immediate crisis issues and proceed with a referral to another therapist could further trigger feelings of loneliness and abandonment.

Eleanor and Imogene seem to know each other in more than a casual way. Overlapping relationships are not uncommon in places where professionals interact socially and in rural or small communities. However, ethics dictate that caution and strict confidentiality be used at all times, since failure to do so can be a source of potential conflicts. Accepting a request to help a friend or close acquaintance in a therapeutic relationship may precipitate a breakdown of therapeutic boundaries (IIIA), leading a client to terminate therapy prematurely or have other unforeseeable negative circumstances. As Adleman and Barrett (1990) put it, "Overlapping relationships do contain potential hazards for boundary violations and ethical missteps" (p. 89).

Is Eleanor having difficulties letting go of her practice? Her decision to see Imogene instead of referring her to another therapist brings up the question of motives. For Eleanor, retiring from work after 20 years of practicing could be traumatic. The ability to help others and the satisfaction of helping a person progress and take control of her life is what attracts many to become therapists. It would be important for Eleanor to be aware of her vulnerability and needs (IVD). She is responsible for practicing ethically but also for monitoring her own feelings (IVB). By understanding her own needs, she could avoid the risk of hurting her client.

The vignette suggests that Eleanor once had a similar life situation. Self-disclosure in a feminist therapeutic situation is valuable if it will help the process (IIB). However, this was not self-disclosure chosen by Eleanor. Imogene's prior knowledge of Eleanor's personal history appears to be harmful, since Imogene seems to be using the information to manipulate Eleanor to see her as a therapist. The reader does not know what Eleanor's supposedly similar experiences are and how she has dealt with them, but painful life experiences can interfere with the therapeutic process unless the therapist monitors herself carefully and seeks consultation, supervision, and personal therapy so as not to let her own issues interfere with the therapeutic session (IVB). (Gloria M. Enguídanos)

IMPLICATIONS

The five cases presented in this section were intended to highlight some of the ethical considerations that arise in working with older women and women of the "sandwich generation." In general, the responses focus more thoroughly on issues of multicultural awareness, power relationships, and overlapping relationships, rather than on age-related issues. This is not surprising, since aging and ageism represent relatively new and unexplored topics that feminist therapists are only beginning to address. Although the respondents varied somewhat in their particular emphasis, very little disagreement occurred among them about the ethical issues in these cases.

"Ignoring societal ageism is a form of ageism on the therapist's part." This comment by Jeanne Adleman in Case A represents a key to establishing ethical guidelines in work with older women. In Cases A and B, each respondent addresses the ethical issues involving power differentials, which frequently occur in working with women in late life, but does not explicitly relate these issues to the client's age.

Case B illustrates the overlap of aging and ethnicity and the importance of recognizing specific ethnic values and attitudes toward old age. Although both respondents note the importance of respecting the client's ethnic value system, Enguídanos' response goes further in stressing the need to determine the client's specific cultural and personal background before making any generalized assumptions about her value system.

Case C deals with possible elder abuse between an elderly mother and her middle-aged son, both in need of supportive services. Overlapping relationships among therapist, elderly client, and caregiver are not unusual and present challenging ethical issues. The respondents present two different approaches to this complex situation. Williams sees the family as the client unit and the therapist as both evaluator and case manager. Lerman sees the son as the presented primary client and urges clarification of the therapist's role in a situation where the needs of two family members might be at odds. She sees a need to differentiate between the therapist as therapist, as evaluator, and as case manager. Williams seeks a solution that would keep the family unit together and at home with supportive services, while Lerman looks for a protected placement for both mother and son, together or separately. Both respondents caution against imposing their own middle-class standards on this family.

Case D illustrates, perhaps more than any other, the dilemma of balancing the awareness of the client's generationally determined value system with an age-affirming approach that is based on treating the client as if she is still able to change or at least to respond positively to new ideas. Had the client been younger, might the respondents been less cautious about exposing her to the kind of information and strategies that are routinely offered to battered and oppressed women? The respondents argue forcefully against imposing the therapist's solutions on the client (IIA), indeed, a key concept in feminist therapy. Leeder also cautions against making the ageist assumption that this client would be too old for new information or for change. Lerman recognizes that a gradual change in the client's attitude might be affected through lengthy therapy and sees this situation as ripe for client advocacy.

The Feminist Therapy Code of Ethics appears weak and not sufficiently clear about the ethical responsibility to protect the welfare of the client when the client's own value system appears to accept her own oppression and victimization. Further clarification is needed in differentiating between providing alternative options and perspectives on the one hand and using the therapist's power to impose the therapist's value system on the other. Additionally, is it more difficult to fully understand or even to challenge a client's value system when the client is old enough to be perceived as a mother figure?

The Feminist Therapy Code of Ethics also does not deal clearly enough with the potential conflicts of interest that can arise in a benign situation, such as between the needs of the older caregiver and her or his patient or an abusive situation such as between the perpetrator of elder abuse and her or his victim.

Case E was intended to draw attention to the ethical issues confronting the aging therapist. Both respondents recommend therapist consultation and self-examination, but again, they do not specifically identify the age-related aspects of the therapist's dilemma. The respondents focus more on the issues of self-disclosure and overlapping relationships that are also in the picture.

The old, especially older women, are mistreated and neglected in many ways in Western societies today, as this section delineates. But, *this need not be the case*. Each person, whatever her or his chronological age, has the ability to alter this situation. Feminist therapists in particular can provide guidance and leadership to alleviate some of the problems of aging. The authors recommend, therefore, at the minimum, the following action agenda:

1. Examination of individual beliefs concerning aging and recognition of possible ageist bias in actions.
2. Development of positive, affirming theories about aging that include understanding of the older woman's continuing personal growth abilities.
3. Reassessment of existing theories on aging for sexist and ageist assumptions.

4. Augmentation of research on older women from the older woman's perspective with ample opportunity for her voice to be heard.
5. Integration of older women's issues in feminist therapy training, discussions, and writings.
6. Provision of more explicit attention to monitoring therapists' lack of information and ageist bias in future revisions of the Feminist Therapy Code of Ethics.

RESPONDENTS

Jeanne Adleman, MA, is an educator-turned-feminist-therapist born in 1919 who has taught and supervised teacher training at several universities and now maintains an active consulting practice in San Francisco.

Gloria M. Enguídanos, PhD, originally from Puerto Rico, is a licensed psychologist working at California State University in Hayward, where she also teaches in the Women Studies Department.

Elaine Leeder, MSW, CSW, MPH, PhD, is Associate Professor and Chair of the Sociology Department at Ithaca College and author of *Feminist Therapy with Abuse in Families: Bringing in the Community*, published (1994) by Springer.

Hannah Lerman, PhD, is a psychologist in private practice in Los Angeles, currently working primarily with the chronically mentally ill and older persons in board and care facilities, and a founding member of the Feminist Therapy Institute.

Elizabeth Friar Williams, MS, teaches psychotherapy at New College in San Francisco (after practicing in New York City for many years) and is the author of *Notes of a Feminist Therapist* and the forthcoming *Off the Couch: Voices of Feminist Therapy*.

REFERENCES

Adleman, J., & Barrett, S. E. (1990). Overlapping relationships: The importance of the feminist ethical perspective. In H. Lerman & N. Porter (Eds.), *Feminist ethics in psychotherapy* (pp. 87–92). New York: Springer.

American Psychological Association. (1992). Ethical principles of psychologists and code of conduct. *American Psychologist, 47*(12), 1597–1611.

Goldhaber, D. (1986). *Life-span human development* (pp. 6–57). Orlando, FL: Harcourt Brace Jovanovich.

Gould, R. L. (1978). *Transformations.* New York: Simon & Schuster.

Gutmann, D. (1977). *A survey of drug-taking behavior of the elderly* (National Institute of Drug Abuse, Services Research Administration Report). Washington, DC: National Institute on Drug Abuse.

Kirkland, R. I. (1994, February 21). Why we will live longer and what it will mean. *Fortune,* pp. 66–78.

Knight, B. G. (1992). *Older adults in psychotherapy: Case histories*. Newbury Park, CA: Sage.

Levy, S. M., Derogatis, L. R., Gallagher, D., & Gatz, M. (1980). Intervention with older adults and the evaluation of outcome. In L. W. Poon (Ed.), *Aging in the 1980s: Psychological issues* (pp. 41–61). Washington, DC: American Psychological Association.

Moody, H. R. (1992). *Ethics in an aging society*. Baltimore: The Johns Hopkins University Press.

Park, D., & Cavanaugh, J. (Chairs). (1993). *Vitality for life: Psychological research for productive aging, HCI Report II. APS Observer Special Issue*. Washington, DC: American Psychological Society.

Pollock, G. H. (1987). The mourning–liberation process: Ideas on the inner life of the older adult. In J. Sadavoy & M. Leszcz (Eds.), *Treating the elderly with psychotherapy* (pp. 3–29). Madison, CT: International Universities Press.

Russo, N. F. (Ed.). (1985). *A national agenda to address women's mental health needs*. Washington, DC: American Psychological Association.

Siegel, R. J. (1993). Between midlife and old age: Never too old to learn. *Women and Therapy, 14*, 173–185.

Siegel, R. J., & Sonderegger, T. B. (1990). Ethical considerations in feminist psychotherapy with women over sixty. In H. Lerman & N. Porter (Eds.), *Feminist ethics in psychotherapy* (pp. 176–185). New York: Springer.

Sonderegger, T. B., & Siegel, R. J. (1987). *Issues in psychotherapy with older women*. Paper presented at Fourth National Forum on Aging, Lincoln, NE.

Weisbord, M. (1991). *Our future selves: Love, life, sex, and aging*. Berkeley, CA: North Atlantic Books.

TWELVE

Therapist Self-Care: A Proactive Ethical Approach

Natalie Porter

THERAPIST SELF-CARE: A PARABLE

Once upon a time, there lived a feminist therapist with a deep love for and commitment to her work. People came from near and far to seek her counsel, both as clients and students. Because the feminist therapist saw the beauty and potential in each client and student, she rarely refused a request to provide therapy, supervision, consultation, or training. After some time, she had more work than she knew what to do with—but her clients were so eager, her students so brilliant, her workshop audiences so stimulating that she pressed on.

Her friends would call, but she no longer had time to visit with them; she dropped out of her peer supervision group because she was frequently out of town when they met; and she began to shave the time allocated to her clients and supervisees in order to see all of them. Complaints did not come easily to her devoted clients and students, but one by one, complain they did. The therapist was outraged: "Why are they not more appreciative of my Amazonian efforts to see them at all? How ungrateful!"

One day, the therapist awoke and discovered that she did not want to go to work: "After all, my clients are not as motivated as they once were, my students not as bright, and workshop participants seem harder to please." The therapist felt distracted and bored with it all, and sadly, she realized that she had lost a most valuable treasure—the love of her work. She decided to seek the advice of a very wise woman who had mentored her a long time before. Upon hearing her story, the wise woman advised her: "Walk to a remote hill each evening and watch the sun set. Talk to a friend each day. And sing or dance at least once a week."

The feminist therapist felt disappointed with this lesson. She had expected to receive brilliant interventions meant to overcome her clients' resistances. Nevertheless she followed her mentor's advice because she felt desperate. Magic began to happen—not right away, but soon enough. Clients got better again; students got smarter and more enthusiastic. Most important, the therapist regained her love for her work and for those around her. She felt very much better.

THERAPIST SELF-CARE:
A FEMINIST ETHICAL IMPERATIVE

The inclusion of therapist self-care issues is one of the most innovative aspects of the Feminist Therapy Code of Ethics. It exemplifies the proactive, educational, and preventive ethical approach feminist therapists have advocated (Lerman & Porter, 1990). No other code refers to self-care issues. The inclusion of self-care issues as an ethical imperative is based upon a common assumption about therapy: that therapist well-being is positively related to the client's therapeutic outcome. A healthy therapist is viewed as possessing appropriate boundaries with clients, objective insight into their dynamics, control over behaviors that might interfere with the therapeutic role, and a capacity to model effective functioning and coping. Poor therapist self-care is associated with increased personal vulnerability, reduced self-monitoring, poorer judgment, and, as a result, greater risk of ethical breaches (Keith-Spiegel & Koocher, 1985).

The incorporation of self-care responsibilities into feminist therapy ethics is in contrast to traditional ethical philosophies. Traditional codes, framed in a legalistic fashion, tend to be fragmented and reactive, focusing on the definitions of violation per se (Lerman & Porter, 1990). Concepts such as "self-care" are not considered in the traditional Hippocratic framework, although the American Psychological Association has given some attention to the concept of the "impaired professional" in recent years. After an ethical violation has been committed, a professional ethics body may connect the therapist's improper behavior to impaired functioning and recommend actions to remediate the impairment. Unfortunately, by the time this happens, there are injured parties. To the victims this approach may appear as analogous to shutting the barn door after the cows are out.

Feminist ethical perspectives have attempted to develop a preventive and more holistic system. In the case of self-care responsibilities, the link between self-care and client outcome is specified.

The therapist must monitor the factors that could contribute to ethical violations prior to, and separate from, the commission of an ethical violation per se. The focus is on creating a positive environment rather than merely a harmless one. Education and prevention become the objectives because the potential causes of abuses are monitored as well as the abuses themselves. The therapist is educated not only about what constitutes ethical breaches with clients but about the risk factors that may precipitate these abuses. Ironically, this approach seems to have become more appealing to traditional ethics boards. Informal conversations with executive and ethics board members of various state associations often lead to discussions about whether state ethics committees would be better off changing their roles to encompass prevention and education rather than enforcement, given the rising costs associated with increasing litigation around ethical complaints (H. Lerman, personal communication, 1990; W. Spaulding, personal communication, October 1993).

DEFINITIONS OF THERAPIST SELF-CARE

Faunce (1990) defined therapist self-care as the integration of physical, mental, emotional, and spiritual well-being. This definition overlaps with Maslow's (1968) concept of self-actualization, the striving for optimal growth and development in one's own personal and professional life.

Faunce (1990) asserted that health in the therapist fosters health in the client: the more self-actualized the therapist, the greater the client's potential for growth. She included actions with clear feminist underpinnings in her definition, such as challenging constricting roles; searching for expressions of spirituality congruent with a nonhierarchical and nonpatriarchal perspective; pushing for understanding of how one's biases, attitudes, or values interfere with the realization of her own and her clients' potential; and working toward a variety of relationships that foster self-fulfillment in all persons.

The standard of therapist self-care may also be approached in a less idealized fashion. This author takes the perspective that the feminist therapist is responsible to take "good enough" care of herself to ensure that she does no harm to her clients. This standard of self-care has emanated from the beliefs and existing research that lack of self-care results in ethical violations, such as dual relationships (Lerman & Rigby, 1990; Rigby-Weinberg, 1986). The therapist is responsible for recognizing her own vulnerabilities and caring for them outside of the therapy relationships in ways that do not interfere with the well-being of her clients. The by-products of poor self-care include isolation, self-deception, poor judgment, grandiosity, and an increased risk of getting one's needs met through the therapeutic relationship. Self-care may take the form of support groups, peer supervision or consultation, psychotherapy, exercise class, adequate leisure time, antiracism consciousness-raising groups, spirituality groups, and so forth.

Therapist self-care serves three primary functions.

1. It protects the client by reducing the risk factors associated with ethical violations, particularly ones involving power and boundary issues.
2. It enhances therapy with the client by promoting and modeling growth and well-being.
3. It protects the therapist from occupational hazards such as burn-out and therapeutic miscalculations by defining the balance that must be negotiated between the therapist caring for self and caring for others.

THERAPIST SELF-CARE PROTECTS CLIENTS

Faunce (1990) stated that therapists violate boundaries when their own needs have gone unmet. Feminist therapists, in linking the personal to the professional, would view poor self-care as a forerunner to client abuse. Ethical violations can occur because of inattention to one's own personal and psychological well-being or difficulties, including loss, isolation, neglecting relationships with family and friends, or overwork. Violations may include boundary violations, power abuse, and inappropriate types of emotional involvement.

Boundary Violations

Lack of self-care fosters a range of boundary violations with sexual exploitation at the extreme end of the continuum. Therapist sexual contact with a client is more likely the outcome of a therapist displacing her unmet needs onto the therapy setting than a purely predatory act. More therapists cross boundaries, such as becoming sexually intimate or inappropriately friendly with clients, by interpreting positive emotions as romantic love or unique friendships than for consciously exploitative motives (Rigby-Weinberg, 1986). Nevertheless, the outcome harms the clients. The therapist still needs to be accountable for these acts, even when the intent may have been the result of self-deception from being out of touch with one's own needs (Lerman & Rigby, 1990).

Other types of boundary violations may not appear as severely exploitative or harmful to clients as sexual exploitation, but may, in fact, be seriously damaging to the therapeutic relationship, to the trust levels of the client, or to her self-esteem and ability to use therapy productively. These abuses may include the therapist gratifying her own needs rather than those of her client. The therapist may accomplish these violations by inserting her own needs and desires into the therapy relationship in what would seem to an objective observer as more of a reciprocal than therapeutic relationship. The therapist might maintain this imbalance through too much self-disclosure or self-disclosure that is not helpful to the client, or through role reversal in which the client becomes the caretaker for the therapist. The therapist may begin to alter the therapeutic relationship by permitting an expansion of the limits of therapy in order to create a "special" relationship between herself and her client. The therapist may also subtly manipulate the content of therapy, conveying greater interest and pleasure in certain topics, for example, those representing unresolved issues for the therapist.

Power Abuses

Poor self-care contributes to power abuses with clients. Therapists may exercise a greater control over their clients as they project their own unresolved conflicts onto them. They may elevate their feeling of power or status by living through the achievements of successful or well-known clients. Confidentiality may be threatened when a therapist channels her needs for self-importance into name dropping. Therapists who feel vulnerable or marginalized in their own lives may expect compliance and passive acceptance from the client.

Inappropriate Emotional Involvement

The therapist may gratify herself by fostering excessive dependency— by becoming "invaluable" to the client who begins to turn to the therapist for every decision and for every emotional stressor, treating each of them as a crisis. This behavior may permit the therapist to feel intimate with and needed by her clients, especially if her own life lacks relationships satisfying these needs. Therapists can also use overinvolvement in client lives as a way to avoid difficult or painful issues in their own lives. Overinvolvement may be analogous to other forms of workaholism.

The therapist's lack of self-care may also be expressed through the therapist's emotional unavailability to her clients. Overwork, preoccupation with difficult life events, or unresolved issues may hamper her emotional accessibility. This response may represent a chronic pattern or a reaction to a recent event, such as loss of a loved one. The therapist may relate to her client in an overly detached and distanced way that breaches the empathic connection between the two. The client is thereby hampered in her work.

Emotional overinvolvement may also take the form of overidenti- fication with the client's issues. The therapist may be unable to evaluate her own countertransference and may distort or misinterpret her client's concerns as well as be unable to maintain objectivity or neutrality in the client seeking her own solutions.

THERAPIST SELF-CARE ENHANCES GROWTH IN CLIENTS

The focus on self-care comes out of the connection that feminists make between how therapists behave toward themselves, how therapists behave toward their clients, and how clients behave toward themselves (Faunce, 1990). Therapist self-care fosters client self-care. Faunce con- sidered the therapist as the role model for the client; the therapist validates the importance of the client's needs, feelings, and thoughts by attending to her own needs, feelings, and thoughts. She demonstrates effective and assertive strategies in meeting these needs.

Self-care is necessary to accomplish the type of self-monitoring described by Adleman (1990). The conditions of respect, which facili- tate the client's, and the therapist's, achieving authenticity in the relationship, require self-monitoring. The therapist must be able to understand her or his emotional responses to the client and the origin of these responses to foster growth in the client. Self-care uses peer support and consultation groups to explore unresolved issues that pro- voke discomfort in the therapist. These groups may range from antira- cism groups to ones that focus on greater personal, relational, or spiritual awareness.

THERAPIST SELF-CARE PROTECTS THE THERAPIST

Perhaps one of the most important reasons to delineate self-care as an ethical mandate is that it recognizes that the therapist must balance her own needs against those of the client. This paradigm shifts away from one where the therapist must only be concerned with care of the client, regardless of the cost to the therapist. Therapists must function adequately to meet client needs, and at times, this standard may result in the therapist's needs being considered as important as those of the client.

Competing needs can become a salient issue in rural or small communities or whenever political, social, and therapeutic communities overlap, such as in feminist, lesbian, or ethnic minority communities. The mandate for self-care implies that when overlapping relationships occur, the appropriate solution is not always for the therapist to drop out of a community activity in favor of the client but to negotiate these issues based on the self-care needs of the therapist as well as the client. For example, a therapist, who views her attendance at a monthly feminist reading group as a major social or intellectual event, does not automatically drop out when her client joins. Instead, the therapist might negotiate with her client to have the client find or start another group.

Many therapists have operated with the assumption that all sacrifices must be born by them, regardless of the impact on their lives. Feminist ethics dictate that therapist self-care issues must be considered with the premise that martyrdom begets poor care of clients, not sainthood. This negotiation is also an important therapeutic task in that it models the therapist taking boundary and self-care issues seriously and arriving at mutually considered solutions. Boundary and self-care negotiations may be some of the most therapeutic transactions between therapist and client.

The following dilemmas depict a continuum of self-care issues. They range from self-care problems that have not yet involved client abuse but could to cases where serious ethical violations have occurred. Although other ethical violations may exist in these examples, the self-care issue is specifically addressed.

DILEMMA A

Nancy and Lynette have been friends and colleagues for several years. Both are therapists in private practice. Nancy has suffered several losses in the past two years, including the death of her father. She is a talented African-American therapist in a community with a large African-American population, and her services are in constant demand. She is active in the community as well, volunteering on several boards and committees for youth projects.

Nancy seems to have coped with the loss of her father by immersing herself in her work. She is unavailable whenever Lynette tries to see her, and Lynette fears that Nancy is becoming increasingly isolated. When they do talk, Nancy's clients are central to their conversations; the theme often centers around Nancy's importance to her clients. Nancy continually focuses on her dedication and instant accessibility to them. She appears to have a conde-scending attitude toward therapists not as dedicated as she is. Client crises are beginning to take up many of her evening hours. Nancy looks increasingly tired and depressed but claims she feels terrific. Lynette wonders about the self-care issues involved, how to approach Nancy, and her responsibility in doing so.

RESPONDENT 1

From the perspective of feminist ethics, this is a somewhat complex case. On the one hand, there seems to be clear evidence that Nancy is not adhering to the feminist ethical guideline for appropriate self-care. From Lynette's perspective, the lack of self-nurturance is damaging to Nancy as a person, as a therapist, as a colleague, and as a friend. It is critical that feminists continue to address the deep internalization of women's historical care-taking roles and the ethical implications of noncon-sciously filling these roles. Nancy is apparently unaware of the damage and potential damage she is doing to her clients and to herself.

At the same time, both cultural and racial issues need to be taken into consideration in this case. The Feminist Therapy Code of Ethics is explicit in stating the need for the feminist therapist to be "aware of the meaning and impact of her own ethnic and cultural background." The code applies, of course, to both Nancy as the African-American thera-pist, and to Lynette in whatever role she plays in intervening with Nancy. The experience of being African-American compounds the phenomenon of internalized oppression and the inhibition of making direct requests for comfort and support. These needs are often indirectly satisfied by giving to others and indirectly justified through a conde-scending attitude toward less self-sacrificing colleagues.

This case reveals the importance of mutual process, which is highly emphasized in the Feminist Therapy Code of Ethics. Any intervention on Lynette's part that is not in the spirit of mutuality and that by-passes the critical importance of relevant self-disclosure is likely to have a negative impact on Nancy. Furthermore, the reality that Lynette and Nancy have a personal as well as professional relationship impacts this case. The ethical guidelines pertaining to the "complexity and conflict-ing priorities inherent in overlapping relationships" must be acknow-ledged and dealt with in mutual process. The active nature of a mutually empathic process is likely to permit Nancy's experiencing of the unre-solved feelings of loss underlying her self-sacrifice and self-aggrandize-ment. Mutual process also permits the cocreation of alternative behav-iors. Addressing the ethical issues in this situation is likely to be mutually empowering for both Lynette and Nancy and is essential for the preser-vation of therapeutic competence. (Maryhelen Snyder)

RESPONDENT 2

Nancy has suffered several losses in the past two years. Self-care questions would be: How has Nancy coped with these significant losses in her life? How is she getting the support she needs? Is she in therapy, or is she utilizing the support of peers or colleagues?

There are several pieces of information mentioned in Nancy's case that raise concerns about self-care issues. Nancy has not discussed the losses she has experienced or how she is doing with Lynette, her friend and colleague. She has been unavailable when Lynette has attempted to make contact with her. When Nancy does talk to Lynette, she avoids the personal, focusing only on her clients, her instant accessibility to them and their crises. These behaviors suggest overinvolvement with her work to avoid personal issues/needs. Nancy claims that she feels terrific in spite of looking tired and depressed.

The self-care concerns that are raised, if not addressed, certainly could become more serious problems of professional and ethical competence for Nancy. Her lack of self-care and her increased dedication to her clients could result in poor boundaries, poor clinical judgments, and possibly unethical behavior. It does not appear that Nancy is caring for herself in her own life or outside of her work with clients. The fact that Nancy may not be soliciting the support of peers and colleagues only serves to increase the risk of poor clinical decisions or a reliance on her clients to meet her emotional needs. Thus, Nancy may be at risk for exploiting her clients to get her own emotional needs met. For example, Nancy may be fostering dependency, encouraging crises, or after-work involvement with clients in order to avoid her own personal issues. Nancy appears to be fostering this dependence by not setting clear boundaries for her clients, a practice possibly having an even more detrimental impact on her more disturbed clients.

Another important issue to consider in this case is the fact that Nancy is a renowned African-American therapist whose services are in constant demand and who also is active in her community. It may be part of her cultural or familial background to continue to present a strong and competent facade even if she is suffering considerable stress and depression over the circumstances of the past two years. Boyd-Franklin (1993) stated that African-American women sometimes feel compelled to carry the weight of the family or the world on their shoulders. They think they have to be strong even when their own mental health needs are compromised. For Nancy, showing any weakness in a community in which she is known and respected for her community work may be a significant threat to her personal and professional esteem. It is likely that Nancy's dedication to her work and her community are sources of self-empowerment. Thus, her decision to immerse herself more in her work may be her way (cultural or familial) of coping with her personal losses. From her dedication and commitment to her work, she derives a feeling of self-empowerment. It would take someone with some cultural sensitivity to address her lack of requests for help and her cultural and familial views on how one copes with personal adversity. Although Nancy is competent, her self-perceptions as an African-American therapist and as an African-American woman may need to be addressed in addition to the self-care issues. (Diana M. Valdez)

DILEMMA B

Ana is a psychologist on the staff of an urban mental health institute. She is one of three Latina, bilingual professionals among a staff of 20 that serves primarily Latino clients, many of whom are monolingual, Spanish-speaking. Ana is viewed in the community as a skilled and knowledgeable leader. The institute has received several contracts with state agencies to serve Latinos. Ana primarily provides the services for these contracts, frequently in collaboration with non-Spanish-speaking team members.

Ana is finding her work more arduous as the contracts increase. Although the agency has promised to hire bilingual staff, they recently hired one of their former interns who only speaks English. Ana is called upon not only to provide her own evaluations but to translate and explain the cultural contexts to the other therapists/evaluators. She is falling behind in her work because of the amount of time she spends assisting others. The administration has sent her a memo recently complaining about the lateness of her reports. Ana recently discovered that the Anglo administrator of this contract is receiving a significantly higher salary than she is, although the contract would not have been awarded without Ana's involvement.

Ana is becoming increasingly frustrated and angry. She is beginning to miss work because she feels too tired and listless to go in. She is becoming more impatient and detached in her work with clients. Her work is falling farther behind. She feels consistently devalued in her role.

RESPONDENT 1

The ethical guidelines for feminist therapists specifically state (IVB, D) that a feminist therapist needs to recognize her own personal needs and engage in ongoing self-care activities. It appears that Ana has failed to do so and as a result has allowed herself to be used in inappropriate and stressful ways by her agency. Ana needs to focus on empowering herself, as she probably does her clients, to look at her own work environment, identify the stressors for her, and develop goals for reducing them.

Ana seems to be feeling abused, overworked, and devalued by her administration. Unresolved feelings of anger are often the precursors to depression. Consequently, if Ana does not go about identifying these feelings and addressing the etiology, she will be at risk for not working effectively with her clients.

Ana is being exploited by her agency in that they have not hired a sufficient number of bilingual professionals. In fact, the agency has failed to keep a promise to her and uses her to help other non-Spanish-speaking therapists, while seemingly making no allowances for the impact on her own workload. Ana might talk to other Latina bilingual professionals to determine whether they have had similar experiences. They might communicate their concerns together to the administration. If the Latina staff is not valued, then one wonders about the administration's attitudes toward the Latino clients they serve.

Empowering herself to question, confront, and demand change from the administration when she feels abused is an important part of her self-care. Ana might suggest that a committee of Latina and non-Latina therapists be formed to review the agency's practices and to make recommendations to the administration. Ana might also make a proposal that she be used as a consultant to the non-Spanish-speaking staff and administration and be provided a salary increase commensurate with new responsibilities. At the same time, her clinical responsibilities could be reduced. If concerted efforts to change the actions of the agency fail, Ana may need to consider whether she wants to continue working there.

Ana may benefit from some brief psychotherapy for herself where she can focus on her feelings about work and explore the antecedents of and alternatives to this situation. She may, for example, have ambivalent feelings about taking care of her own needs or about being assertive with authority figures. Ana needs to first understand why she has allowed herself to be treated by her agency in this particular manner. Ana could also use her own treatment to begin to think of ways that she can effect change in her work environment, picking ones that seem to be most comfortable for her yet most effective in reaching her goals. Although specific approaches are varied and will not be listed here, support from other bicultural or bilingual peers at work may be very helpful and supportive. (Helen Jackson)

RESPONDENT 2

Ana is caught in a bind that women typically find themselves in: wanting to do good for others without recognizing the consequences to themselves. The bind is even more complex in this situation because it could appear to both Ana and her colleagues that the agency's commitment to serve the Latino community pivots on Ana's Latina heritage. Thus a self-care issue becomes a political issue.

The agency promised to hire more bilingual staff but has not honored that commitment. The most pressing need, more bilingual staff, has been compromised. The staff, with support from Ana, should have protested the hiring of the former intern who is not bilingual.

As Ana shoulders the increased pressures, because that's what good, efficient professionals do, she cooperates in keeping the issues blurred. Meanwhile, the administration has taken advantage of her interest and dedication to helping the agency's Latino clients. Ana needs help, either from peers, supervision, or therapy to deal with the issues.

There is also a subtle thread of racism here. Ana, a Latina, appears to stand alone against a white administration that criticizes her for not being more efficient, rather than acknowledging her contributions.

A move toward better self-care for Ana would keep the political issues central and rally collegial support around these issues. The issues impact on everyone, not just Ana.

She could begin by discussion with the other bilingual staff members. Together they should involve the rest of the staff. Until the staff takes a position, Ana should take a firm stand about new clients and about not translating for co-workers or helping them understand the cultural context of their clients. She could suggest in-service staff cultural-awareness training be provided by an outside facilitator.

It is difficult and unwise for Ana to protest these issues alone because that would heighten her isolation, which augments her depression, as well as her anger and frustration. Facing this situation alone reinforces feeling oppressed, whereas group action engenders empowerment and keeps the ethical/political issues central. (Joan Hamerman Robbins)

DILEMMA C

Christine is a therapist in a Midwestern university town with a closely knit core of feminist and lesbian university faculty, therapists, and other professionals. This group, including Christine, started a biweekly pot-luck and support group for lesbian women and activists. The group has grown beyond the original group and includes women from all walks of life.

Christine has found the event to be an important support for her. It has helped her maintain a balance in her life and prevented isolation, given the scarcity of feminist therapists in the community. She considers it one of the most valuable sources of support in this small community.

One of Christine's long-term clients showed up at the last pot-luck. This is a woman with few social supports and friendships. Christine believes the group would be good for her client but is torn because she thinks it is too much of a boundary violation for both of them to attend. She would suffer a significant loss by dropping out of this group she helped originate 18 months ago but recognizes its potentially positive impact for her client.

RESPONDENT 1

There are both interesting similarities and differences in this dilemma with issues occurring with people of color. For some cultures (American Indian and some Latino), the therapist's participation in a community group in which her clients are present would be seen as a positive sign that the therapist is not aloof or elitist. This belief is particularly true of a therapist on a reservation or in an ethnic minority rural community, such as a migrant worker community. For those therapists, participation in religious/spiritual ceremonies, community activist groups, the local school, or youth groups are seen as positive. However, dual relationship issues and lack of support for the therapist can also occur in large cities among therapists who are people of color and especially among therapists of color who are gay or lesbian.

The faculty and other professionals in Christine's small community do not have the same ethical and therapeutic restrictions regarding socializing with clients that she does. This restriction is particularly important with clients with severe relationship problems, clients who tend to become dependent upon authority figures, or clients who cannot handle knowing too much about their therapist. This restriction is also important for therapists who have not been trained to have the flexible but clearly defined boundaries needed to work in a small community. It also applies in communities (in this country, usually white communities) that do not have established roles for their healers. The community members in such communities do not have a clear idea of how to integrate, yet protect, their local therapist. Traditional American Indian and indigenous Central American and Mexican communities have prescribed social and working roles for their healers of which everyone in the community is aware. The same is true of the role of preachers or ministers in small African-American communities.

Christine's major mistake was in not preparing for this dilemma when organizing the group. In a small town, any open group is bound to include a conflict of boundaries sooner or later. Her feminist sensibilities might have inhibited her from suggesting a closed group. In her desire to be egalitarian, she ignored a small but crucial difference between her profession and the other professions represented by the group members. In addition, not discussing the potential ethical dilemma with the other organizers of the group could also represent (1) a disregard or minimizing of the need for ethical standards, (2) a naive denial on her part that it could ever happen to her, (3) a lack of trust in the other women in the organizing group to take her issue seriously, or (4) a failure to take her own ethical and self-care needs seriously.

It is interesting that Christine is considering dropping out of the group without raising the issue publicly. If she did so, she would be depriving the community that she values of the opportunity to engage in some creative problem solving to address the needs of all its members. She would risk slipping into a "martyr" role that would not provide for her needs. Raising the issue, with the help of the other therapists in the group, could be a valuable learning experience for all members as they discover the safety parameters needed for people in therapy as well as therapists. (Melinda A. Garcia)

RESPONDENT 2

This dilemma frequently occurs in small communities, whether geographic communities or communities of small groups with common issues. There were some actions that might have reduced the probability of this particular ethical dilemma. The founders of the original support group included faculty, therapists, and other professionals, in a small, Midwestern town. The founding mothers might have anticipated boundary problems with either students, in the case of faculty, or clients in the case of the therapists. They could have developed a system for dealing with this situation if or when it developed.

It appears that Christine has spoken to her client about the need for social supports and friendships. At this time, Christine could also have discussed this group and potential boundary problems in both women attending it. Christine would have been modeling the importance of taking care of herself as well as the appropriateness of setting boundaries in tight communities (IVD).

Since the client has already attended one of the pot-luck support groups, it is necessary for Christine to address the issue with her client immediately. There is a relationship of trust as well as a history of working through difficult issues with each other in therapy, since this is a long-term client. Addressing this current problem would seem a natural part of an ongoing, therapeutic relationship. It is a way of educating the client about boundaries and, at the same time, giving Christine the chance to talk about her concerns and discomfort (IIB). This would be an appropriate self-disclosure and one that would benefit the therapeutic relationship. At that point, it would be very important for Christine and her client to take a look at what other solutions might be available for the client to meet her social needs. (Kathleen Gates)

DILEMMA D

Diana is a therapist with a private practice in a rural community. She primarily provides therapy to adult women in an office adjacent to her home, where she lives with her partner of two years. She has been working with a client, Karen, for almost three years. Karen experienced extensive intrafamilial sexual and emotional abuse as a child. She began therapy suicidal and depressed with few friends and difficulty in maintaining employment. She has worked hard in therapy and has not made a suicide attempt in more than one year. She returned to college and has achieved so well that she is considering graduate school. Karen met Diana's partner, Casey, in a class and they developed a friendship. Diana became aware of the friendship when Casey informed her that she was ending their relationship in order to pursue one with Karen. Casey moved out of their home and began to date Karen. Diana is devastated by the loss of her relationship. Karen thinks that her progress would be jeopardized by switching therapists. She does not show much awareness of the impact of her behavior on Diana or Diana's pain. She stated that the relationship between Diana and Casey must have already been poor if Casey were so willing to end it. Diana does not know what her responsibilities are to her client who insists on maintaining the therapeutic relationship.

RESPONDENT 1

This situation with its interpersonal betrayals has developed into a repetition of Karen's childhood sexual and emotional abuse. Karen may be unconsciously replicating her childhood abuse, whereas Casey may be acting out her anger against her former partner. Casey may be exploiting Karen or naively believe that this relationship has nothing to do with anger toward Diana. At the very least, neither Karen nor Casey has a sense of feminist sisterhood as they pit one woman's loyalty against the other.

Karen, as the client, does not have an obligation to have insight into her therapist's pain. However, her lack of awareness, including her expectation that her therapist can deny her feelings and continue on as if nothing had happened, indicates that she still has a long way to go in understanding her own history and its reenactment in the current triangle. It may be true that her progress would be jeopardized by switching therapists, but that is not Diana's responsibility, beyond, perhaps, making an appropriate referral.

Diana, while trying to be the good mother who does not abandon her charge, must nevertheless ethically be concerned with her own self-care. She cannot expect to be a good therapist if she attempts to overlook her own emotional pain. In doing so, she would not be presenting herself as a very effective role model for the behavior and process that her client would ideally achieve. Her resentment at what has happened, whether it be directed toward Karen or Casey, is unlikely to be so well contained that it will not have an effect on the therapeutic relationship. For example, Karen, having become involved in this new relationship, would probably want to discuss both the problems and the pleasures with her therapist and that cannot be someone who was personally affected by the development of the relationship. One option that might have been available early in the relationship between Karen and Casey would have been for Diana to propose to Karen that she make a choice between continuing in her therapy with Diana, which she says is important to her, or to continue in her relationship with Casey. It is questionable that this is still a viable option once Casey has made the break in the relationship by moving out, because the breach will have seriously affected the countertransference.

Diana's ethical responsibility for self-care is primary now, so that her feelings of devastation from the loss of this relationship do not adversely affect her other therapeutic relationships. (Joan R. Saks Berman)

RESPONDENT 2

Diana needs to recognize and act on the principle that she is worth at least as much as anyone whose therapy she facilitates. Therefore, continuing as Karen's therapist is not an option. Remaining sessions should focus on closure and preparation for referral to a therapist of Karen's choice.

Simultaneously, if Diana does not already have a colleague support group, she should find one within commuting distance of her home as soon as possible. She may also want to find a therapist in addition to the support group. To assure her privacy and confidentiality, it should be in a larger town where it is not as likely that "everybody knows everybody else's business."

The vignette about Diana and Karen does not provide information about the demographics of their community. Most rural communities at best tolerate lesbians and at worst are very hostile to them. Consequently, issues of race, class, sexual orientation, and other excuses to discriminate will inevitably influence additional actions Diana may need to take.

Most important is the realization that Diana's first responsibility is to herself and her own wholeness. Diana can not adequately discharge her responsibility to her client unless she first takes responsibility for her own well-being. She might even consider a short vacation and have someone else cover her practice until she regains her perspective.

In no way is this an occasion for self-flagellation or guilt. These sorts of overlapping relationships and chance contacts outside of therapy are intrinsic to rural life. One cannot expect empathy or insight from one's clients. The expectations and limits of contacts outside of therapy need to be made clear at the outset, though most traditionally prescribed behaviors for therapists are not applicable to small towns and rural areas.

Solo practice of medicine, psychiatry, social work, or psychology in these settings is not recommended. Collegial consultants and a support network are essential to therapist self-care. (Ruth Peachey)

IMPLICATIONS

The cultural aspects of these dilemmas increased their complexity. The social pressures on, and the exploitation of, the therapists in these vignettes shaped the therapists' responses as well as their perceptions of their options. The respondents varied in the extent to which they emphasized cultural factors or social structures as influencing the therapists' responses. Respondents emphasized both individual responsibility in creating and solving the dilemma or a broader cultural perspective, where community expectations and workplace exploitation were viewed as major factors. Ethnicity of the respondent did not necessarily predict whether they emphasized personal responsibility or cultural explanations.

In the first two dilemmas, respondents recommended a combination of individual and social support to achieve changes. In the second dilemma, the respondents agreed that social support would not be sufficient. They recognized the need for an organized political response to combat the workplace's exploitation of Ana, a bilingual/bicultural therapist. They also recognized Ana's dilemma. Her attempts at self-care may place her job in jeopardy. Ana must rely on collective action in order not to increase her own vulnerability within an exploitative environment.

The last two scenarios represented cases where the self-care issues would be seen as preventative. There were no clear ethical breaches by the therapists. These cases have been included because they demonstrate the future potential for ethical breaches when self-care is not attended to in the present. They also demonstrate possible differences between traditional therapy approaches, where putting the client first at all costs is frequently advocated, and feminist therapy, where the therapist must balance her own self-care needs with those of her clients.

Traditional therapists may be likely to resolve Dilemma C by dropping out of the support group and Dilemma D by continuing to see the client, while working out their own "countertransference" issues in their own therapy. The feminist ethical perspective provides a different framework. The therapist is mandated to attend to her own well-being, which in the long-term could be compromised by too much self-sacrifice. Women and ethnic minority therapists are too much on the line already to ignore when they need to set limits. These limits may seem "uncaring" to therapists working in larger communities with more resources and more buffers between their lives and those of their clients.

Lest it appear that feminist therapists advocate bailing out of difficult situations, invoking self-care as a reason to avoid mutual process with clients, the respondents of Dilemma C clearly delineated the therapist's responsibilities. They both cited their concern that the therapist did not adequately anticipate or prepare for the dual relationships conflict that appeared. They both advocated the use of mutual process in resolving this issue, implying that the needs of both therapists and clients would be taken into account in a mutually empowering process. The respondents for Dilemma D recognized that therapists must not minimize the consequences of their own pain and betrayal in their work with clients. They implied that clients are best protected when therapists realistically acknowledge their own limitations. What appears as client concern in traditional schemas may actually mask denial and grandiosity on the part of the therapist.

The inclusion of self-care as an ethical imperative presents a thorny dilemma itself. Where lies the boundary between the promotion of proactive, preventative, and self-regulatory therapist behavior and punitive, puritanical, and intrusive external monitoring of therapist behavior? What is the balance between the therapist's individual rights and the client's well-being? For example, is a therapist who smokes unethical under the Feminist Therapy Institute guidelines? Is she unethical if she smokes privately, because her self-care is obviously compromised, or only if she smokes in front of the client? Must the therapist be continually striving for optimal health and well-being, or can her responsibilities be limited to ensuring client well-being, for example, to a "well enough" standard of self-care?

The ethical decision-making model provides one framework to deal with these questions. The model does not exemplify a rigid, moralistic, or perfectionistic ideal but promotes the analysis of areas in which behaviors may be jeopardizing client care or relationships, either in the present or in the future. The feeling-intuitive process presented in the model is in itself a model for self-care as well as a model for mutual process, advocated by several of the respondents. The model balances therapist and client perspectives, validates feelings, recognizes the need to appraise the impact on the therapist as well as the client, and promotes mutual problem solving. This model, by promoting these activities, is in fact promoting therapist growth and care.

RESPONDENTS

Joan R. Saks Berman, PhD, a clinical psychologist at the Albuquerque Indian Hospital, specializes in domestic violence, sexual trauma, and dissociative disorders.

Melinda Garcia, PhD, a clinical and community psychologist in private practice in Albuquerque, NM, specializes in the training and delivery of culturally competent services to diverse populations.

Kathleen Gates, MA, is in private practice in Duluth, MN, and in northwestern Wisconsin, where she specializes in dissociative disorders.

Helen Jackson, PhD, is Clinical Assistant Professor of Psychiatry at the University of New Mexico, in private practice in Albuquerque and serves on the New Mexico Psychology Association's Ethics Committee and the State Board of Psychology Examiners.

Ruth Peachey, MD, recently retired as a consultant in research and social psychiatry, continues to support work with battered women incarcerated for killing their abusers in Kentucky and Tennessee.

Joan Hamerman Robbins, LCSW, is in private practice in San Francisco where she specializes in working with women and couples and is the author of *Knowing Herself: Women Tell Their Stories in Psychotherapy* (1990).

Maryhelen Snyder, PhD, Clinical Director of the New Mexico Relationship Enhancement Institute, was guest editor for the special issue on feminist ethics for the *Journal of Feminist Family Therapy* (1994).

Diana M. Valdez, PhD, is Assistant Professor in the Department of Psychiatry at the University of New Mexico School of Medicine with clinical interests in the areas of culture and psychotherapy and forensics.

REFERENCES

Adleman, J. (1990). Necessary risks and ethical constraints: Self-monitoring on values and biases. In H. Lerman & N. Porter (Eds.), *Feminist ethics in psychotherapy* (pp. 113–122). New York: Springer.

Boyd-Franklin, N. (1993, August). *Clinical psychological treatment of women of color—Family therapy*. Paper presented at symposium conducted at the American Psychological Association Convention, Toronto, Ontario.

Faunce, P. S. (1990). The self-care and wellness of feminist therapists. In H. Lerman & N. Porter (Eds.), *Feminist ethics in psychotherapy* (pp. 185–194). New York: Springer.

Keith-Spiegel, P., & Koocher, G. P. (1985). *Ethics in psychology: Professional standards and cases*. New York: Random House.

Lerman, H., & Porter, N. (Eds.). (1990). *Feminist ethics in psychotherapy*. New York: Springer.

Lerman, H., & Rigby, D. N. (1990). Boundary violations: Misuse of the power of the therapist. In H. Lerman & N. Porter (Eds.), *Feminist ethics in psychotherapy* (pp. 51–59). New York: Springer.

Maslow, A. H. (1968). *Toward a psychology of being* (2nd ed.). Princeton, NJ: Van Nostrand.

Rigby-Weinberg, D. (1986, March). *Sexual involvement of women therapists with their women clients*. Paper presented at the Eleventh National Conference of the Association for Women in Psychology, Oakland, CA.

THIRTEEN

Looking toward the Future

Elizabeth J. Rave
Carolyn C. Larsen

Therapists who have their clients' best interests as their primary concern must act in an ethical manner. Practicing ethically is about doing a client no harm. Although the moral imperative has always been there, the legal incentives for ethical therapy have strengthened as consumer rights have become entrenched in North American societies. Consumers of therapy services are more apt to know they have recourse if they feel treatment has been unethical. Some states require that therapists make the avenues of client recourse available to clients from the beginning of treatment. In the area of sex between therapist and client, many states now consider such behaviors illegal. Victims of such behavior, as well as therapists, were instrumental in getting these laws passed. Over 15 years ago, Keith-Spiegel (1979) talked about why sex with clients is "a stupid thing to do." Many of her points emphasized that clients are bolder than ever in seeking redress for poor treatment, that feminism in psychology has increased, that the profession takes ethical complaints seriously, and that insurance companies turn on unethical therapists. These points remain valid not only with respect to sexual activity but about unethical behaviors in general. In other words, not only is ethical behavior the right thing to do for clients but it is wise business practice as well.

Even though the topics addressed in this book are wide ranging and central to women's concerns, they are not inclusive of all possible topics. New issues emerge, and new questions develop from experiences and research. For example, there are ethical issues surrounding the birth control method using RU-486 and the medical techniques allowing older women to bear children. The profound reorganization of the work force and the impact of technologies on work, health care, communication, and knowledge are all potential areas for future ethical consideration. The following discussion touches on the ethical implications of some of these developments as well as suggests what remains to be done in the areas covered by this book.

DECISION-MAKING MODEL

The Hill, Glaser, and Harden ethical decision-making model acknowledges the role of the affective domain in making ethical decisions. The feelings of the therapist, the client, and perhaps others involved with the ethical situation are used as valid and valuable information. This domain may be extremely difficult to include when writing about decision making, but its importance in the decision making itself should not be minimized. A consultant would be especially helpful in facilitating therapists determining the role affect might be playing in decision making.

Being a feminist therapist makes ethical decision making more complicated in some ways. The Feminist Therapy Code of Ethics recognizes that the therapist needs to take into account not only feminist ethics but also the ethical codes of other professional organizations to which the therapist adheres. When the two codes are in conflict, it is up to the therapist to determine which ethical principle does the least harm to the client. Little direction is given in the FTI Code, however, to help the therapist make these choices. The Hill, Glaser, and Harden model may facilitate resolving those conflicts. Building on their model to develop guidelines for therapists' prioritizing and resolving conflicts between ethical principles would be most helpful for practitioners.

CONFIDENTIALITY

Confidentiality between client and therapist is the foundation of trust in the therapeutic relationship. Some of the directions in which managed health care is moving put that cornerstone of trust between client and therapist in jeopardy. Increasingly, decisions about who will receive therapy for how long and with whom are being decided by people outside the therapeutic professions. Diagnoses and sometimes progress reports are required by third-party payers. These are business decisions, not therapeutic decisions. Therapists are losing their professional decision-making rights to determine in consultation with the client the label, frequency, duration, and type of therapy to be provided.

Even *who* will do therapy is often determined by what credentials an insurance company will recognize as acceptable for reimbursement for services. Many insurers pay only for services by traditionally trained

therapists and not all trained therapists are eligible for payment. The type and level of graduate degree are often dictated by insurance carriers. The payment schedule both in fee per session and in total amount payable within a specified time frame is often set by nonprofessionals. As these decisions are moved out of the professional's power, it is the client as well as the therapist who loses.

Maintaining confidentiality between therapist and client is essential to developing a trusting relationship in successful therapy. As institutional systems are encroaching on more and more aspects of therapy, ability to maintain confidentiality is eroded. While it is important for therapists to be accountable, increasingly that accountability is to managers and insurance companies outside the usual professional boundaries. The loss of control over who has information and how it is used is a critical concern.

Technology has also created difficult problems for maintaining confidentiality of information. As information is stored and transmitted by computers and fax machines, it becomes harder and harder to maintain control over information. The loss of control creates serious ethical problems in keeping information about clients confidential and in informing clients about risks associated with confidentiality loss (Cram & Dobson, 1993). Anecdotal references have already appeared in newspapers about individuals accidentally receiving confidential medical records via their fax machines (Lacitis, 1994) when senders dialed the wrong number.

For feminist therapists, the situation is particularly painful. The problem becomes how to comply enough with new requirements to help clients have access to services but how not to be coopted by the increasingly restrictive system. Maintaining feminist principles of practice becomes more difficult within agencies and institutions as well as in private practice. As more decisions are taken out of therapists' hands, one has to wonder whether it will even be possible for private practitioners to survive.

Feminist therapists have to consider if and how to protest these and other changes that may develop and how to educate the public about the impact of the changes on the therapeutic process. Certainly all change is not bad or bad for therapy. What is important is for professionals to maintain control over their practice, regardless of its setting, and to be part of a consultative process so decisions are not made that contravene effective practice.

CONTINUING CONCERNS

As Ballou points out in an earlier section, the label put on a mental health condition determines how therapists and others think about the

client. Although the smallest profession in numbers, psychiatry holds tremendous influence in the field. Perhaps the greatest influence of all is in naming. For all practical purposes, the American Psychiatric Association through the *Diagnostic and Statistical Manuals* (DSM) determines what labels are used by the remainder of the helping professions. Insurance companies, for example, use DSM labels to determine eligibility for payment.

Before DSM-III-R was published, considerable action was taken by feminists within the psychiatric community as well as from outside. As a result of organization and questioning by a wide variety of mental health practitioners, two proposed personality disorders, late luteal phase dysphoric disorder and self-defeating personality disorder, were listed only as research categories rather than as diagnostic categories in DSM-III-R (American Psychiatric Association, 1987). Unfortunately, the process of developing categories remains fairly closed (Caplan, 1987, 1991; Caplan & Gans, 1991; Gallant & Hamilton, 1988). Unless more permanent changes occur in the process, future manuals will be developed by a small group of psychiatrists. Action taken did have some impact on the process of developing DSM-IV (American Psychiatric Association, 1994). The two research categories mentioned above have not become diagnostic categories. The process, according to the American Psychiatric Association, was more open, and there was at least minimal representation from related mental health professions.

The area of labeling and naming is wide open for social action. Training institutions teach students about the DSM and what the categories or labels mean but rarely include discussion about how the labels are derived, the type of research if any that determines labels, or any evaluation of the labels themselves. Each related professional organization would do well to have a task force or permanent committee established to consider how best to affect the DSM process or how to develop its own diagnostic system, which might more accurately reflect the clients it serves.

Biaggio and Greene expand the discussion of overlapping relationships into more subtle behaviors. Although most therapy ethical codes now include prohibitions against sexual contact between therapists and clients, not everyone agrees that sex in a mental health–related setting between people with power differentials is a negative experience for the person of lesser power. Recently ("Professors' Group," 1994) news stories appeared about a group of professors and students who have organized to promote the right of professors to have sex with students. Headed by a sociologist, the nationwide group with a membership of 70 students and current and former professors is dedicated to the principle that professors have the right to have sex with willing students. The group strategizes by e-mail on the Internet raising questions concerning how

the real identity of the participants can be known. The story also pointed out that there are many critics of this group and their purpose.

Even though most academic institutions have sexual harassment policies, there still is a need for training sessions with academicians about sexual harassment. There are some professors and supervisors who do not recognize the significance of power differentials between themselves and students. In psychology and related fields where they are modeling professional interpersonal relationships while living them with students, it is crucial for professors and supervisors to understand power differentials. One of the most difficult areas remains how to approach colleagues who are misusing power with students to meet their own needs. These areas are also ripe for social action.

Violence against women and children seems entrenched in Western societies. Feminists have been at the forefront in raising consciousness about violence and establishing preventive and treatment programs. Feminist therapists need to continue social action in these areas. The risks of taking power away from the client by acting for the client and the risks of overlapping relationships in social change activities are many. It would be very helpful for practitioners to have guidelines to direct them in these activities.

It is almost a truism in the field to say that a therapist must care for self before caring for clients. Unfortunately, the discussion has not gone much beyond the truism. Porter's section brings specific issues to the forefront and includes suggestions on approaching an impaired colleague. The next step may be to develop guidelines for the therapist to determine whether the need for intervention is necessary. What kinds of questions, for example, would be helpful for a therapist to ask herself or himself to see whether outside facilitation is appropriate?

LEARNINGS FROM OTHER PROFESSIONALS

A contentious ongoing issue for feminist therapists involves evaluation of information from nonfeminist sources. Much of the research done by medical professionals starts with questions from a patriarchal framework. In fact, until recently most medical research used small samples of male subjects only. Results were then generalized to females and to all humans regardless of their ethnicity, socioeconomic status, and other life factors. In their section, Liburd and Rothblum discuss the implications of the hierarchical and paternalistic medical model. However, questions remain. How do feminist therapists deal with results from medical research that affect their clients' mental and physical health? For example, because the knowledge regarding obesity and coronary problems or diabetes comes from medical research with males, should it be ignored? Or is the feminist therapist doing a serious injustice to clients by not including that information when appropriate during therapy? One role of feminist therapists should be to facilitate clients' interpretation of medical data, as well as data from other patriarchal researchers.

Another illustration involves information gleaned from work with male batterers. Lesbian feminist therapists have been in the forefront of recognizing same-gender battering. How can the data about male batterers be evaluated and applied to female batterers without making false assumptions? For example, therapists working with male batterers frequently describe them as charming and charismatic. Therapists working with battered women frequently describe them as being depressed and demonstrating low affect. Are the same characteristics common in same-gender batterers and victims? A therapist working with lesbian batterers and survivors has the responsibility of knowing how to evaluate information gleaned from working with heterosexual batterers and survivors before applying that information to their clients. Making similar mistakes with lesbian batterers and survivors that were made with their heterosexual counterparts would be an unnecessary and harmful delay in effective treatment.

An ethical concern involves the dissemination of knowledge. Feminists historically have been diligent in illustrating how the patriarchal system omits women in all facets of society. One clear way is through developing and keeping new knowledge and technological tools. For example, when women were kept out of higher education, they were deprived of information about advances in knowledge. The current technological explosion with all of its advances offers major challenges to feminists. Therapists who work in institutions, academia, or higher-priced private practices are more apt to have access to new technologies and be able to share information relating to clients very readily. Individuals who work with limited-income clients may not.

If women only respond to e-mail or faxed messages, they are layering the communication process by only communicating with others who have the equipment. Access to information affects personal decision making, and it is important for feminists to work toward women's involvement in the original spread of information as well as decision making. Thinking about privilege and responsibility may be appropriate in dealing with the technological future. To avoid making the same mistakes men have made and been criticized for under a patriarchal model, feminists need to take special care to include women in all stages of communication. It would be ironic indeed if feminists were charged with exclusivity by other women.

DIRECTIONS FOR THE CODE

With the rapidly changing complexions of populations in Canada and the United States, is the FTI Code sufficient? Or does it need to more directly reflect therapists' responsibilities for knowledge and awareness about racism, multiculturalism, and diversities? As awareness of world populations increases, therapists need to become more proactive in acquiring self-knowledge.

Medicine and pharmacology are becoming more involved in therapy as new drugs are developed. At minimum, feminist therapists need to educate themselves about medical and mental health advances. Therapists often have clients who are receiving medication. Not only does the therapist need to understand the potential impact of the medication on the client's functioning but also to be able to communicate knowledge about medication effects to the client when appropriate. At this point, the FTI Code does not address the issue of drugs in the treatment of mental health. The current debate in the American Psychological Association involving the right of psychologists to prescribe drugs makes drug-related issues even more pertinent to feminist therapists.

As health care systems change, methods of and qualifications for payment are changing. As insurance companies determine the type and length of treatment, more interference by outsiders in treatment occurs. Now that fee payment is becoming ever more complex with more and more players and decision makers, is the FTI Code inclusive enough for contemporary monetary issues? Perhaps there is need for specific references to money as a significant aspect of power differential and for providing access to therapy.

Many contemporary issues relate to the aging population. How can feminist therapists who have not reached a certain age be cognizant of the issues surrounding that age? Ageism is one of the most subtle and pervasive forms of discrimination, and feminist therapists are not immune to it. Individuals certainly can understand the effects of aging intellectually but may not be able to understand the impacts emotionally until they are older themselves. The emphasis on youth in Western societies may hinder individuals from fully understanding the impact of aging. To do so would be to acknowledge one's own aging, a particularly painful process if one is even minimally engaged in appearing youthful. Perhaps the elder members of FTI should suggest changes in the Code that address issues surrounding aging specifically rather than generally.

Younger populations present different mental health and ethical issues. Some diagnostic categories, medications, and treatments are specific to children, for example. Feminist therapists, including family therapists, who work with children need training specifically related to developmental and other issues. Additionally, therapists should understand the impact of their own experiences during development as they affect therapeutic liaisons with children. Because adults have ultimate responsibility for children, therapists may have difficulty in determining how and when to involve children in decision making. Feminist ethical guidelines for working with children would be a welcome addition to the field.

One focus of this book has been the diversity of feminist therapists and their approaches to ethical dilemmas. The bottom line is that most feminist therapists responded in similar ways to the same scenarios. The process of thinking through the dilemmas may have been different, but the end results were very similar. The therapist's age, affective responses, experiences, socioeconomic level, ethnicity, geographic location, living conditions, sexual preference—all these and other idiosyncratic characteristics may have contributed to the different routes therapists took to get to the same destination. The unifying factor that directed the course, that focused the destination so to speak, may be feminist philosophy. Regardless of the type of feminist belief system each espouses, all respondents identify themselves as feminists.

Would behaviorist therapists take different routes but end at the same ethical destination? Would humanistic therapists? Or psychoanalysts? Would psychodynamic therapists? Additionally, would any or all of those therapists respond differently to ethical dilemmas than feminist therapists? These questions are ripe for additional research and exploration.

Ethical codes of professional organizations assume that all members should respond in similar ways to ethical dilemmas regardless of their theoretical backgrounds. The accuracy of that assumption has not been empirically demonstrated. Even questions about gender differences in ethical decision making generally remain unasked and unanswered. Those dilemmas are subjects for further exploration.

Finally, just as feminism itself is committed to social change that improves the lives of people, it is incumbent upon feminist therapists to be actively involved in social change. Working with one client at a time is not sufficient to meet the criteria of active social change. Each feminist therapist needs to continually evaluate herself and her behaviors to determine how well she is being a social change agent.

REFERENCES

American Psychiatric Association. (1987). *Diagnostic and statistical manual of mental disorders* (3rd ed., rev.). Washington, DC: Author.
American Psychiatric Association. (1994). *Diagnostic and statistical manual of mental disorders* (4th ed.). Washington, DC: Author.

Caplan, P. J. (1987). The psychiatric association's failure to meet its own standards: The dangers of self-defeating personality disorder as a category. *Journal of Personality Disorders, 1*, 178–182.

Caplan, P. J. (1991). Delusional dominating personality disorder (DDPD). *Feminism and Psychology, 1*, 171–174.

Caplan, P. J., & Gans, M. (1991). Is there empirical justification for the category of "self-defeating personality disorder"? *Feminism and Psychology, 1*, 263–278.

Cram, S. J., & Dobson, K. S. (1993). Confidentiality: Ethical and legal aspects for Canadian psychologists. *Canadian Psychology, 34*, 347–363.

Gallant, S. J., & Hamilton, J. A. (1988). On premenstrual psychiatric diagnosis: What's in a name? *Professional Psychology, 19*, 271–278

Keith-Spiegel, P. (1979, September). *Sex with clients: Ten reasons why it is a very stupid thing to do.* Paper presented at the 87th Annual Convention of the American Psychological Association.

Lacitis, E. (1994, August 14). "Like it or not you can't always be of assistance." *Seattle Times*, p. L1.

Professors' group seeks the right to sleep with consenting students. (1994, July 24). *Seattle Times*, p. L3.

Index